The complete guide to food for sports performance

The complete guide to food for sports performance

A guide to peak nutrition for *your* sport

Second edition

Dr Louise Burke
with Michael McCoy

ALLEN & UNWIN

For my family,
and for the Frickers, my Canberra family

Figures by Valda Brook
Chapter opening pictograms by Hand Graphics

First published in 1992
Second edition 1995
Allen & Unwin
9 Atchison Street,
St Leonards NSW 1590 Australia
Phone: (61 2) 8425 0100
Fax: (61 2) 9906 2218
E-mail: frontdesk@allen-unwin.com.au
Web: http://www.allen-unwin.com.au

National Library of Australia
Cataloguing-in-Publication entry:

Burke, Louise.
    The complete guide to food for sports performance.

    2nd edn.
    Bibliography.
    Includes index.
    ISBN 1 86373 916 5.

    1. Athletes—Nutrition. I. McCoy, Michael. II. Title.

613.711

Set in 10.5/11.5pt Cheltenham, Linotron 300
by Graphicraft Typesetters Ltd, Hong Kong
Printed by Australian Print Group, Maryborough, Vic

10 9 8 7 6 5 4

Forewords

What I eat has always been important to me. I like to think that I was a little ahead of my time in the sports world, not just in realising the connection between nutrition and sports performance, but in putting this into practice in my daily life. During my athletic career, I have seen sports nutrition develop greatly, both in terms of the specialised knowledge now on offer, and the interest generated amongst athletes.

As Director of the Australian Institute of Sport, I was in daily contact with athletes from a variety of sports and recognised great differences in the demands and lifestyles of their athletic commitments. It is clear that the time has come to address the special needs of each group individually. *The Complete Guide to Food for Sports Performance* provides a leap forward in this direction. As well as providing an up-to-date review of sports nutrition theory, this book looks at nutrition from inside the athlete's world. A range of sports including swimming, distance running and gymnastics have been examined with detail and insight, raising nutritional issues that can be applied to many other sports as well. The practical advice will be appreciated by athletes of all levels, and provides an important bridge between ideas and action. Any athlete who has had to travel overseas, to eat out in a restaurant with friends, or to carbohydrate load before an event will know that choosing food well is often a challenge.

The Complete Guide to Food for Sports Performance is a welcome addition to an athlete's library.

Robert de Castella
Former Director of the Australian Institute of Sport
and champion marathon runner

It is a great honour to be invited to write a foreword to a text that will go a long way toward reducing one of the many risk factors associated with elite athletic performance.

I have no great knowledge in the areas of nutrition and diet, and as a coach, I am convinced that athletes and coaches do not sufficiently use the expertise and knowledge of those around them with this training.

The author of this book has this knowledge, has used it herself as a triathlete, and is now endeavouring to categorise all sports so that other athletes can get the most benefit from it.

Travelling to swim meets and training camps both in Australia and overseas has given Dr Burke a sound 'hands-on' understanding of how individual athletes think and work. Her advice to team members under my control in both individual and group situations has made a major contribution in giving athletes focus in the correct areas, and the rationale and incentive to keep that focus.

Years ago, even though I held world records, this sort of information would certainly have enhanced my performance as a competitor. We were then instructed not to drink fluids at all on competition days—dehydration was not considered at all; the rationale was that with no fluid intake you would be lighter and not have so much weight to drag through the water. What this did to our metabolism is anyone's guess!

I would have swum every major meet having eaten steak, eggs and chips, believing I needed protein to build muscle. Of course, now we know that if you don't have the muscle by race day, all the protein in the world eaten on that day will not help. Furthermore, I cannot recall the word 'carbohydrate' ever being mentioned.

There are few issues more clouded by misinformation on diet and its effects than athletic performance. Millions of dollars are spent by athletes each year in the hope that some fad diet—rarely based on sound nutritional requirements for the sport followed—or the diet followed by the current champion, will be the easy way.

There is no easy way—in this day and age, we must seek out and respect those who have proven knowledge, and then use it to our best advantage and to help us keep focused.

The task of athletes and coaches today is to eliminate any risk factors that detract from performance, and to maximise potential. This book is a very sound and sincere effort to give you the opportunity to reach your goals.

Terry Gathercole AM
Former senior coach, Australian Institute of Sport,
ex-world record holder breast stroke
Swimming Coach of the Year 1991

Contents

Useful hints and checklists   x
Case histories   xii
Tables   xiii
Figures   xv
Acknowledgements   xvi
Introduction   xvii

Part I Principles of sport nutrition   1

1 Training nutrition: the principles of everyday eating   3
   1.1 *Enjoying a variety of food*   4
   1.2 *Reducing fats and oils*   7
   1.3 *Increasing your carbohydrate intake*   14
   1.4 *Looking after your electrolytes*   26
   1.5 *Replacing your daily fluid losses*   28
   1.6 *Using alcohol sensibly*   33

2 Fine tuning—how much and when?   37
   2.1 *Energy*   37
   2.2 *Carbohydrate*   43
   2.3 *Protein*   44
   2.4 *Vitamins*   47
   2.5 *Iron*   52
   2.6 *Calcium*   54
   2.7 *Timing of meals*   59

3 Matters of physique—losing and gaining   61
   3.1 *Desirable body-fat levels*   61
   3.2 *Assessment of body fat*   62
   3.3 *Losing body fat*   65
   3.4 *Low-energy consumers*   70
   3.5 *Making weight*   75

3.6	*Bulking-up*	76
3.7	*The high-energy diet*	76
4	**Competition nutrition**	79
4.1	*A checklist of fatigue factors*	79
4.2	*General preparation for competition*	81
4.3	*Carbohydrate loading for endurance events*	83
4.4	*The pre-event meal*	87
4.5	*Sugar prior to the event?*	90
4.6	*Fluid intake during events*	92
4.7	*Endurance events—fluid and food intakes*	94
4.8	*Sports drinks—the rebirth*	102
5	**Eating to recover**	107
5.1	*Restoring fluid and electrolyte balance*	107
5.2	*Replacing glycogen stores*	110
5.3	*Other recovery issues*	115
5.4	*Putting it all together—practical considerations*	116
5.5	*Multi-event competitions*	119
6	**Pills and potions**	122
6.1	*Why do athletes use supplements?*	122
6.2	*Dietary supplements in sport*	122
6.3	*Nutritional ergogenic aids*	125
6.4	*How do you prove something works?*	132
6.5	*Making your own decision about ergogenic aids*	136
Part II	**Sports nutrition in action**	137
	Introduction	139
	Triathlon	140
	Swimming	151
	Cycling	163
	Distance running	172
	Middle distance running	189
	Jumps, sprints and hurdles	198
	Strength sports—Olympic weightlifting, powerlifting and throwing events	208
	Bodybuilding	218
	Wrestling and boxing	234

Gymnastics and diving   242

Rowing   263

Australian Rules Football   275

Rugby League   286

Soccer and field hockey   296

Basketball and netball   306

Tennis   315

Golf   327

Cricket   340

Skiing   350

Index   365

Useful hints and checklists

Checklist for peak training nutrition   4
Encouraging food variety   6
Reducing intake of fats and oils   10
What do we mean by 'percentage fat'?   12
Emphasising nutritious carbohydrate-rich foods in your diet   24
Increasing your fibre intake   25
Using sugar well   26
Using salt wisely   28
Monitoring fluid balance during training   29
Looking after fluid needs in training   33
Using alcohol sensibly   36
Putting more vitamins per mouthful in your diet   49
An iron boost   53
A calcium boost   58
Meal timing   59
Typical reasons for athletes wanting or needing to lose body fat   65
Healthy fat-loss plan for athletes   67
Successful and sustained loss of body fat   69
Low-energy consumers   73
'Making weight'   75
Achieving a high-energy intake   77
Competition preparation diet   81
Preparation for general sports competition   82
A 'modified' carbohydrate loading program   85
The pre-event meal   89
Pre-event meal ideas   91
Fluid intake during general sports competition   95
Intake of carbohydrates and fluids during endurance events   100
Recovery after prolonged strenuous exercise   116
Eating well in a cafeteria-style dining hall   161
Finding alternatives for high-fat carbohydrate foods   187
Factors associated with runner's diarrhea   193
How to evaluate dietary advice   221

Signs of eating disorders   250
Dealing with eating disorders   252
Special issues in vegetarian eating   260
Steps to quick and healthy cooking   292
Checklist for a well-stocked pantry and fridge   294
Recipe books based on high-carbohydrate, low-fat eating   295
A guide to take-aways   314
The travelling athlete   321
Non-perishable food supplies for the travelling athlete   326
Eating well in a restaurant   332
How to meet your nutritional goals in a restaurant   334

Case histories

The dangers of being too strict with your diet   146
Eating and drinking during endurance events   148
Achieving a high energy diet to overcome fatigue   158
Eating in a communal dining hall   159
The Tour de France   169
Calcium, stress fractures, and menstrual irregularity 179
Iron deficiency   182
Carbohydrate loading   185
Runner's trots—diarrhea and gut upsets during exercise 192
Pritikin eating   194
Eating and drinking over a day of competition events   202
Assessing your eating patterns   203
Bulking up—gaining muscle mass   213
Food or supplements?   215
Exploring nutrition myths   226
Examining a scientific article about sports supplements 230
Losing weight/making weight for competition   237
Making weight in boxing   239
Eating disorders in athletes   248
Understanding daily changes in body weight   251
Vegetarian eating   257
Achieving a high-energy diet   268
Losing weight and gaining energy—the light-weight's dilemma 271
Using alcohol well in sport   281
Losing weight—a male perspective (1)   282
Learning to cook   290
Injury and weight gain   301
Pre-event eating   303
Weight loss through reorganising eating behaviour   311
Take-aways   312
The travelling athlete   319
Tournament nutrition   323
Eating in restaurants   331
Losing weight—a male perspective (2)   344
Fluid intake during cricket   347
Examining the high-fat theory   358
The international athlete   362

Tables

1.1 Glycemic Index of some common carbohydrate-rich foods 19
1.2 Typical estimated sweat losses and fluid intakes of elite athletes in training 31
1.3 Problems and solutions for good fluid intake practices during training 32
2.1 Basal Metabolic Rate for reference adults 40
2.2 Average activity levels expressed as multiples of BMR 40
2.3 Estimated daily energy allowances for growth, pregnancy and breastfeeding 40
2.4 Estimated energy cost of activity 41
2.5 Ready reckoner of carbohydrate-rich foods 45
2.6 Ready reckoner of protein-rich foods 47
2.7 Vitamins: where to find your recommended dietary intake 50
2.8 Iron-rich foods for the optimal training diet 54
2.9 Calcium-rich foods for the optimal training diet 57
4.1 A typical plan for carbohydrate loading 86
4.2 Common food and fluid choices used in endurance sports 98
4.3 Analysis of some common sports drinks 102
5.1 Examples of 50g carbohydrate snacks 114
5.2 Nutritional practices for various competition schedules 120
6.1 Dietary supplements and their uses in sport 124
6.2 Some popular nutritional ergogenic aids for which there is some scientific support 127
6.3 Some popular nutritional ergogenic aids that are currently under review 129
6.4 Other popular nutritional ergogenic aids that have not yet passed the 'proof' test 131
A triathlete describes his daily diet to a dietitian 147
Sample high-carbohydrate (high-energy) eating plan for a swimmer 159
Average daily intake of Tour de France cyclists 170
A female distance runner's diet before and after counselling 182
Dietary intake of runners carbo-loading for a marathon 185
Nutrient analysis of a typical day's eating for a 78kg hurdler 206
Nutrient intake from food and supplements 216
Weight-loss diet for a boxer 240
A day in the life of a rower 269

Food for sports performance

A day in the life of a light-weight sculler   272
Weight-loss diet for a sculler   273
Healthy weight-loss diet for a footballer   284
Comparison of low and high-carbohydrate food selections   284
Healthy weight-loss diet for a cricketer   346

Figures

1.1 Food is a complex mixture of chemicals 6
1.2 The food pyramid 7
1.3 What is energy? 9
1.4 The fat content of food 15
1.5 Carbohydrate foods 23
1.6 Alcohol content of common drinks 35
2.1 How to predict your daily energy requirements 38
2.2 Energy balance 42
2.3 Complementary vegetable proteins 48
2.4 Risk factors for amenorrhea 55
3.1 Sites for taking skinfold measurements 64
4.1 The 'modified' carbo-loading program 84
4.2 Concentration and volume of drink necessary to supply fluid and carbohydrate needs 104
5.1 Daily recovery from prolonged exercise 111
5.2 Short-term recovery after prolonged exercise 113
6.1 Cost of protein—supplements versus food 133
6.2 Cost of amino acids—supplements versus food 134

Acknowledgements

Many athletes, coaches, and sports dietitians provided the inspiration and information for this book. Thank you to all who participated in the project, particularly those from the Australian Institute of Sport.

Special greetings go to my colleagues from the sports nutrition program at the AIS—Vicki, Mareeta, Prue, Liz and Greg. Professor Peter Fricker, Fearless Leader of Sports Medicine, has provided most of the words of wisdom and cups of tea that I have enjoyed during my five years at the AIS. There are many wonderful coaches here, but only one Coach. To these people I owe much of my productivity, enjoyment of life and, on occasions, sanity.

The heights, weights and skinfold data were collected using the Telford technique described in Chapter 3. A 'typical' physique was calculated only for sports where sufficient numbers of athletes have been tested, with 'typical' being represented by the mean ± one standard deviation of group value. The data were kindly supplied by the Department of Physiology at the Australian Institute of Sport and the South Australian Sports Institute. Thanks to Sarah Woolford (SASI) and to Lynn Gunning and David Pyne (AIS) for providing this material. The Australian Rules football data was taken from *Footy Food* by Lorna Garden.

This book would not have been possible without Dr Mike McCoy, who helped with the research on the individual sports, and without all those who proofread and commented on the chapters. Drs David Pyne, Ron Maughan and Dave Martin were particularly patient and dedicated to this task.

Introduction

There have been many exciting developments in sport since the first edition of this book was released. In Australia we have finished celebrating the announcement of the Sydney 2000 Olympic Games and are now committed to a program that will produce the most spectacular Games the world has seen and the most successful results that our athletes have ever achieved. Nutrition is an integral part of this plan—from the organisation of the dining hall in the Athlete's Village, to education programs that will ensure that all of our athletes train and compete with the benefits of a winning diet.

There have been some developments in the science of sports nutrition. New studies have shown ways in which nutrition strategies can help the athlete to train more effectively and recover more efficiently. In the competition setting there are some new ideas to help reduce the onset or effects of fatigue, and to produce a winning performance. Whether you are aiming for Sydney 2000, or just hoping to do a personal best in your local competition, these strategies can be part of your plan.

As before, this book will take a practical and individual approach to sports nutrition—recognising that each sport has specific nutritional interests and requirements arising from its particular training and competition program. The second edition of *The Complete Guide to Food for Sports Performance* presents an updated summary of nutrition for athletes—transforming science into practice, and taking a real-life approach to the special nutritional needs and lifestyles of various sports.

Note

Metric units are used throughout the book:

$$1 \text{ kilogram (kg)} = 2.2 \text{ pounds}$$
$$100\text{g} = 3.5 \text{ oz}$$
$$250\text{g} = 8.8 \text{ oz}$$
$$1 \text{ litre (L)} = 35.2 \text{ fl. oz}$$
$$100\text{ml} = 3.52 \text{ fl. oz}$$
$$1 \text{ kilojoule (kJ)} = 4.2 \text{ calories}$$

I Principles of sports nutrition

1 Training nutrition: the principles of everyday eating

Although what you eat before a big event may appear important, it is actually your training diet that holds the most potential to influence sports performance. Consider the many hours that you commit to training each year, to prepare yourself for an event that will last only a fraction of this time—perhaps even only seconds or minutes.

Just from the time angle alone, your everyday diet has most opportunity to make an impact on your body. But more importantly, remember that it is training that lifts you to the stage from which you will compete, and that your diet will play an important role in helping you along the pathway to maximum improvement.

Daily training will create special nutritional needs for an athlete, particularly the elite athlete whose training commitment is almost a full-time job. But even recreational sport will create nutritional challenges. And whatever your level of sport, you must meet your nutritional needs if the maximum return from training is to be achieved. Without optimal training nutrition, much of the purpose of your training might be lost. In the worst case, dietary problems and deficiencies may directly impair training performance. However, on the positive side, with the right everyday eating plan your commitment to training will be fully rewarded.

So what is the basis of the optimal training diet? There is no perfect combination of foods or single eating plan that will meet the nutritional challenges of every athlete. If you take a quick look at Part II, you will see that nutritional needs and interests vary between sports. And imagine trying to find one meal plan to encompass the food likes and dislikes, not to mention lifestyles, of all athletes! While the focus and details will differ from one athlete to the next, there are certain goals that are common to all sports. The following checklist will rate

3

CHECKLIST FOR PEAK TRAINING NUTRITION

- Can you achieve and maintain a desirable level of body weight and body fat for your sport?
- Do you provide your body with all its nutrient needs, remembering that requirements for some nutrients will be increased by a strenuous training program?
- Do you promote recovery between training sessions with practices that will rapidly replace fluid and fuel stores, and allow the body to recover and adapt to the training load?
- Do you think about the future? Do you take into account the nutrition guidelines for long-term good health? (Not only will this affect the quantity and quality of your own life, but you may be a role model for others who admire your sporting achievements.)
- Does food provide pleasure in your day? Are you able to enjoy social eating opportunities with your family and friends?
- Do you create opportunities in training to try out your competition eating practices (such as the pre-event meal, or eating and drinking during an event)? Practice makes perfect, and identifies many of the problems that could go wrong on the big day.

---

the quality of your training diet. If you are achieving all these goals with your everyday eating plan, then congratulate yourself for having achieved peak training nutrition.

Obviously, peak training nutrition doesn't just happen by chance. Before you can branch into the special and individual areas of sports nutrition, you must start with a dietary structure based on the common ground shared by all athletes. Once you have these principles in place, you can then fine-tune your eating plan to account for your particular nutritional needs and dietary goals. At each level, by knowing more about what is in food and ways to select and prepare it, you are in control of what you choose to eat. You can choose to meet your dietary challenges in ways that are both enjoyable to you, and complementary to your busy schedule. So let's start with the basic principles.

1.1 Enjoying a variety of food

We have a tendency to oversimplify the food we eat—focusing on one or two nutrients it contains such as iron, cholesterol or sugar. We are quick to pin labels on food—for example, we might believe that yoghurt is 'good' for us while chocolate is 'bad'.

In fact, there is no such thing as a 'good' or 'bad' food. Instead, there are good *uses* of a food—if it contributes toward the achievement of your nutritional goals. This depends on what you are trying to achieve and what else you are eating over the day. A chocolate milkshake might be a great afternoon snack for a hungry basketball player with 'hollow legs'. But two milkshakes in a day would blow the kilojoule budget of a tiny gymnast, and at the 30km mark of a marathon, a runner is looking for a different kind of drink.

Taking the 'good' and 'bad' idea one step further, some people think that a 'good diet' is one where all the bad foods have been removed. So they set themselves the task of giving up all the foods they consider 'bad' (often the ones they enjoy the most). Athletes are particularly skilled at this: they are motivated (often obsessively) and good at self-discipline. No pain, no gain—right? It is not unusual to find athletes who 'out-Pritikin' Pritikin, and who eat a very restricted diet from which many foods, and indeed whole food groups have been removed. At best this may bring some mental satisfaction, but at what cost? All the advantages of a varied diet are lost.

The first step in understanding what is at stake is to appreciate how intricate and sophisticated our food really is. Nutrients do not exist in isolation and are not eaten individually. There is more to an orange than vitamin C, and more to meat than protein. As shown in Figure 1.1, food is a complex mixture of hundreds of chemicals (yes, carbohydrate and colourings, protein and preservatives are all chemicals). What's more, each food is greater than the sum of its chemical composition, because once inside the body, the chemicals in a food interact with each other and with the chemicals in other foods eaten at the same time. Although some popular diet books have spread the myth that certain foods shouldn't be eaten in combination, the truth is that the nutritional quality of a meal is often improved by mixing and matching foods together. For example, the iron in cereal foods is better absorbed in the presence of vitamin C, making a glass of orange juice with your breakfast cereal a clever combination.

Enjoying a wide variety of foods, both in your general diet and at each meal, provides the opportunity to sample a little of everything that food has to offer. And although we do not fully appreciate the extent of food interactions at this stage, nutritional variety will provide plenty of potential for good combinations at a meal.

From another angle, a varied diet can be viewed as 'eating in moderation'. A little of everything helps to prevent you from overeating any one food, or overexposing yourself to particular food chemicals (whether they be put there by nature or by a food manufacturer). Since the nutritional problems in developed countries such as Australia and the United States are linked mostly to overconsumption of dietary

Figure 1.1 Food is a complex mixture of chemicals

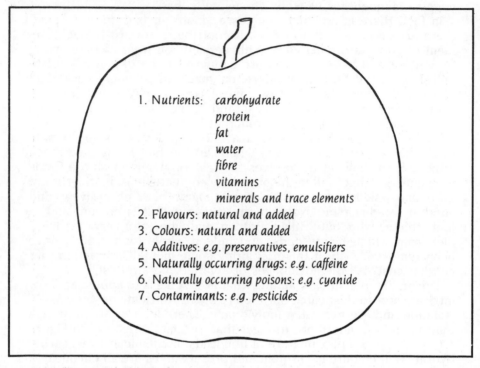

1. Nutrients: *carbohydrate*
   protein
   fat
   water
   fibre
   vitamins
   minerals and trace elements
2. Flavours: *natural and added*
3. Colours: *natural and added*
4. Additives: *e.g. preservatives, emulsifiers*
5. Naturally occurring drugs: *e.g. caffeine*
6. Naturally occurring poisons: *e.g. cyanide*
7. Contaminants: *e.g. pesticides*

HINTS TO ENCOURAGE FOOD VARIETY

- Be prepared to try new foods and new recipes.
- Make the most of foods in season.
- Explore all the varieties of a food. For example, try bread made from different grains other than wheat (rye, multigrain, fruit breads, etc.) and in different forms (sticks, bagels, pita bread etc.).
- Mix and match foods at your meals. Avoid meals made up of just one food type, such as having a fruit-only lunch.
- Think carefully before you banish a food or food group entirely from your diet. Maybe some features do not fit in with your nutritional goals or the dietary principles in this chapter. However, consider what other value the food may have—in particular which other nutrients it could supply. There may be ways to reduce or modify your intake, rather than discard the food totally.

Figure 1.2 The food pyramid encourages variety, but gives priority to some foods

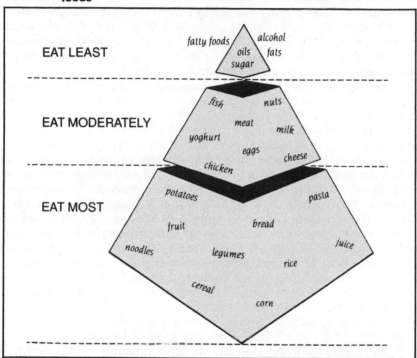

EAT LEAST — fatty foods, oils, sugar, alcohol, fats

EAT MODERATELY — fish, nuts, meat, milk, yoghurt, eggs, cheese, chicken

EAT MOST — potatoes, pasta, fruit, bread, noodles, legumes, juice, rice, cereal, corn

compounds, eating a wide variety of foods is a good way to keep your intake of all food components within healthy levels.

Last, but by no means least, a varied diet offers greater opportunities for flexibility, enjoyment and adventure with food. A major reason that we eat is for pleasure and social interaction, and unnecessary restrictions to your diet will mean an unnecessary sacrifice of this. While optimal training nutrition is about choosing 'a lot of what you need', 'a little of what you fancy' is also part of dietary balance. The food pyramid (Figure 1.2) is a model for the good use of food. Certain foods should be emphasised in your eating program, forming the 'base' of your meals and snacks. However all foods can be part of the scheme—with less nutritious foods claiming a small role at the 'tip' of your dietary plan.

1.2 Reducing fats and oils

The good news about fats (and oils) in food is that they provide a concentrated source of energy (otherwise known as kilojoules), and

7

make meals tasty, satisfying and rich in texture. They can also supply essential fatty acids and fat soluble vitamins—both important to your health and fitness. The bad news is that too much of a good thing is not necessarily better, and a high fat intake can cause problems. Unfortunately, a high fat diet is second nature to most Australians, with fats and oils providing about 35 per cent of our total energy intake, and some individuals consuming higher levels again.

Looking at long-term health considerations, there is ample evidence linking a high-fat diet with problems such as coronary heart disease, and some cancers. With this in mind, nutrition guidelines have been set for the whole population, recommending that fat intake be reduced by a quarter, to less than 30 per cent of total energy.

While athletes also have their future health to consider (life does go on after the Olympic Games), they are understandably more interested in the here and now, and the role of dietary fat in sports performance. The verdict on this front is that although dietary fats and oils are the most concentrated source of food energy, they do not provide the major source of fuel for exercising muscles. Instead, body carbohydrate stores provide the critical energy source for strenuous activity—critical firstly because below a certain level of supply, intense exercise cannot be maintained, and secondly because the body carbohydrate stores are exhausted in hours and must be continually replenished from carbohydrate in the diet. Body fat stores, on the other hand, is in plentiful supply even in the leanest of athletes, and could supply fatty acids for hours and days of exercise.

So while a high-fat diet may not directly influence sports performance, the disservice to an athlete comes from the displacement of kilojoules which could have come from carbohydrate foods. The energy from fat contributes heavily to an athlete's daily kilojoule budget without taking care of the muscle's fuel needs.

Another point to consider is that fats and oils have twice the energy density of protein and carbohydrate (that is, more than twice the kilojoules per mouthful). This means that high-fat foods make it easy to overeat your daily energy requirements. What's more, there is some evidence that high-fat diets are especially efficient in promoting increased body fat stores, independently of the amount that you eat. All in all, high-fat eating can lead to a high-fat body!

On the other hand, a lower-fat diet can help to prevent you gaining body fat, as you have to eat more mouthfuls to reach your energy needs. And when weight loss (loss of body fat) is on the agenda, cutting back on fat intake is the most effective way of reducing your kilojoule intake and reducing your body fat levels.

Figure 1.3 illustrates the concept of energy in food.

So how much fat should an athlete eat? This question is best answered by first determining your daily kilojoule requirements for protein and carbohydrate. The remaining kilojoules can be then filled in

Figure 1.3 What is energy?

FOOD ENERGY *– per gram*

FAT *–37 kilojoules (9 kilocalories)*
ALCOHOL *–29 kilojoules (7 kilocalories)*
PROTEIN *–17 kilojoules (4 kilocalories)*
CARBOHYDRATE *–16 kilojoules (4 kilocalories)*

*To the dietitian, energy means fuel for all
the body.
Energy in food comes from carbohydrate,
fat, protein and alcohol, and is measured in
units of kilojoules (kJ) or kilocalories (Cals).*

To convert: 1 Cal = 4.2 kJ

*To the athlete, energy means 'get up
and go' and vigour for exercise.
The most important <u>muscle</u> fuel is body
carbohydrate, which is stored from the
carbohydrate in food.*

with fat. For most athletes, as for the rest of the community, cutting
back fat and oils to less than 30 per cent of total energy intake is a
suitable goal. For athletes whose kilojoule needs are in short supply
(small eaters and those trying to lose weight), it may be necessary to
cut back the fat intake to 15–25 per cent of total energy intake to
allow for other nutrient needs. A similar ratio might be suitable for
some endurance athletes with heavy daily training schedules, to make
way for their large requirements for carbohydrate energy.

The important point to remember is that dietary fat should not be
left out altogether. Some nutrition books (and many athletes) have
tried this approach, attempting to reduce fat to less than 10 per cent
of the diet or even no fat at all. This might sound like good economy,
but in real life it is impossible to achieve without sacrificing variety
and its benefits. Small amounts of fat are found in many important
foods, and fat 'headhunters' will eventually pay for cutting them out
of their diets. Stick to the moderate angle: trim the excess and enjoy
the valuable.

A last word on the different types of fat in food. There is much that is still being learned about the role of various chemical forms of fat and oils in food—saturated, monounsaturated, polyunsaturated, cholesterol and so on. A good nutrition textbook can fill you in if you want to pursue this further. However, the best advice overall is probably to make up your total fat quota with a little of each type.

HINTS FOR EATING LESS FATS AND OILS

Protein and dairy foods

- Choose lean cuts of meat, chicken, fish and seafood. Get to know your butcher/fishmonger well, or examine the packaged trays in the supermarket. If meats are labelled, go for those that are 90 per cent fat-free and above.
- Choose non-oil varieties of canned fish, or carefully drain off all the oil.
- Look for new types of processed meats with a lower fat content (95 per cent fat-free or above). Avoid high-fat sausage and luncheon meat products.
- Whatever the protein—meat, fish, chicken, egg or a combination of these—make the total serve accompany a meal rather than be its star attraction. Make use of low-fat or non-fat dairy products such as skim and low-fat milks, ricotta and cottage cheese, and low-fat yoghurt.
- The highest-fat dairy protein food is cheese (30–40 per cent fat by weight). Even reduced-fat hard cheeses are quite high in fat (around 25 per cent fat by weight). Use these in preference, but limit the serve—e.g. a slice in a sandwich or a sprinkle on a pizza. Some hard cheeses and cheese slices boast a 7–10 per cent fat content by weight. These are the best choice. In terms of fat content, nevertheless you may prefer to use small amounts of richer tasting cheeses in some situations.

Cooking

- Become a whizz with low-fat cooking methods. Grill, bake on a rack or in foil, barbeque, microwave, steam, or 'dry fry' with a non-stick frypan with a smear of oil.
- Invest in a good non-stick frypan and/or wok. At most, you may need to brush with a small amount of oil, or a non-stick spray to guarantee that food will not stick and burn. Stir-fries are a quick and nutritious way to cook.

- Replace roast vegetables and chips with 'dry baked' items. Cut potatoes (or pumpkin, carrot etc.) into desired chips or chunks. Spray or brush the tray to stop sticking, and then brush the chips with a little oil and some herbs. Bake in a hot oven. Oven-baked fries (96 per cent fat-free and above) are another alternative to greasy chips.
- While pastries are high in fat, phyllo (filo) pastry is a low fat alternative for pies or pasties. Brush a little oil on the top sheet, but it is unnecessary to put oil or butter between each sheet.
- Cook with reduced fat ingredients. You can often find an alternative for high-fat ingredients—e.g. plain yoghurt instead of cream, skim milk instead of full cream milk.

Desserts and sweets

- Low-fat yoghurts and light fromage frais, or a little low-fat icecream (96 per cent fat-free and above) make quick and nutritious desserts, or a topping for other desserts.
- Make custards or rice pudding with reduced-fat milk, or fruit-based desserts (e.g. baked apples, fruit in filo pastry).
- It is possible to make reduced-fat versions of muffins, cakes and puddings. You can make your own from 'healthy' recipe books or modify your favourite recipes to reduce the amount of butter, margarine, oil or other high-fat ingredients. There are a number of commercial brands of these items now appearing on supermarket shelves.

Processed foods

- Many processed or baked foods are high in hidden fats and oils. Identify these and find lower fat substitutes—e.g. scones or bagels instead of croissants, low-fat icecream instead of icecream or cheesecake.
- Learn to read labels to estimate the fat content of packaged foods (see following box). Try to choose those that are lower in fat—for example, if you can calculate the ratio of fat to energy in a food, stick to those in which less than 30 per cent of kilojoules come from fat.
- Beware of labels that say 'lite' or 'light'. This does not necessarily mean light in fat or kilojoules. In fact, it may simply mean light in salt, colour or flavour.
- 'Low cholesterol' is another misleading term, since foods can still be high in oils and kilojoules without containing cholesterol. Learn to read all the label.

- Enjoy chocolate, biscuits, pastries and rich cakes as a treat. If you go for quality in the foods that are special to you, you won't mind a smaller quantity.

Snack foods and take-aways

- Snack foods such as chips, corn chips, and nuts are high in fat—as well as being very 'moreish'. Keep away from the bowl when these foods are served. Many brands of pretzels provide a low-fat alternative.

- You can make your own low-fat snacks by popping corn (with minimal oil), or by toasting strips of pita bread to make 'chips' for dips. Raw vegetables can also be chopped into bite-size snacks.

- Take-aways are high in fat—especially if fried, battered or in pastry. Hopefully, they do not make up a big part of your diet. When having take-aways, choose the lower-fat types or order a small serve only (add other nutritious foods to make up the rest of the meal).

WHAT DO WE MEAN BY 'PERCENTAGE FAT'?

1 *Percentage fat by weight*

Food manufacturers usually talk about the fat content of food by weight: The percentage of fat by weight is the number of grams of fat in a hundred grams of a food.

For example:
Cheese may be 35% fat—meaning that there are 35g of fat in 100g of cheese

Sometimes this information is inverted, and the manufacturer may talk about the 'fat-free' content of the food.

For example:
A brand of turkey ham may be advertised to be '95% fat-free'. This means that the product contains 5% fat by weight, or 5g per 100g of ham.

So what % of fat is good or bad?

Remember, no food by itself is good or bad. And the fat content of food must be judged according to the 'Big Picture'. This includes:
— What is the total nutritional value of the food?
— How much is a typical serve of the food?
— What is the fat content of the rest of your diet?

Since the energy content of fat is much greater than the other nutrients, and since the weight of a food can be made up of many other things (including water), sometimes the percentage fat by weight can be misleading.

For example:
Whole milk contains 4% fat by weight. However, the overwhelming weight of milk is water (89%), with carbohydrate (4%) and protein (3%) making up the rest.

When the energy contribution of the three nutrients is calculated, fat comes out as 52% of total energy!

Also, we need around 500–1000g of milk (or equivalent in other dairy products each day) to meet our daily calcium needs. Drinking this much of a 4% milk could contribute 20–40g of fat each day. Changing to a 2% or non-fat milk may not look like a big change, but it can mean a big drop in total fat intake for the day.

Many foods such as meats and dairy products are now available in a range of fat contents. The 'best' fat content for each food will be individual to the food and individual to your diet.

Knowing the percentage fat by weight, and knowing what quantity you eat of the food, could allow you to calculate the number of grams of fat this food has supplied. This information, of course, is only useful if you know what sort of a daily target your total fat intake should achieve.

A reduced-fat diet of 25–30% fat might allow 40–50g of fat per day on a 6400 kilojoule (1500 Calorie) budget, or 80–100g of fat per day on a 12 800 kilojoule (3000 Calorie) budget.

Most people do not need or want to calculate every gram of fat they consume and total it up towards a daily total. This represents a whole lot of unnecessary work, and makes it tempting to forget the Big Picture of nutrition because you are too focused on fat. However, these calculations might be useful, like in the case of the milk above, to work out whether it is useful to switch to a food with a reduced fat content.

2 Percentage fat by energy

Nutrition experts are more interested in the percentage of the energy (or kilojoules) in a food that comes from fat. This is also quoted as the percentage fat, but is quite a different number and a different concept. It provides a common denominator for comparing foods with widely different nutritional composition, and helps to pinpoint whether the fat content of a certain food is likely to be over-represented in our kilojoule budget. (Figure 1.4 shows how to calculate the percentage fat by energy in a food.)

We have already said that the fat content of our diets should be less than 30 per cent of total energy, and for some athletes 15–25 per cent of total kilojoules. Although this is not a hard and fast rule, it is generally a good idea to choose individual foods that contain less than 30 per cent of their energy as fat, especially where these foods have a significant role in your diet. But remember that it is hard and unfair to judge a single food! It is often better to judge the percentage fat of the combination of foods in a meal or snack, rather than pick on one food by itself.

So, do you need to count or calculate percentage fat in everything you eat?

No. Even though this section shows you how to make the calculations if you want to, we have already said that it is unnecessary to do this for every food and every meal. For most athletes, a reduced-fat diet can be achieved by following the food habits outlined in the previous Hints section. However, on occasions you may need to judge the fat content of a processed food, or weigh up the claims that a manufacturer makes about the fat content of its product and then the information in Figure 1.4 and this section will help.

When you need to be especially careful about fat intake (for example, on a fat-loss program, or when you need to maximise carbohydrate intake for heavy training), these skills may also help you to cut back a little further.

1.3 Increasing your carbohydrate intake

Carbohydrate foods play a vital role in exercise performance. The critical source of fuel for exercising muscles comes from your body's carbohydrate stores—in the form of blood glucose (a small amount), and glycogen stored in the liver and muscles (larger stores, but still only sufficient for up to about 90 minutes of continuous intense exercise). These stores must be continually refilled from the carbohydrate in your diet, and obviously the more you exercise the greater your dietary carbohydrate needs will be.

Figure 1.4 How can you tell the fat content of food?

HINT ONE: *Read the ingredient list on the label.*
These are listed in descending order:
- *If fat is in the 'Top Three', or listed several times by various names, then this food is probably high in fat.*
- *Fat may be hidden under the following aliases: vegetable fat, vegetable oil, animal fat, shortening, lard, cream, butter, margarine, copha ...*

HINT TWO: *Look for fat content of the food by weight. Nutrition information may be provided in a Nutritional Contents box on the product label, or you may need to consult a book of Food Composition Tables or reputable "Kilojoule Counter" book. Sometimes the manufacturer may make some claim about the fat content (or 'fat free' content) on the label. This information may help you to work out how many grams of fat your typical serve of this food will add to total daily fat intake. See last box for interpretation.*
- *Multiply the number of grams of fat in a serve by 37*
Divide by total kilojoules in the same serve
Multiply by 100
(For kilocalories, multiply by 9 and divide by Cals)

Example: Super chocolate cake — 50g serve

$$\text{Fat - energy ratio} = \frac{8 \times 37 \, kJ}{795} \times 100$$

$$= 37\%$$

- *Try to choose foods with less than 30% of energy from fat.*

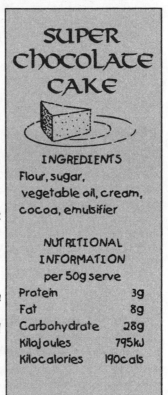

SUPER CHOCOLATE CAKE

INGREDIENTS
Flour, sugar, vegetable oil, cream, cocoa, emulsifier

NUTRITIONAL INFORMATION
per 50g serve

Protein	3g
Fat	8g
Carbohydrate	28g
Kilojoules	795kJ
Kilocalories	190cals

PRODUCT OF AUSTRALIA

Currently, carbohydrate provides about 40–45 per cent of the total energy in the Australian diet. For the athlete a general target of 50–60 per cent is set, with higher levels again for endurance athletes and those undertaking lengthy daily training sessions. With carbohydrate making such a large contribution to total energy needs, the most important food choices will be those that can supply additional nutrient value. After all, your peak training diet must achieve a number of other goals as well as contribute to muscle glycogen stores.

Are all carbohydrate foods the same?

When we talk about 'carbohydrate foods' we should really be using the term 'carbohydrate-rich' foods, to remind us that the overwhelming majority of these foods provide other nutrients and dietary needs, as well as being a good source of carbohydrate. Since such a variety of foods fall into the carbohydrate-rich classification it is not suprising that they are NOT all the same. Unfortunately, until recently we have not done justice to the diversity of carbohydrate-rich foods and their individual features.

Traditionally, carbohydrate foods have been classified in terms of the chemical structure of the carbohydrate molecule—being 'simple' carbohydrates (or sugars) of one or two molecules, or 'complex' carbohydrates (or starches) made up of thousands of sugar molecules joined together.

In addition, the following qualities have been given to each type of carbohydrate:

- Simple carbohydrate foods are less nutritious because they don't contain much in the way of vitamins or other nutrients, whereas complex carbohydrate foods contain plenty of important nutrients.
- Simple carbohydrates or sugars cause a rapid rise in blood sugar levels, followed by a rapid fall which leaves you feeling tired. Complex carbohydrate foods are absorbed more evenly into your body and create a gentle blood glucose curve.

You've probably guessed that simple carbohydrate foods got a 'bad' reputation while the complex carbohydrate foods were the 'good' guys. Now that you've read this, forget it! New nutrition research and a closer examination of food composition shows us that these statements should be confined to the bin reserved for 'old wives' tales'.

There are many features of carbohydrate-rich foods that could be considered, but for the purposes of sports nutrition we will confine ourselves to the following three: total nutritional value, effect on blood glucose and practical issues. Note that a number of carbohydrate-rich foods may be able to supply the same amount of carbohydrate to an athlete's diet, but in any given situation certain carbo-rich foods may have an advantage. Different situations have different demands—so it's all about 'horses for courses' rather than 'good' and 'bad' carbohydrate-rich foods.

Total nutritional value
While a system describing the nutritional value of foods will always be arbitrary, we can try to simplify carbohydrate-rich foods into categories of 'wholesome' and 'refined'. 'Wholesome' relates to the content of carbohydrate and other nutrients compared to the total energy content—and most of the time athletes will be after maximum nutritional value for the kilojoules they eat. 'Wholesome' carbohydrate-rich foods can also be described as those providing valuable amounts of vitamins, minerals, protein or fibre for a moderate kilojoule intake. 'Refined' carbohydrate-rich sources include foods that have been processed to remove much of their original nutritional value, or foods in which fat and sugar add lots of kilojoules to dilute the total nutrient–energy ratio. Figure 1.5 provides examples of carbohydrate-rich foods which might fall into the 'wholesome' and 'refined' categories.

Figure 1.5 also illustrates the problem with the old 'simple' versus 'complex' carbohydrate story; foods which technically fit into these structural categories do not necessarily fit the expected nutritional value picture. Just as some carbohydrate-rich foods based on 'simple' carbohydrates provide a valuable source of fibre and vitamins (for example, fruit), there are 'complex carbohydrate'-rich foods that contain little in the way of fibre, vitamins or minerals (for example, a Danish pastry). There are also carbohydrate-rich foods that contain significant amounts of both 'complex' and 'simple' carbohydrates (for example, a cake containing both flour and sugar), thus muddying the traditional classification line.

In the peak training diet, 'wholesome' carbohydrate-rich foods should be the number one choice. Not only will these provide the fuel for training and competition, but they will also help to provide the nutrients that keep your body well-tuned (e.g. fibre, vitamins, minerals). Hints are found in the following table, but the most important requirement is a change of attitude. Many of the wholesome carbohydrate-rich foods are items that we have made an afterthought in our eating habits. Become creative with these foods so that they become the number one part of your meals and snacks. You'll know you're on the right track when you start planning your evening meal: 'Maybe I'll have a rice dish or some stuffed potatoes (with some meat)', rather than 'I'll roast a leg of lamb or defrost some steak from the freezer'.

Effect on blood glucose
We've already mentioned the theory that 'simple' carbohydrate foods cause rapid highs and lows in blood sugar, and that 'complex' carbohydrate foods keep blood sugar levels even. However, recent nutrition

research has shown that this is a myth; in fact, each carbohydrate-rich food has a unique effect on blood glucose and other body metabolism, and this effect is quite unconnected to its 'simple' or 'complex' form. Blood glucose changes that occur after eating a food are related to the speed with which the food is digested and absorbed. Many factors in food influence this—including the type and amount of fibre in a food, the way in which complex carbohydrate molecules are joined, and even the physical form of the food (whether it is thick and sticky, in whole pieces or mashed up, hot or cold). You can't predict how a food will affect blood glucose levels—you can only measure the results.

In fact, a ranking system has been created to compare individual carbohydrate foods according to their actual blood glucose responses. This system, called the Glycemic Index, compares blood glucose measurements taken when carbohydrate-rich foods are consumed in a standard test. The food is eaten, first thing in the morning, in a serve that provides 50g of carbohydrate. The resulting blood glucose curve is compared to the response that occurs when 50g of pure glucose is consumed. A standard food (by convention either pure glucose or white bread)—which produces a high curve—is given the value of 100. So foods which produce a similarly high rise will have similar values, while a 'flat' and even response will have a low value.

Table 1.1 provides a list of the measured Glycemic Indices of some common carbohydrate-rich foods compared to a glucose standard. While this is an arbitrary line, 'high Glycemic Index' foods are generally considered to have a GI of above 70, while 'low Glycemic Index' foods are those with a GI of 50 or below. (The moderate GI foods— 50–70—are usually lumped in with the high GI group.)

You will notice that some foods have unexpected GI levels. Did you think that sugar would have a really high GI, or that bread and potatoes would be low GI foods? And what about the similar values scored by white bread and wholemeal bread? It's just more evidence of the need to throw out our previous ideas about the value of 'simple' or 'complex' carbohydrates.

In some areas of nutrition, particularly in the prevention and treatment of diabetes and high blood fat levels, the Glycemic Index has been used to design eating patterns that manipulate favourable blood glucose levels. In the next few years, we might learn that there are some areas of sports nutrition that might be aided by being able to control or produce a certain blood glucose response. In the later competition chapters of this book, you will see some early research that suggests that the high Glycemic Index carbohydrate-rich foods are most appropriate for recovery of muscle glycogen stores after strenuous exercise. It is also possible that low Glycemic Index foods will be helpful at other times, or for athletes who experience problems with large blood sugar highs and lows. For the present, the nutritional

Table 1.1 Glycemic Index of some common carbohydrate-rich foods

	Food	GI
High Glycemic Index (>70)	Glucose	100
	Cornflakes	84
	Cocopops	77
	White rice, boiled	88
	Sunbrown quick rice	80
	Instant mashed potato	83
	Baked potato	85
	Sports drink/Lucozade	95
	Jelly beans	80
Moderate Glycemic Index (50–70)	Sucrose	65
	Honey	58
	White bread	70
	Wholemeal bread	69
	Pancakes	70
	Weet Bix	70
	Sustain	68
	Mashed potato	70
	Boiled potato (whole)	56
	Boiled potato, new (whole)	62
	Basmati or doongara rice	58
	Bananas	60
	Watermelon	72
	Sultanas	56
	Soft drink	68
	Cordial	66
	Orange juice	52
	Icecream	61
Low Glycemic Index (<50)	Fructose	20
	Porridge	49
	All Bran	42
	White pasta, boiled	41
	Wholemeal pasta, boiled	37
	Baked beans	48
	Lentils	30
	Kidney beans	27
	Oranges	40
	Apples	36
	Apple juice	41
	Chocolate	49
	Flavoured yoghurt	34
	Vitari	28

Note: The GI values for these carbohydrate-rich foods have been derived from studies which observed the effects of these foods on blood glucose, where the intake of pure glucose has been given the value of 100. Since the applications of GI to sport are not fully known, this list is not complete. Rather, it is intended to show you that different carbohydrate-rich foods impact on blood glucose in a manner that might not be predictable from other features of the food.
Source: Dr Jennie Brand-Miller, 1995

value angle will probably continue to be the most important one, but stay tuned for more information about the Glycemic Index.

Practical issues

It doesn't matter how good a food looks on paper. Food doesn't become 'nutrition' until a person has actually eaten it. And sometimes there are factors that stand in the way of athletes eating the amount of carbohydrate they need, when they need it. For a start, an athlete may simply not like a food (for example, how would *you* fare if brussels sprouts were found to contain a magic ingredient for sports performance?).

Furthermore, as you progress through this book you will find that factors such as appetite, availability of food and stomach 'fullness' can sometimes stand in the way of eating adequate carbohydrate—especially in situations before, during and after exercise. Some carbohydrate-rich foods will be more practical than others to consume in these special circumstances. For example, at times you may need to find a carbohydrate source that is easy to consume when you are on the move, or one that is less fibrous and filling when gastrointestinal issues must be considered. Sometimes the search is on for a portable and non-perishable choice that can travel with you to a training or competition venue. Since it is important to be realistic in matching nutritional advice to an athlete's busy lifestyle, there are many sections in this book devoted to the 'practical' carbohydrate-rich foods that suit various situations.

While some 'practical' carbohydrate-rich foods may also be wholesome, there may be times or situations where practical issues take priority over the total nutritional value of a food. This is all part of dietary balance. You will also find that special sports products have been formulated to match some specific nutritional needs of the athlete —particularly those immediately before, during or after exercise. Products such as sports drinks, sports bars and liquid meal supplements have been specially manufactured to make the athlete's nutritional goals easy to achieve.

Throughout the rest of this book you will see a variety of carbohydrate-rich foods used in the diets of athletes. The various features and characteristics of the foods will be matched to the immediate priority of the situation and the overall balance of the eating plan.

What about fibre?

A good reason for choosing wholesome carbohydrate-rich foods is that they often provide a good source of fibre—a nutrient that has enjoyed a resurgence of interest in the last 20 years. However, despite the early publicity, there's a lot more to the fibre story than sprinkling bran on your cornflakes or eating oatbran muffins by the truckload.

Fibre is not one substance, but rather is a family of compounds. The different types fall into various categories such as 'soluble fibre', 'insoluble fibre' and the more newly recognised form of 'resistant starch'. Different types of fibre exert different effects on the digestion and metabolism of food in the body. These include aiding digestion, regulating blood glucose and blood cholesterol levels, and reducing the risk of some cancers. Fibre is also useful in making food and meals filling—an invaluable aid when you're cutting back on kilojoules to lose body fat.

Fibre is found in fruit and vegetable foods—or more precisely, fibre occurs naturally in these foods. Quite often the processing of food removes much of the fibre—not just in the food factory, but in the restaurant or in your kitchen. It is not uncommon for people to eat processed food minus its fibre, then buy bran or a fibre supplement in the belief that this is 'healthy'. Apart from the waste of money, it is unlikely that you will purchase all the types of fibrous compounds found in the original product. The best guideline is to eat fibre as it naturally occurs in the variety of foods that you eat. This will ensure that you get a mixture of the fibre types, and that the quantity of fibre varies with your energy and nutrient intake.

Like anything else, too much fibre has its disadvantages. As previously mentioned, some fibres add bulkiness and volume to foods, making meals filling. This can be a friend to those with low-energy requirements, but can make life difficult for athletes with heavier energy needs. For them, high-fibre eating may exceed the stomach 'comfort' limit. Too much fibre intake, or a sudden increase in fibre intake, can also lead to flatulence and diarrhea. Fibre-rich foods may not be the best choice just before training or competition. So be guided by a sensible amount and variety of fibre intake. Most times you will be pleased to enjoy the fibre that naturally occurs with your carbohydrate-rich foods. However, know the limits and the times for limiting!

And finally, to sugar!

Sugar has suffered some confusing publicity. On the one hand it is labelled 'pure, white and deadly' and blamed for all manner of health problems; on the other it is hailed as a 'natural part of life' and even an 'energy food for athletes'. Who is telling the truth?

Sugar is the popular name for sucrose, the most commonly occurring simple carbohydrate in the Western diet. Of all carbohydrate-rich foods, it is the most refined, being extracted from sugar cane and purified to remove all other compounds—including any other nutrients. In all forms, sugar and related substances such as honey, glucose and fructose, provide carbohydrates and kilojoules and little else. You've probably heard the term 'empty Calories' (or 'empty kilojoules').

To be fair, sugar contributes to, rather than causes, health problems. And these problems relate to excessive sugar intake and to association with other unhealthy eating habits (e.g. excessive fat intake and inadequate fibre intake) rather than sugar alone. All Australians—and athletes in particular—are advised to increase their intake of carbohydrate-rich foods. However, there are very few people who would need to increase their intake of sugar, since this is an activity that most of us have well-mastered—in fact, in some cases too well. The current intake of sugar in Australia is almost a kilogram a week, or about 20 per cent of total energy intake. This represents an overstatement of the need for sugar in the diets of most people, and is the reason that one of the dietary guidelines for Australians is 'Eat less sugar and sugary foods'.

Sugar intake is well-linked to tooth decay. On the other hand, some wholesome carbohydrate-rich foods which are sticky and cling to the teeth after eating, can also be involved in this process. Looking after your teeth is not just a matter of choosing healthy foods, but making sure that teeth are brushed or cleaned after eating.

A chief problem with sugar is the company it keeps. Sugar is a compact and delicious form of kilojoules that is easily overeaten, but this becomes a particular problem in the case of sugar-coated fats such as chocolate, cakes and icecream. And this combination of high kilojoules and fat, in many cases minus fibre, vitamins and minerals, is where the potential for overuse and subsequent health disadvantages lies.

So, what is the role of sugar and sugary foods in the peak training diet? Using sugar well is a matter of choosing:

- the right amount (many of us could afford to cut back on our present intake, especially where kilojoules are in short supply)
- the right type (watch the fat–sugar combinations), and
- the right occasions (situations calling for practical considerations such as compactness or low-fibre content).

While sugar and sugary foods generally fall into the category of 'less wholesome' or 'refined' carbohydrate-rich foods, they often come out well in the 'practical' and enjoyment classifications. Being compact, they can be added to a wholesome carbohydrate meal to boost the total carbohydrate content without adding extra bulk. And it is rare to find someone who doesn't like chocolate!

In the everyday training diet, when the big picture of your nutritional goals is important, sugar and less wholesome carbohydrate-rich foods should provide a small part of total energy intake. Even so, there may be occasions for treats, or for specialised 'practical' uses of these foods (e.g. a sports drink during and after a prolonged training session). We shall see later, that in many competition settings, overall nutritional goals may take a lower priority to more practical and specialised uses of carbohydrate-rich foods. In these situations, sugary foods may have a greater role to play in providing carbohydrate to the athlete.

Figure 1.5 Carbohydrate foods

REFINED CARBOHYDRATES	WHOLESOME CARBOHYDRATES	
• sugar • honey, jam • syrups, toppings • glucose, fructose • soft drinks, cordial, flavoured mineral water • sports drinks, high carbohydrate supplements (carbo-loaders) • sweets, chocolates • high-fat cakes, pastries, biscuits and desserts (high fat and sugar)	• fruit • fruit juice • canned fruit • dried fruit • milk, yoghurt, fromage frais • liquid meals (Sustagen Sport, Exceed Sports Meal, Gator-Pro) • low-fat cakes, biscuits, desserts (scones, pancakes, special recipes, etc.)	SIMPLE CARBOHYDRATES
• pastry • chips • crisps, Twisties, etc. • high-fat cakes, pastries, biscuits and desserts	• breads, muffins, bagels, etc. • pizza bases • breakfast cereals • pasta and noodles • rice and other grains • starchy vegetables (e.g. potatoes, corn) • legumes (e.g. lentils, baked beans) • low-fat cakes, biscuits, desserts (scones, pancakes, special recipes, etc.) • dry biscuits and rice cakes	COMPLEX CARBOHYDRATES

Carbohydrate foods can be classified according to the chemical form of the carbohydrate—but a better classification system rates the total nutritional value of the food. Note that some foods, such as cakes, contain significant amounts of both simple carbohydrate (sugar) and complex carbohydrate (flour).

HINTS TO EMPHASISE NUTRITIOUS CARBOHYDRATE-RICH FOODS IN YOUR DIET

- Be prepared to be different. A typical Western diet is *not* a high carbohydrate diet. You will need to plan ahead, be organised, and on occasions 'stand away from the crowd'. Hopefully however, your high-carbohydrate diet being the blue-print for healthy eating, other people will follow your lead.

- Plan each meal around a carbohydrate food, making it the centre of attention and adding the rest of the meal around it—for example, add filling to a sandwich, sauce to pasta, topping on breakfast cereal. Otherwise, take your traditional meal, cut the protein serve in half and add a generous serve of carbohydrate foods (bread rolls, potatoes, rice, etc.) to fill up more than half the plate.

- Choose breakfast cereals from the low–moderate sugar, high-fibre range. Look out for toasted mueslis—they are high in fat. Make your own muesli recipe or use the commercial toasted varieties as a sprinkle on top of other cereals.

- Enjoy the sweetness and variety of fruit at meals and snacks. Fresh is usually the most nutritious form—but make good use of juices and dried, canned and stewed fruits.

- Explore bread in all its forms—pita, bagels, rolls, crumpets, damper and fruit bread to name but a few. Go for thick-sliced loaves, or bread rolls to increase the bread part of the sandwich.

- Cakes, muffins, slices and puddings can be high in fat. Scones and pancakes are a great choice—or experiment with reduced-fat recipes for wholemeal cakes, muffins, and wholemeal puddings. Modify your own recipes or find low-fat commercial varieties (e.g. Pritikin style).

- Other low-fat carbohydrate desserts include non-fat fruit yoghurts, light fromage frais, and low-fat icecream or ice-desserts. Otherwise, make your own recipes based on fruits.

- Many icecream shops now sell soft-serve yoghurts, icecreams and ice-desserts that are high in carbos and low in fat. Many taste like a creamy indulgence!

- Become versatile with pastas and noodles in all their shapes and sizes. Eat them plain as a side dish, or add a low-fat sauce and make a meal. Rice can also be used in this way—with main dishes including paella and fried rice (dry-fried of course).

- Try legumes (kidney beans, lentils, chick peas, etc.) in pasta sauces and casseroles to replace some or all of the meat, fish or chicken. Make a hearty soup or bean salad a meal in itself.

- Make the most of starchy vegetables—potatoes, corn, peas, etc. Baked potatoes and corn on the cob can pep up a meal, and stuffed potatoes make a delicious main meal.
- Note that other vegetables, particularly salad vegetables, are good sources of fibre as well as some vitamins and minerals. However, they are not good sources of carbohydrate by themselves and should be eaten with other carbohydrate foods at the meal.
- Low fat 'carbo shakes' can be made with skim milk, fruit and ice cubes. Low fat icecream and non-fat yoghurt are optional extras for a creamy drink. Commercial liquid meal supplements are also available.
- Be adventurous with your cooking. Vegetarian and 'healthy' recipe books can provide clever ways of making cereals, grains and vegetables the focus of a meal.

HINTS FOR INCREASING YOUR FIBRE INTAKE

- On most occasions choose foods with the fibre content left intact by:
  - selecting wholegrain breads and breakfast cereals, wholemeal pastas and brown rice
  - enjoying some of your fruits and vegetables raw—for example, fresh fruit, salads, crunchy vegetable sticks, fruit salad, whole fruits blended into 'smoothies'. Eat the skins and seeds where appropriate.
  - cooking fruit and vegetables lightly, leaving them a little crisp rather than overcooked. Again, leave the skins on where appropriate.
- Cook with wholemeal flour. You may find that many of your recipes can be made with wholemeal flour, or a mixture of half white and half wholemeal.
- Experiment with vegetarian recipes or ideas. Try legumes and other types of grains and cereals.
- There is probably no need for added fibre, such as unprocessed brans, unless they are part of a whole food recipe.

HINTS FOR USING SUGAR WELL

- Look at the total amount of sugar that you eat. Let it accompany rather than dominate your total carbohydrate menu.

- When weight loss is desired, take a stronger hand to reduce sugar intake and save the kilojoules for more nutritious carbohydrate foods.

- Enjoy sugar-coated fat foods as a treat. Think of chocolate, icecream, and rich cakes as 'fun' foods rather than 'energy' foods, and give them a special rather than a regular place in your eating plan.

- Use sugar as an addition to your base of nutritious carbohydrate foods—such as a little jam on toast, syrup on pancakes, soft drink with a meal. But, don't let it take over the show.

- Apart from times when a carbohydrate drink is specifically required for your sports performance, stick to water, low-joule drinks and plain mineral water.

- Good ways to cut back the extra sugar are:

  — gradually cut back what you add to your coffee or sprinkle on your breakfast cereal

  — look for 'unsweetened' and 'no-added-sugar' brands

  — experiment with recipes to cut back the added sugar

  — make use of low-joule artificial sweeteners, especially where energy needs are tight. Of course, treat such sweeteners with respect—you can overdo the use of these as well.

  — learn to read labels in order to recognise sugar by its other names (sucrose, fructose, corn syrup, glucose, etc.).

- Care for your teeth by eating sugary foods as part of a meal, and try to have your toothbrush around when sticky foods are eaten (or drunk) by themselves.

1.4 Looking after your electrolytes

Salt is sodium chloride, with the sodium portion of more interest to us here. Sodium is the most important electrolyte found outside the body's cells (potassium is its opposite partner within the cells). The sodium concentration helps to regulate blood pressure and volume, and assists in balancing the distribution of fluid and nutrients between the inside and outside of cells. When the sodium concentration falls outside its normal range, the delicate balance is disturbed and cell function can be crippled.

Your body has a fairly sophisticated system (involving, amongst other things, your kidneys and thirst drive) to regulate how much sodium and water is taken in, and how much these and other electrolytes (potassium, chloride, etc.) are excreted in urine. Electrolytes, particularly sodium, are also lost in other body fluids—the most important being sweat. Massive losses of sweat can potentially deplete the body's electrolyte stores, so the body cleverly adapts, with training and acclimatisation to a hot environment, by diluting sweat and thus conserving electrolytes. It then expects you to replace nett losses through your diet. In this way, within a broad range of challenges the body can manage its electrolyte levels quite well.

However, the life of an athlete isn't always a series of gentle challenges, and it is probable that you throw your body into some extreme situations at times. Electrolyte balance can be threatened either by heavy consumption of electrolytes or by severe losses. The usual problem is overconsumption, and the usual culprit is sodium. In fact, the Australian diet has almost made excess salt intake an art form.

Sodium, like the other electrolytes, is found naturally in many foods. However, our dietary patterns have completely distorted sodium intake, through the addition of large amounts of salt to our foods and our meals. Other sodium compounds include MSG (monosodium glutamate), sodium bicarbonate, and some vitamin C tablets (sodium ascorbate). The kidneys battle hard with the excessive intake of sodium—however, one in five people will go on to suffer high blood pressure in later life. Excess salt also interferes with calcium balance and can contribute towards low bone density for those at risk. Since we don't always know who is at risk for these problems until it is too late, healthy nutrition guidelines encourage all Australians to curb their salt habits.

There is a much smaller possibility that salt depletion will occur, if massive sweat (and sodium) losses are not adequately replaced. Theoretically, this could happen if an unacclimatised athlete exercised furiously in a hot climate, replacing sweat losses with plain water or other low-sodium fluids. In real life this happens rarely. A sports drink during and after long, sweaty sessions, or a little salt at the next meal will help to replace both fluid and electrolyte levels. It should be noted that today's sports drinks contain a relatively small amount of sodium, in the concentrations that can replace fluid and electrolytes simultaneously and in balance.

The need to replace sodium and electrolytes during exercise will be discussed in Chapter 4, which looks at competition strategies. Your training sessions should follow a similar protocol, especially where they mimic the demands of strenuous competition.

One final word. Salt tablets are not necessary at any level or at any time. They provide more salt than the body can handle in one hit, and can provoke sodium–fluid imbalances, and frequently nausea and vomiting. Far from preventing or curing muscle cramps, they can be a disadvantage—even a danger—to your exercise performance.

HINTS FOR USING SALT WISELY

- Never take salt tablets.
- In general, there is little need to add salt to your food, either in cooking or at the table. Go easy also with salty sauces and flavourings (for example soy sauce, stock cubes and vegemite).
- Experiment with herbs, spices, lemon juice and other salt-free flavourings to make your meals tasty.
- Reduce your intake of salty snack foods, processed foods and take-aways.
- Learn to read labels to check the salt content of processed foods. Look for new varieties with reduced salt or low sodium content.
- Make this campaign a gradual process, and your taste buds will gradually adapt (and even thank you!).
- After lengthy training sessions in hot weather, you may be wise to drink a sports drink or add a little salt at your next meal—particularly until you adapt to the conditions.
- Practise competition plans for sports drink intake during training—especially during prolonged intense sessions. Practice makes perfect!
- Sports drinks contain a little sodium for important reasons—to assist with rehydration processes. Their sodium content is only a small part of your dietary intake; the majority of heavily-training athletes who benefit from the use of sports drinks, need not be concerned about them being 'too salty'.

1.5 Replacing your daily fluid losses

Water is your most important nutrient. The effects of dehydration are quickly felt and affect not only performance, but at times can endanger your life itself. The needs and strategies for fluid intake during exercise will be covered in Chapter 4: Competition. However, while athletes have become more aware of fluid needs in the competition arena, many completely forget about the training situation. It is an essential part of your training nutrition to look after day-to-day maintenance of fluid balance. Unfortunately, thirst is not a good indicator of what you need: you will have to work out what you are up against in your own training schedule, and plan your fluid strategies accordingly.

MONITORING FLUID BALANCE DURING TRAINING

A pair of accurate digital scales can help you to determine the success of your fluid intake strategies during training.

1 Since you will be using them to measure changes in body weight over time, it is important that you 'standardise' conditions of weighing. For example: have the scales on a level surface and the same surface each time.
2 Weigh yourself each time in minimum clothing (i.e. your underpants or bathers) and towel-off before weighing. Being wet will artificially increase your weight, especially if you are wearing sweat- or water-soaked clothing.

Depending on the length and intensity of training sessions, the acclimatisation of the athlete, and the environmental conditions, daily sweat losses can be considerable. In some cases, athletes will face greater dehydration threats in training than they will ever encounter in competition. Swimmers, for instance, can train for hours in a warm pool and incur significant sweat losses, yet never become dehydrated in a 100 metre race!

It is especially tricky to comprehend dehydration in training when there is no visible proof of sweat. Swimmers are already wet, so how can they notice it? A cyclist might come home quite dry from a road session, because the sweat evaporates quickly in the passing wind.

One way to get an idea of your nett fluid loss is to weigh yourself before and after the session—each kilogram lost is roughly equal to a litre of fluid that must be replaced.

The following box shows you how to make simple calculations to monitor sweat loss and your success in replacing this fluid during training. While the effects of dehydration will be discussed in more detail in the competition chapter, remember that it is important to maintain fluid balance during training as well. After all, you want to get the best out of each session that you do! It is not necessary to do these calculations at each session, but it is useful to monitor how well you are doing every now and again. A change in weather or a change in training is often a good time to reassess your goals and whether your strategies measure up. The calculations will estimate the rate and total of sweat loss during a session (letting you plan how much fluid you need to have on hand and how often you need to drink), as well as estimating percentage dehydration at the end of training (telling you not only how well you did today, but what you need to replace before the next training session). Try to keep below the 1–2 per cent dehydration mark—more about that later.

3   Accurately measure: a = pre-training weight (kg)
b = post-training weight (kg)
c = amount of fluid consumed during the session (L) (either know the volume of your drinking bottle and how much you consumed, or weigh the bottle before and after; 1000ml or 1 Litre water = 1000g or 1kg)

4   Estimated total sweat loss during training session (d)
= body weight change (a – b) + fluid intake during training (c)

5   Estimated sweat rate per hour during session
$$= \frac{\text{total sweat loss (d)}}{\text{length of training}}$$

6   Level of dehydration at end of session
$$= \frac{\text{body weight change}}{\text{body weight at start of training}} \times 100$$
$$= \frac{(a - b)}{a} \times 100$$

Of course, if you eat any food or go to the toilet during the training session these factors (and weight changes) will need to be taken into account. For this calculation we will keep things simple.

Our athlete weighs 65.4kg before training: a = 65.4kg
After 1.5 hours of hard running in summer,
his post-exercise weight is 63.9kg   b = 63.9kg
He drank 500ml of fluid during the session   c = 0.5L = 0.5kg

Calculations:

Sweat loss (kg or L)   = a – b + c
= 65.4 – 63.9 + 0.5kg
= 2.0kg or 2000ml (remember 1L or 1000ml = 1kg or 1000g)

Sweat rate (ml/hr)   = 2000ml/1.5hr
= 1333ml/hr

Percentage dehydration $= \frac{(a - b)}{a} \times 100$
at end of session
$= \frac{(65.4 - 63.9)}{64.5} \times 100$
= 2.3%

Table 1.2   Typical estimated sweat losses and fluid intakes of elite athletes in training

Athletes	Temperature at training	Sweat loss (ml/hr) average (range)	Fluid intake (ml/hr) average (range)	% Dehydration end of session average (range)
Male soccer	20–28°C	925ml (200–1580)	401ml (0–1025)	1.2% (0–2.9)
Female netball players	20–28°C	720ml (460–965)	430ml (145–850)	0.8% (0–1.7)
Male basketball players	20–28°C	1350ml (970–2105)	765ml (305–1160)	1.0% (0–2.1)
Male rowers	32°C	1980ml (990–2915)	960ml (410–1490)	1.7% (.5–3.2)
Male rowers	10°C	1165ml (430–2000)	582ml (215–1265)	0.6% (0–2.3)
Female rowers	32°C	1390ml (740–2335)	780ml (290–1390)	1.2% (0–1.8)
Female rowers	10°C	780ml (360–1550)	405ml (145–660)	0.5% (0–2.0)

Table 1.2 shows real-life calculations for sweat losses and fluid intakes of some athletes training at the Australian Institute of Sport. Note that on average, the athletes kept their dehydration levels below 2 per cent—but the range shows us that some athletes did not meet their fluid intake needs well.

Another feature of training, unlike competition, is that conditions may not make fluid intake easy and accessible. There are no aid stations, and sometimes no trainers to bring out a water bottle to you. And if you are doing your long weekend run in the hills or cross-country, you are unlikely to come across a tap or a shop!

Table 1.3 lists some of the factors standing in the way of adequate fluid intake during a training session—and ways around these problems. With motivation and some creativity you can usually solve, or at least improve the situation.

Looking after your fluid needs during training will mean better training (and greater improvement) as well as good practice for competition. You will be learning both to 'stomach' fluid while on the move, and to tolerate various sports drinks. And although the leading runners in the marathon make it look easy on television, there is quite a skill to grabbing a drink from an aid station and getting it all into your mouth without losing a stride.

You will also need to look at your fluid intake between training sessions to ensure that fluid levels have been fully restored. In most cases, water will be sufficient since your basic need is to replace fluid. However, fluids can also contain other nutrients, and depending on your individual situation, this can either be a useful way of supplying energy and other nutrients or a trap for overconsuming kilojoules.

Table 1.3 Problems and solutions for good fluid intake practices during training

Problem	Solution
No fluid available at training venue.	Take your own water bottle with you to training—you may have to fill it up before you go.
Hard to carry fluid with you if you are on the move during training (e.g. running).	• Look for special belts that can carry your water bottle, or for a special bottle with a 'hand grip handle'. • Plan a drink stop or two along the course—you may be able to organise your route to go past a tap or your own fluid station. Either stop for a drink or top up the bottle you are carrying.
Your style of exercise makes it difficult to drink without stopping or reducing the pace (e.g. rowing, kayaking, sailing, cycling, running).	• Be prepared to stop or slow down at regular intervals to drink. Although this may spoil your rhythm for a minute, it will eventually pay off by improving the total quality of your training. • Try a 'bikestream' or similar device—a drinking pouch with a tube that delivers fluid straight to your mouth. Not only is this 'hands free' drinking, but it will allow you to stay in your desired cycling or sailing position. Since the drinking pouch is under pressure, you don't even have to suck on the straw—just bite on the valve for a squirt of fluid.
You don't like the taste of water (or your sports drink).	If you don't like plain water, add a dash of lemon or lime juice, low-joule cordial (no carbos or kilojoules), or drink cordial or sports drink (adds carbos for a long training session). There are many sports drinks on the market—find one with a taste that you like.
You forget to drink when you are concentrating on your training.	• Organise some set drink breaks ahead of the training session and stick to the plan. • Set your watch to 'beep' at set intervals to remind you to drink.
You don't know how much fluid you need to consume.	Do a couple of fluid balance checks during typical training sessions (see box p.30) to calculate typical sweat losses under various training and environmental conditions. Ideally, aim to replace about 80% of fluid losses during the session. If this is not feasible or practical, do the best job you can, and be prepared to rehydrate well after the session.
You think you need to 'train tough' so that you learn to cope with heat and dehydration.	You can't learn to tolerate dehydration—just like a car can't learn to tolerate an empty radiator. This is 'training stupid' rather than 'training tough'. Staying well hydrated will mean better training and greater improvements.

HINTS FOR LOOKING AFTER FLUID NEEDS IN TRAINING

- Form a plan to look after your fluid needs. Don't leave it to good luck.
- Start a training session well-hydrated. On hot days, have an extra drink just before you start.
- Make fluids available during training sessions, especially during long sessions in hot weather. See Table 1.3 for solutions to fluid intake problems.
- Include dress rehearsals of competition strategies—practise with the type, quantity and frequency of fluid intake that you intend to use during your event.
- Fully rehydrate between training sessions. Helpful strategies include keeping a jug of fluid in a prominent place that will remind you to drink.
- If you need a guide to your fluid deficit (and how much fluid should be replaced) after an exercise session, compare your pre- and post-body weight. See box, page 30.
- Choose fluids that will help you meet other nutrition goals and be careful with the energy considerations. In most cases, water will be adequate. A sports drink or cordial will provide extra carbohydrate and may be useful during or after lengthy training sessions.
- Monitoring morning bodyweight is a useful way to pick up chronic dehydration (often a sign of overtraining).

Since liquids do not give you the same feeling of fullness as solid foods, it is usually easier to drink kilojoules than to eat them. This strategy can be useful for an athlete who needs help to meet massive daily energy needs, or who could benefit from carbohydrate intake straight after exercise but feels too tired or nauseous to eat. In other chapters you will see how drinks such as sports drinks, fruit juices and even soft drinks can provide a carbohydrate during and after exercise, and how 'liquid meals' can be made from low-fat milkshakes or special commercial supplements (such as Sustagen Sport, Gator-Pro or Exceed Sports Meal). However, when your kilojoule needs are tight, you should concentrate on drinking water and low-energy fluid to replace fluid losses and save your kilojoules for food.

1.6 Using alcohol sensibly

Alcohol can be an enjoyable part of most lifestyles, including that of an athlete. It is hard to think of a celebration without champagne—

33

and hopefully you will have many sports successes to celebrate! The issue with alcohol is how well you use it, and unfortunately in some sports alcohol is used very badly.

A nutrition text book will warn you about the health and social consequences of excessive alcohol intake, including its contribution to our annual road toll. For most athletes, however, tales of liver cirrhosis are hard to comprehend. But alcohol intake doesn't have to reach this level of abuse before it affects sports performance. With this in mind, we shall consider alcohol intake solely from the exercise viewpoint.

The immediate effects of drinking alcohol include dilation of blood vessels (vasodilation) and depression of the central nervous system. As a result, you will feel a little flushed (losing more heat through your skin) and your sensitivity will be dulled. So, while you think you are giving a great performance (be it in the disco or on the playing field), in fact your judgement, co-ordination and vision will be impaired. Effects will be related to the quantity of alcohol that you drink, and your individual tolerance (note that females tend to have poorer tolerance). However, most people will experience an effect after 20–30g of alcohol is consumed, and the effects will increase with the amount that is drunk. Figure 1.6 illustrates the alcohol content of various drinks.

Alcohol is not good for fluid replacement—in fact, it acts as a diuretic and may cause dehydration. And despite what you may have heard about beer and 'carbo-loading', alcoholic drinks will not fuel up your muscle glycogen stores. The kilojoules in alcoholic drinks come from alcohol, *not* carbohydrate, and alcohol is high in kilojoules— 29 kJ per gram (see Figure 1.3). In addition, alcohol may interfere with glycogen synthesis.

The bottom line is that alcohol should not be consumed just prior to or during exercise (and this includes heavy intake on the night before sport). The penalties include dehydration, poor fuel stores, impaired skills, and a greater threat of hypothermia in a cold environment (heat losses though the skin will interfere with normal temperature regulation).

After exercise, alcohol intake should not compromise rehydration and refuelling needs. But, once these priorities are taken care of, there is only one other reason that could prevent athletes enjoying a couple of drinks. This issue, often forgotten in the post-match cheer, is the vasodilatory effect of alcohol and its impact on tissue damage. Remember that you ice and elevate soft tissue injuries and bruising to constrict blood flow to the injured parts. The injured athlete who consumes alcohol immediately after the event may cause extra swelling and bleeding, delaying recovery, and in some cases even exacerbating the extent of the damage. The most sensible pathway for an injured athlete to take is to avoid any alcohol in the 24–48 hours post-exercise.

Figure 1.6 Alcohol content of common drinks

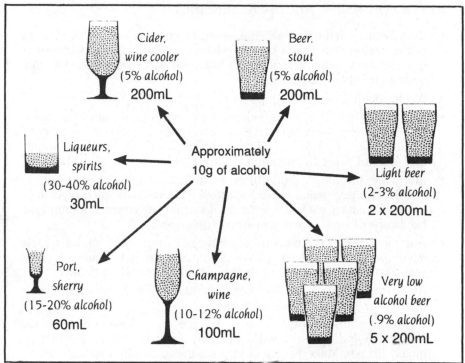

So should an athlete worry about occasional alcohol binges—or perhaps the weekly post-match 'wind-down'? The answer is that even a single episode of excess intake will cause some damage—in particular it will delay recovery and adaptation after exercise, and perhaps lengthen injury time. Slow recovery could be crucial if your next competition is a day, or even a week away, and catches you at less than your full capacity. Even if competition is some time away, you should consider whether your next training sessions will be disrupted, and whether you can afford this.

The real problem with alcohol occurs when drinking binges are repeated, as is often seen after weekly matches in team sports. Repeated alcohol binges will slowly but surely erode your skills, your fitness and your sports career. And that is a fact—even if everyone on the team does it and it appears to be normal (or desirable) behaviour. Another thing to remember is that alcohol is a high-kilojoule source of poor nutritional value. Heavy consumption and binge periods will

HINTS FOR USING ALCOHOL SENSIBLY

- If you choose to drink alcohol, learn to enjoy a couple of glasses per occasion. It is much better to have a couple of drinks throughout the week, than save up for a binge on Saturday night (or after your competition).
- Avoid alcohol in the 24 hours prior to competition.
- Be wary of dehydration after consuming large amounts of alcohol, as well as the increased risk of developing hypothermia in cold environments (e.g. skiing). Take precautions if you have consumed any alcohol prior to training sessions (including the night before).
- Enjoy alcohol after competition, without causing damage to yourself or your performance. Rehydrate and refuel with carbohydrates before you start with alcoholic drinks, then set yourself a limit and be aware of how much you have consumed.
- Don't get caught up in group drinking situations. The advice which accompanies drink-driving laws in your state may be a useful guide (see Figure 1.6 for a guide to the alcohol content of drinks).
- Avoid any alcohol for 24 hours post-exercise if any soft tissue injuries or bruising have occurred.
- Use tricks to make the alcohol go further. Drink low-alcohol beers, mix your wine with mineral water and order half-nips of spirits in mixed drinks. Make plenty of non-alcoholic drinks available, both as thirst-quenchers and as an enjoyable alternative to alcohol. This could include fruit juices, plain mineral water, and soft drinks, as well as special non-alcoholic cocktails.
- If you need to restrict your energy intake, treat alcohol as a luxury item. There are more nutritious ways of consuming kilojoules.

lead to weight gain. Have you noticed how much heavier you are on your return from the end-of-season trip?

Alcohol is not 'sweated out' or 'exercised off'—these are just more of the locker room tales that help to sustain alcohol misuse in sports. It is a drug that, at high levels, causes damage to many organs and tissues in your body. The only way to prevent this from happening is not to drink to excess.

Having said all this, alcohol can be a small part of a healthy diet. A drink after a hard day's training can help you relax, and a few drinks can add sparkle to social occasions. If you choose to drink, make it work for you, rather than pull your sports potential back to the level of those who would have you believe that 'team bonding' (getting drunk together) is all that sport has to offer.

2 Fine tuning— how much and when?

Now that the basic principles are in place, it is time to start accounting for your individual characteristics, and to plan for your specific needs. You must calculate your requirements for the various nutrients, and then arrange these within your energy budget. And of course, you will need to consider how best to arrange your food intake over your busy day—to gain nutritional advantages as well as meet your schedule of commitments.

2.1 Energy

How many kilojoules should I eat each day? This is a question frequently thrown at dietitians—and athletes expect an answer to three decimal places. Such precision is impossible, because your body is a unique energy system with its own tally of energy needs. In a nutshell, you need enough energy to be you!

The major factors that make up your total energy requirements are:

- Your basal metabolic rate (BMR)—the energy required just to keep your body functioning. This varies with age (decreasing as you get older), with body mass (increasing with a larger body mass), with body composition (increasing with greater muscle mass and decreasing with greater fat stores), and gender (greater in men than women). Metabolic rate is determined and altered by many other factors as well.

    Obviously, this energy need will vary greatly between people, and can be a great source of frustration and discouragement to those who 'drew the short stick'. We all know those lucky people who can eat food by the truckload without gaining a gram of body fat (due to an inefficient metabolism which 'wastes' food energy), while others horde every kilojoule they are presented with (efficient metabolism) and gain a kilo just by smelling a box of chocolates!

Figure 2.1 How to predict your daily energy requirements

STEP ONE:	Find your basal metabolic rate (BMR) using Table 2.1.
STEP TWO:	Rate your everyday activity level. You can either rate the activity level of your life (minus sport activities) then add the energy cost of your sport separately (step 4) or rate your daily activity in total. If you are exercising less than 3 times a week, and your sessions are low to moderate in intensity, it may be easier to rate your daily activity in total.

If you are rating your non-exercise activity level, note that many athletes are relatively inactive outside their training or competition sessions (either sleeping or doing low-level work or study).

Use Table 2.2 to choose an activity level for your total day, or your total day minus exercise.

STEP THREE:	Multiply your BMR by the activity level factor.
STEP FOUR:	Estimate the energy cost of your training/competition/exercise using Table 2.3. Multiply the hours you spend in exercise each week, by the approximate energy cost of the specific task. Divide the weekly total by 7 to get a daily average. Add this to the total generated by Step 3.
STEP FIVE:	If you are growing, pregnant or breast feeding, add the energy cost (see Table 2.4).
EXAMPLE:	Mary is a 20-year-old basketball player and weighs 60kg. She trains 3 nights a week — an hour of running (@ 5 min per km) and plays one game each week, averaging 20 minutes of court time each game. Her lifestyle outside basketball is light-moderate in activity (e.g. walks to University and between classes).

Step 1	BMR	= 5755 kJ (Table 2.1)
Step 2	Activity level factor	= 1.6 (Table 2.2)
Step 3	5755 x 1.6	= 9208
Step 4	Exercise each week	= 3 x 60 mins x 52 kJ/min + 20 mins x 35 kJ/min (Table 2.3)
	Exercise/day	= 10060/7 = 1437 kJ
	Total daily energy expenditure	= 9208 + 1437 kJ = 10,645 kJ
Step 5	No energy required for growth etc.	
	Therefore, Mary's estimated daily energy requirements	= 10,645 kJ/day (2546 Cals/day)

- Growth, including pregnancy and breast-feeding. Children and adolescents may need plenty of additional kilojoules to provide for new bone and body tissues as they grow.

- Muscular work. While some athletes hold jobs that involve heavy manual labour, for the most part it is exercise, and particularly the training schedule, that adds a significant contribution to total energy needs.

So how can you tell what your total energy requirements will be? An approximation can be made using tables that calculate average figures for each of these major factors. Remember, however, that individuals vary quite remarkably around average figures, and that the purpose of doing such a calculation will be to find a ballpark figure for your expected energy requirements. See Figure 2.1 for instructions on how to calculate your estimated energy needs. Don't be surprised or disappointed if your estimation doesn't seem to match exactly your usual energy intake from food. (After all, you probably don't earn the average wage in this country either.)

Most of the time, we want to be in energy balance (this is when we match our energy requirements with a similar intake of energy from food). Your body has a buffer for this energy balance equation. The body's fat stores provide an energy reserve to store extra kilojoules when you consume more than you expend, or to make up the deficit when the reverse is true. This is how you gain or lose weight from body fat. (See Figure 2.2.)

Even when you are in energy balance (neither gaining or losing body fat), you will not necessarily have to eat *exactly* the same number of kilojoules as you expend for that day. In the short term—say over a couple of days—there may be little correlation between your energy input and requirements. However over a period of a week or more, the energy balance equation should be maintained with considerable precision.

This gives you a way of fine-tuning the assessment of your energy requirements. If you can record your total food intake for a week, accurately and honestly, without changing things just because you are watching yourself, then an assessment of your energy intake will give you a closer estimation of your energy requirements (energy intake equals energy requirement, right?). Remember, you must be following your usual habits, and neither gain nor lose body fat over this time. A dietitian can instruct you how to undertake this task, and will make an expert analysis of the results. (The dietary analysis can also tell you about your intake of carbohydrate, protein, vitamins and minerals, making it a valuable exercise.)

Your energy requirements are individual and specific to you. In general, the largest energy requirements are reported by athletes who are young, growing, large, with plenty of muscle mass, and who

Table 2.1 Basal Metabolic Rate for reference adults

		Daily energy (kilojoules/day[a])			
	Your body weight	10–18 yrs	18–30 yrs	30–60 yrs	over 60 yrs
Men	55kg	6824	6360	6295	5155
	60kg	7195	6675	6535	5400
	65kg	7565	6990	6775	5645
	70kg	7935	7305	7015	5890
	75kg	8305	7620	7255	6135
	80kg	8675	7935	7495	6380
	85kg	9045	8250	7735	6625
	90kg	9415	8565	7975	6870
Women	40kg	5140	4515	4900	4275
	45kg	5420	4825	5070	4465
	50kg	5700	5135	5240	4845
	55kg	5980	5445	5410	5035
	60kg	6260	5755	5580	5225
	65kg	6540	6065	5750	5415
	70kg	6820	6375	5920	5605
	75kg	7100	6685	6090	5795

Note: [a] Kilocalories can be calculated by dividing by 4.2
Source: *Recommended Nutrient Intakes*, NHMRC, Australia, 1990

Table 2.2 Average activity levels expressed as multiples of BMR

Activity level	Males	Females
Bed rest	1.2	1.2
Very sedentary	1.3	1.3
Sedentary/maintenance	1.4	1.4
Light	1.5	1.5
Light–moderate	1.7	1.6
Moderate	1.8	1.7
Heavy	2.1	1.8
Very heavy	2.3	2.0

Source: *Recommended Nutrient Intakes*, NHMRC, Australia, 1990

Table 2.3 Estimated daily energy allowances for growth, pregnancy and breastfeeding

	Additional daily energy (kilojoules/day[a])	
Boys and girls	10–14 yrs	+8kJ per kg
	15 yrs	+4kJ per kg
	16–18 yrs	+2kJ per kg
Pregnancy	Trimesters 2 & 3	+850–1000kJ
Breastfeeding		+2000–2400kJ

Note: [a] Kilocalories can be calculated by dividing by 4.2
Source: Adapted from *Recommended Nutrient Intakes*, NHMRC, Australia, 1990

Table 2.4 Estimated energy cost of activity (kilojoules/minute)

Activity		Your body weight				
		50kg	60kg	70kg	80kg	90kg
Aerobics	*beginners*	22	26	30	34	39
	advanced	28	33	40	45	51
Badminton		20	24	28	33	37
Ballroom dancing		11	13	15	17	19
Basketball		29	35	40	46	52
Boxing	*sparring*	46	56	65	74	84
	in ring	29	35	40	46	52
Canoeing	*leisure*	9	11	13	15	17
	racing	22	26	30	34	39
Circuit training		22	26	30	34	40
Cricket	*batting*	17	21	24	28	32
	bowling	19	22	26	30	34
Cycling	*9km/hr*	13	16	18	21	24
	15km/hr	21	24	28	33	38
	racing	35	42	49	56	63
Football		28	33	39	44	50
Golf		18	21	25	28	32
Gymnastics		14	16	19	22	25
Hockey		18	20	24	29	33
Judo		41	49	57	65	73
Running	*5.5 min per km*	40	49	57	65	73
	5 min per km	44	52	61	70	78
	4.5 min per km	48	55	65	75	85
	4 min per km	54	65	76	87	98
Skiing	*cross-country*	35	42	49	56	63
	down hill (easy)	18	21	25	29	33
	down hill (hard)	29	35	40	49	55
Squash		44	53	62	71	79
Swimming	*freestyle*	33	40	46	52	59
	backstroke	36	43	49	56	63
	breast stroke	34	41	47	54	61
Table tennis		14	17	19	23	26
Tennis	*social*	15	17	20	23	26
	competitive	37	44	50	58	65
Volleyball		10	12	15	17	19
Walking	*10 min per km*	21	26	30	35	39
	8 min per km	25	30	35	40	45
	5 min per km	44	52	61	70	78

Adjustment for occupational activity—adjust total daily energy allowance

	50kg	60kg	70kg	80kg	90kg
Minimum daily activity (e.g. bedridden, wheelchair)	−2000	−2400	−2800	−3200	−3600
Heavy labouring job	+2000	+2400	+2800	+3200	+3600

Notes: All figures are approximate values only.
Kilocalories can be calculated by dividing kilojoule values by 4.2
Source: Adapted from: *Recommended nutrient intakes*, NHMRC: Australia, 1990
Katch F.I. and McArdle W.D., *Nutrition, Weight Control and Exercise*, Lea and Febiger: Philadelphia 1988

Figure 2.2 Energy balance

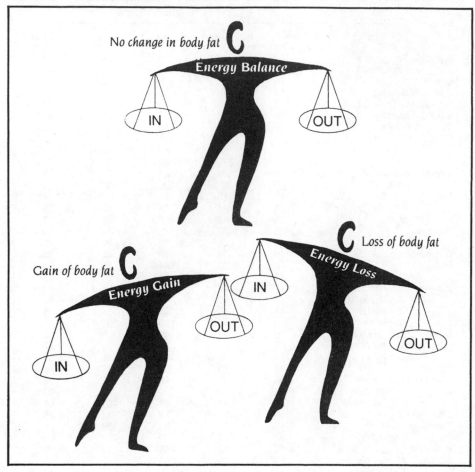

undertake lengthy high-intensity training sessions each day. Into this category we might put growing teenage basketballers, heavyweight rowers, marathon runners and triathletes. On the other hand females will be expected to have smaller energy requirements, and a tiny athlete who does little training (or training that is skill-based rather than energy-intensive) will be the typical small-energy consumer. Female gymnasts and ballet dancers are good examples.

These generalisations are by no means hard and fast. You should not be surprised if your predicted (tables) and estimated (food diary) energy requirements are quite different from other athletes—even those in the same sport as you. The most important thing is that they are right for you.

Once you have an idea of your daily kilojoule budget, your next task is to see how you can 'spend' it wisely to ensure that you cover your requirements for the following important nutrients.

2.2 Carbohydrate

Your carbohydrate requirements are estimated on the basis of muscle glycogen needs, to replace the fuel that you burn up in daily exercise. This will depend on the amount of training (or competition) that you undertake each day, and the size of your muscles.

A general estimation of the daily carbohydrate needs of various athletes is as follows:

General sports activity (up to 60 minutes of training per day or unlimited low-intensity training)	5–6g of carbohydrate for each kg you weigh
Moderately training athletes (60–120 minutes of intense or lengthy medium-intensity exercise)	6–8g of carbohydrate for each kg you weigh
Endurance training (over 120 minutes of intense training per day)	8–10g of carbohydrate for each kg you weigh
Extreme exercise—(5–6+ hours of intense daily exercise—e.g. cycle tour)	10g+ of carbohydrate for each kg you weigh

So a female basketballer (60kg) whose daily training added up to 30–60 minutes of actual exercise would have approximate carbohydrate needs of 300–360g per day. A 65kg triathlete training strenuously for 3–4 hours each day should aim for 585–650g of carbohydrate each day to replace carbohydrate stores. Look at Table 2.5 for a ready-reckoner of carbohydrate content of various foods. According to this guide, our triathlete would need to eat around 40 'serves' of carbohydrate foods each day—for example 2 large bowls of cereal (8 serves), 12 slices of bread (12), 8 pieces of fruit (8), 3 cups of juice (6) and 3 cups of cooked pasta (6)!

Clearly, carbohydrate will take up most of the kilojoules in your diet. In fact, it is estimated that carbohydrate may account for the following percentages of total energy intake:

43

General and moderate training level	50–60 per cent of total energy
Endurance training	50–70 per cent of total energy
Restricted energy diet (low energy consumers and weight loss diets)	60–70 per cent of total energy

While these figures are only a general guide, they reflect how far you may need to change your dietary patterns from a typical Australian diet (currently providing 40–45 per cent of energy as carbohydrate).

Do you need to count up your carbohydrate intake each day? For most athletes this is probably an unnecessary task. The food hints summarised in Chapter 1.3 should help you form habits that will increase your carbohydrate intake to the 50–60 per cent energy mark. Athletes who have to push their carbohydrate and total kilojoule intakes further may be helped by periodically calculating the amount of carbohydrate foods needed, because it is often more than their appetites or typical meal patterns would 'naturally' achieve. In a special situation such as carbo-loading, when you need to maximise glycogen storage, carbohydrate counting will ensure that you achieve your daily target of 8–10g per kilogram of your weight.

2.3 Protein

The protein needs of athletes have been hotly debated for many years. In the red corner, we have strength sports who argue that large intakes of protein are needed for great big muscles! And in the black corner, we have endurance athletes who get so involved in carbohydrate counting that they shun protein altogether. Luckily, in recent years sufficient scientific research has allowed the referee to step into the ring with a final verdict.

And the decision is: protein requirements *are* increased by exercise —firstly to account for the small contribution of protein to muscle fuel, and secondly to account for any extra muscle that is laid down. However, don't go rushing for a protein powder—although protein requirements increase in absolute terms (you may need more total grams), the extra kilojoules in your diet will automatically allow you to eat more protein without having to consciously emphasise protein foods.

In fact, for many athletes, total protein needs will still be met by the general recommendation of 1g of protein per kilogram of body weight— e.g. 60g for a 60kg athlete. But athletes whose daily training sessions are lengthy and intense (burning up a significant total of protein fuel),

Table 2.5   Ready reckoner of carbohydrate-rich foods

Approximately 15g of carbohydrate is supplied by the following foods:

Cereals	bread	1 thick slice (40g)
	bread roll	1/2 average roll (35g)
	muffin or crumpet	1/2 average (35g)
	breakfast cereal	20g = 1/2 to 2/3 cup Weeties or 'light' cereal = 1/3 cup muesli flakes or 'heavier' cereal = 1.5 Weetbix
	rolled oats	1/4 cup (20g)
	untoasted muesli	1/4 cup (20g)
	porridge	3/4 cup cooked (180g)
	scones/pancakes	30g = 1/2 average size
	wholemeal cake (low fat)	25g = 1/2 to 1/3 av. slice
	dry biscuit	25g = 4–6 crackers
	rice cakes	15g = 1.5 cakes
	plain muesli bar or breakfast bar	20g = 2/3 bar
	plain sweet biscuit	20g = 2
	popcorn	20g = 1 cup
	rice	1/3 cup cooked (50g)
	pasta/noodles	1/2 cup cooked (60g)
	tinned spaghetti	1/2 cup (120g)
Vegetables	potatoes	80g cooked (1 medium) 90g mashed (1/3 cup)
	carrots/pumpkin/peas	300g cooked (1.5 cups)
	corn	70g cooked (1/2 cup)
Legumes	kidney, soy beans	1/3 cup cooked (80g)
	baked beans	3/5 cup (150g)
	lentils	1/3 cup cooked (80g)
Fruit	fresh fruit	100–150g piece = medium apple, orange = small banana = 3/4 cup cherries, grapes
	juice	120ml sweetened (1/2 cup) 180ml unsweetened (3/4 cup)
	dried fruit	20g (1.5 Tablespoons)
	canned/stewed fruit	120g sweetened (1/2 cup) 240g unsweetened (1 cup)
	fruit salad, fresh	120g (1/2 cup)
Dairy products	low-fat milk	300ml
	fruit low-fat yoghurt	100g (1/2 200g carton)
	plain low-fat yoghurt	200g (carton)
	low-fat icecream	100g (2 rounded Tablespoons)
	light fromage frais	130g (2/3 200g carton)
Sugary foods	sugar	15g (2 heaped teaspoons)
	jam and honey	20g (Tablespoon)
	plain lollies	15–20g packet
Drinks	soft drinks and flavoured mineral water	150ml
	cordial	200ml
	fruit juice	120–180ml
	sports drinks	200–250ml
	liquid meal drinks	100ml
	carbo-loader drinks	100ml
	low-fat milk shakes/smoothies	120–150ml

Source: NUTTAB 1991–92, Australian Department of Community Services and Health

45

or who are in a muscle gain stage of their programs, will require an increase in their protein allowance. Athletes who are growing will need to cover these physiological requirements as well. The protein requirements for various groups of athletes might be summarised as follows:

General sports activity	1g of protein for every kg you weigh
Strength-training athletes (aim for the high end of range during muscle gain periods)	1.2–1.6g of protein for every kg you weigh
Endurance training athletes (aim for the high end of range for very prolonged strenuous training)	1.2–1.6g of protein for every kg you weigh
Adolescent and growing athletes	2.0g of protein for every kg you weigh
Pregnant athletes	Extra 10g of protein per day in trimesters 2 and 3
Breast-feeding athletes	Extra 20g of protein per day

In general, you should earmark about 12–15 per cent of your total energy intake to meet these recommended levels—the same as most Australians do now. Even at this level, most athletes who eat a high-energy intake will surpass these daily protein amounts. However low-energy consumers may find that 15–20 per cent of their total energy budget is needed.

Protein foods should be chosen with your other nutritional goals in mind—that is, you should choose protein foods with a minimal fat content which are also good sources of other nutrients. Table 2.6 provides a ready reckoner of the protein content of some valuable foods. Lean animal protein foods are able to supply all the body's essential amino acids, as well as calcium (dairy foods) and iron (meats and shellfish). If you look at the vegetable protein foods, you will see that some of these appear as good carbohydrate sources also. The ready reckoner should convince you that it doesn't take half a side of beef to make up your daily protein needs—cereal with skim milk for breakfast, a chicken sandwich for lunch and a small steak for dinner will provide over 60g of protein for a 60kg squash player.

Is vegetable protein as valuable as animal protein? Protein is made from various combinations of small building blocks called amino acids. Some of these amino acids can be manufactured in the body by

Table 2.6 Ready reckoner of protein-rich foods

Approximately 10g of protein is provided by the following foods:

Low-fat animal foods	grilled fish	50g (cooked weight)
	tuna or salmon	50g
	lean beef or lamb	35g (cooked weight)
	veal	35g (cooked weight)
	turkey or chicken	40g (cooked weight)
	game meat (rabbit, venison)	35g (cooked weight)
	eggs	2 small
	cottage cheese	70g
	reduced-fat cheese (11% fat slices)	30g = 1.5sl
	non-fat fruit yoghurt	200g carton
	light fromage frais	150g (3/4 200g carton)
	low-fat milk	300ml
	liquid meal supplements	150ml
Vegetable foods	wholemeal bread	4sl (120g)
	wheat flake cereal	3 cups (90g)
	untoasted muesli	1 cup (100g)
	cooked pasta or noodles	2 cups (300g)
	cooked brown rice	3 cups (400g)
	cooked lentils	3/4 cup (150g)
	cooked kidney beans	3/4 cup (150g)
	baked beans	4/5 cup (200g)
	cooked soy beans or tofu	120g
	nuts	60g
	seeds (e.g. sesame)	60g

Source: NUTTAB 1991–92, Australian Department of Community Services and Health

rearranging the structure of other compounds, while the other amino acids (called the essential amino acids) can only be obtained by eating food. Animal protein foods contain a good variety of amino acids including all the essential ones. On the other hand, plant foods tend to have one or more of the essential amino acids in short supply. This could be a problem if plant foods make up most or all of your diet—for example if you are a vegetarian.

Fortunately however, while one vegetable protein food will contain a good supply of some essential amino acids, while lacking in one or two others, another vegetable protein food will have the reverse problem. By cleverly mixing and matching these foods the total amino acid picture can be achieved. This is known as *complementing* vegetable proteins, and can also be done by mixing a vegetable type with a small amount of animal protein, such as a dairy food. Figure 2.3 shows you which protein foods can complement each other, and some typical examples.

2.4 Vitamins

Helped along by some clever advertising from vitamin supplement companies, most people think of vitamins as the most important nutrients in their diet and the ones most likely to run into short supply.

Figure 2.3 By combining certain food groups, vegetable protein foods are complemented and a first-class protein meal is achieved.

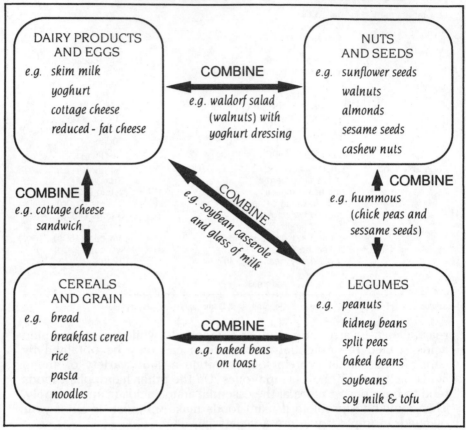

However, the truth is quite different. While an adequate vitamin intake is an essential component of good health and optimal training nutrition it is one of the least likely things to be deficient in the Western diet.

In the correct sense of the word, vitamins do not provide energy— that is, they do not contribute any kilojoules to the body. But various vitamins are involved in the production of energy from fuel stores, by acting as catalysts for metabolic reactions. Vitamins are involved in many other reactions too—including the production of red blood cells, the repair of tissues, and the synthesis of protein. When vitamin levels drop below a certain mark, these body processes will be impaired, and sports performance has been shown to be affected. However, if your vitamin supply is continually maintained, then metabolism will continue unimpeded.

HINTS FOR PUTTING MORE VITAMINS PER MOUTHFUL IN
YOUR DIET

- Enjoy a good range of fruits and vegetables—the more colour the
  better.
- Where possible choose fresh types, especially those in season.
- Frozen vegetables are also a nutritious choice.
- Go for the wholemeal versions of your favourite carbohydrate foods.
- Don't overcook vegetables—keep them crisp by microwaving or
  steaming. If boiling, keep it brief and the water level low.

Nutrition experts have set a recommended intake for most of the
vitamins (known as the Recommended Dietary Intake or RDI). The
RDIs for vitamins are set as a general target, and most peoples' diets
provide intakes well above these levels. A diet that provides less than
the RDI for a vitamin is not necessarily deficient in that vitamin, because quite a large safety margin has been set.

However, if your usual diet consistently supplies you with less than
two-thirds of the RDIs, some expert dietary advice and remodelling is
suggested. The first line of attack will *not* be to take a vitamin supplement, but rather to change your diet to overcome its shortfalls.
After all, because nutrients exist together in food, it is likely that any
diet that is low in one or more vitamins also fails to meet other goals
of peak training nutrition. A vitamin supplement might reverse your
low vitamin intake, but how will it help your high fat intake or your
low carbohydrate supply?

After looking at the population RDIs for vitamins, athletes usually
ask two questions:

- Does heavy exercise increase the requirements for vitamins?
- Will extra vitamins, especially large doses, improve performance
  by making metabolism move faster?

The second question really belongs in the area of supplements and
ergogenic aids (performance boosters), and will be covered in Chapter 6. On the trail of extra vitamin needs, research has not been able
to show that the vitamin requirements of athletes are raised above
the RDI levels. In fact, the RDIs for the vitamins involved in energy
metabolism have been set according to energy intake level. So a higher
energy expenditure already has an inbuilt increase in total vitamin
requirement.

Table 2.7 summarises food sources of each vitamin, with RDIs adjusted for athletes. Where an RDI has not been set for a vitamin, it is

Table 2.7 Vitamins: where to find your recommended dietary intake (RDI)

Vitamins	Daily RDI for adult athletes	Good dietary sources	Examples of RDI from food
Thiamin (vitamin B1)	0.10mg per 1000kJ that you eat i.e. 6 000kJ = 0.6mg 10 000kJ = 1.0mg 20 000kJ = 2.0mg	Pork, liver (& pate) breakfast cereals, wholegrain breads and cereal foods, yeast extract (e.g. Vegemite), legumes	1mg is provided by: 2 slices wholemeal bread + 1 tsp Vegemite + 1 cup Weeties
Riboflavin (vitamin B2)	0.15mg per 1000kJ that you eat i.e. 6 000kJ = 0.9mg 10 000kJ = 1.5mg 20 000kJ = 3.0mg	Liver, dairy products, breakfast cereals, yeast extract, wholemeal breads and cereal foods	1.5mg is provided by: 2 Weetbix + 1 cup skim milk + 2 slices wholemeal bread + 200g carton low-fat yoghurt
Niacin (vitamin B3)	1.6mg per 1000kJ that you eat i.e. 6 000kJ = 9.6mg 10 000kJ = 16mg 20 000kJ = 32mg	Meats/eggs/fish/dairy foods, yeast extract, breakfast cereals, wholegrain breads and cereal foods legumes	16mg is provided by: 2 slices wholemeal bread + 120g lean meat + 1 cup skim milk
Pyridoxine (vitamin B6)	0.02mg per gram of protein that you eat i.e. 50g protein = 1.0mg 100g protein = 2.0mg	High protein foods, wholegrain breads and cereal foods, potatoes, bananas	1mg is provided by: 1 banana + 1 cup Allbran + 100g chicken
Folate	200µg	Green leafy vegies, oranges, wholegrain breads + cereal foods, liver	200µg is provided by: 200ml orange juice + 1 cup spinach
Pantothenic acid	No RDI—widely distributed	Meats/fish/egg, wholegrain breads + cereal foods, legumes	Widely distributed in foods

Biotin	No RDI—some manufactured by gut bacteria	Liver, meats, egg yolks, nuts	—
Vitamin B12	2mcg	Animal foods—not generally found in plant foods.	Small amount of animal foods
Ascorbic acid (vitamin C)	30mg (women) 40mg (men)	Citrus fruits, berries, tropical fruits, tomato, green leafy vegetables, parsley	40mg is provided by: half an orange or 1/2 cup fresh strawberries
Vitamin A	750µg	Liver (& pate), dairy products, some fish, green leafy vegetables, yellow/orange fruits and vegetables (carrots, peaches, spinach etc).	750µg is provided by: 1/2 cup cooked carrots or 1 mango
Vitamin D	Manufactured by the action of sunlight on skin	Butter/margarine, fish oils, eggs	Daily sunlight
Vitamin E	10mg	Wheatgerm and wholegrain cereal foods, nuts, seeds, vegetable oils, margarine, avocado	10mg is provided by: 1 avocado + Tbs peanut butter + 2 tsp polyunsaturated margarine + cup untoasted muesli
Vitamin K	No RDI—some manufactured by gut bacteria	Liver, green leafy vegetables: cabbage, cauliflower, broccoli, legumes	—

Source: *Recommended nutrient intakes, Australia* NHMRC, 1990 assumed that an adequate intake is already taken care of. In terms of vitamin intake, the two biggest assets that an athlete's diet can have are a high energy intake (more food should mean more nutrients), and a wide variety of foods (as you learnt earlier, variety increases your opportunities to get a little of everything you need).

Athletes most likely to run into problems with vitamin intake are those on very restricted diets (e.g. fad diets, strict vegetarian diets, fussy eaters) and those with low energy intakes (low energy consumers and weight loss diets). In these situations, a sports dietitian can help you to maximise your dietary intake, and may also suggest a low-dose vitamin supplement to help fill any remaining gaps.

2.5 Iron

Iron is an important nutrient in sports performance, since it is a component of the oxygen carriers in the blood (called hemoglobin) and in the muscles (called myoglobin). In addition, iron is involved with some of the enzymes that promote exercise metabolism. An iron deficiency will reduce the oxygen supply to muscles as well as slow down some of these metabolic reactions. Obviously, this is not compatible with optimal performance.

Athletes with very low iron stores complain of tiredness and poor recovery from training. If the situation worsens and blood hemoglobin levels become lowered (called anemia) the symptoms become more drastic—severe fatigue, cramps, headaches and often shortness of breath. It is at the anemia stage that there is definite proof of reduced performance. It has been harder to prove that low iron stores, even when the athlete is 'tired', actually reduce performance. Nevertheless, even if low iron stores do not directly cause changes to performance, this condition should be treated to stop the progression to anemia.

Iron requirements for athletes provide a few challenges. Firstly, females need to eat more iron than their male counterparts to account for the blood losses of menstruation. The tricky part is that females usually need to eat less kilojoules than males, and must therefore find more iron per mouthful in their diet.

Secondly, heavy exercise increases iron requirements, by increasing iron losses from the body. Iron can be lost through sweat and gastro-intestinal bleeding—particularly if you take a lot of anti-inflammatory drugs for injuries. Red blood cells are destroyed by continual jarring and impact, whether in contact sports or from pounding the pavements while running. A guide to iron requirements is provided as follows. The upper ranges for the endurance athletes represent the worst-case scenario where an athlete is experiencing iron drain from all exercise-related sources:

General training—males and non-menstruating females	7mg iron per day
General training—menstruating females	12–16mg iron per day
General training—growing adolescents	10–13mg iron per day
Pregnancy (trimesters 2 and 3)	22–36mg iron per day
Endurance training—males (particularly running and other high-impact sports)	7–17.5mg iron per day
Endurance training—non-menstruating females (particularly high-impact sports)	7–17mg iron per day
Endurance training—menstruating females (particularly high-impact sports)	16–23mg iron per day

HINTS FOR AN IRON BOOST

- Include lean red meat or liver (pate, perhaps) in your meals three to five times per week. It doesn't have to be a big serve—perhaps a slice in a sandwich or a handful in your stir-fry. These foods not only contribute heme iron (well-absorbed), but they increase the absorption of non-heme iron from other foods at the same meal. The frequency of eating heme iron may be more important than the total quantity eaten.

- Other sources of heme iron are seafood (especially oysters), darker types of fish, and the dark cuts of poultry (the leg rather than the breast). Like meat, they can be used to enhance the total iron absorbed from the meal.

- Make use of commercial breakfast cereals that have been fortified with iron. Read the label to check the iron content of your cereal.

- If you are not having a heme iron food at a meal, make sure that you have a good source of non-heme iron food—such as eggs, a wholegrain cereal food, some legumes or some spinach/silverbeet.

AND

Combine these non-heme iron meals with a vitamin C food to enhance the iron absorption—for example, orange juice with your breakfast cereal, tomatoes with your spinach omelette.

- Avoid sprinkling wheat bran on your meals. You probably don't need extra fibre in your peak training diet.

- Don't drink strong tea with your meals if you are in a high risk category for iron deficiency.

- Work extra hard on the non-heme mixes and matches if you are a vegetarian, and think about cooking in cast iron pots.

53

Table 2.8 **Iron-rich foods for the optimal training diet**

Food	Serve	mg Iron
Heme iron foods		
liver	100g (cooked weight)	11.0mg
liver pate	40g (2 Tbsp)	2–3mg
lean steak	100g (cooked weight)	4.0mg
chicken (dark meat)	100g (cooked weight)	1.2mg
fish	100g (cooked weight)	0.6–1.4mg
oysters	100g	3.9mg
salmon	100g (small tin)	1.5mg
Non-heme iron foods		
eggs	100g (2)	2.0mg
breakfast cereal (fortified)	30g (1 cup)	2.5mg
wholemeal bread	60g (2 sl)	1.4mg
spinach (cooked)	145g (1 cup)	4.4mg
lentils/kidney beans (cooked)	100g (2/3 cup)	2.5mg
tofu	100g	1.9mg
sultanas	50g	0.9mg
dried apricots	50g	2.0mg
almonds	50g	2.1mg

Source: NUTTAB 1991–92, Australian Department of Community Services and Health

The final complication in the iron situation is that the people who need to eat the highest intakes are often the people who steer away from the most valuable foods. Dietary iron is found in two forms—a special form called 'heme' iron that occurs in some animal foods, and a simpler form known as 'non-heme' iron. Table 2.8 shows the iron content of some common serves of food.

The importance of this classification is two-fold—the heme foods have generally more iron overall and, secondly, the heme iron is well absorbed. By contrast, the non-heme iron is poorly absorbed, and can be further tied up by other factors in food such as tannin (in tea), phytates (in wheat bran and wholemeal cereals) and oxalates (in spinach). Athletes whose diets are based heavily, or solely, on plant iron foods—such as vegetarians or endurance athletes who are keen on carbohydrates only—may find that their iron intake is inadequate and unavailable.

Some special tactics are needed to put an iron boost into the optimal training diet. This will include clever mixing and matching of foods to make use of low-fat heme iron foods, and to take advantage of dietary factors that actually enhance the absorption of non-heme iron—vitamin C and meat/fish/poultry itself.

2.6 Calcium

The best-known function of calcium in the body is its role in bone, since 99 per cent of the body's calcium is in the skeleton.

A growing awareness of osteoporosis has put the spotlight on calcium in recent years. Osteoporosis is typically a process of ageing, more pronounced in women, which leaves bones thinner and more fragile. Remember how your grandmother fell and broke her hip or her arm? An influential factor in loss of bone calcium is thought to be a reduced level of the hormone, estrogen. Estrogen levels fall after menopause in women, causing a rapid decline in bone mass over the next few years.

More recently, there has been some concern about young female athletes who either stop having periods or fail to start them at all. These conditions, known medically as amenorrhea, are also associated with reduced estrogen levels. As a consequence bone mass can be lost at a time when young women should be laying down bone structure for the rest of their lives. While this may mean a higher risk of osteoporosis in older age, some sportswomen may also pay an immediate penalty in the form of an increased risk of stress fractures.

The cause of amenorrhea in athletes is not fully understood. A number of risk factors have been identified although some athletes with these risk factors enjoy regular menstrual function (see Figure 2.4 for a summary). It appears that some females may be more susceptible to particular stresses than others or perhaps that some of these factors combine to put the athlete at greater risk. Whatever the

Figure 2.4 Risk factors for amenorrhea (disturbances to menstrual cycle)

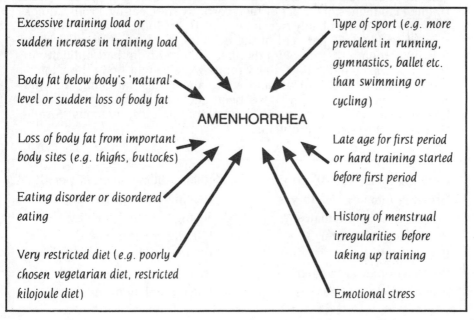

Excessive training load or sudden increase in training load

Body fat below body's 'natural' level or sudden loss of body fat

Loss of body fat from important body sites (e.g. thighs, buttocks)

Eating disorder or disordered eating

Very restricted diet (e.g. poorly chosen vegetarian diet, restricted kilojoule diet)

AMENHORRHEA

Type of sport (e.g. more prevalent in running, gymnastics, ballet etc. than swimming or cycling)

Late age for first period or hard training started before first period

History of menstrual irregularities before taking up training

Emotional stress

cause, failure to establish or maintain regular menstruation should be discussed with a sports medicine doctor. It is important to assess and minimise any effects on bone health. In any case, it is likely that the factors which are causing menstrual problems are also causing other nutritional or training problems. So take it as a sign that a check-up could be overdue.

But back to the calcium story. Dietary factors which help to promote healthy bone calcium levels include (not surprisingly) a healthy calcium intake. Factors that increase the risk of bone loss include low intake of calcium—especially during adolescence and early adulthood —and excessive salt and protein intake. Your peak training diet has already taken care of these last two items, so now it remains for us to protect bone structure with high calcium eating. Think of it as superannuation for your bones—the more bone mass you can store now, the better protected you will be when bone loss occurs in later life. And you may be helping to reduce the risk of stress fractures in your present athletic career. (Of course, stress fractures, as we shall see later in a case history, also reflect the volume of training you are doing, the surfaces and shoes that are involved and how good your biomechanics are. Too much repeated pounding or a hard fall will eventually crack any bone—but soft bones make any situation worse.)

Targets for calcium intake are presented below, with greatest calcium requirements occurring when you are growing, pregnant or feeding a baby, or experiencing low estrogen levels. Table 2.9 provides a list of calcium-rich foods—with emphasis on those that also fit the peak training guidelines of low-fat or high-carbohydrate eating. From a quick glance you can probably see how well dairy foods feature—in fact they provide 60–75 per cent of the calcium in a typical Western diet. It is unfortunate that dairy foods have suffered from bad publicity in recent years. Like red meat, dairy foods were caught up in the cholesterol concerns of the 1970s, and were labelled as 'fattening' and full of saturated fat. They have also been accused by many 'alternative health' followers of causing all manner of allergies, 'mucous' formation and other health problems.

Growing males (12–18 yrs)	1000–1200mg calcium per day
Growing females (12–15 yrs)	1000mg calcium per day
Adult males and females	800mg calcium per day
Pregnancy (trimester 3)	1100mg calcium per day
Breast-feeding	1200mg calcium per day
Post-menopausal women	1000mg calcium per day
Amenorrheic athletes	1000mg calcium per day

Table 2.9 Calcium-rich foods for the optimal training diet

Food	Serving	mg Calcium
Skim milk	200ml (glass)	250mg
Low fat (1–2%) milk (Calcium added)	200ml (glass)	285mg
Reduced-fat cheese (11% fat slices)	20g (1 slice)	160mg
Cottage cheese	100g (1/2 cup)	80mg
Non-fat fruit yoghurt	200g (carton)	350mg
Light fromage frais	200g (carton)	128mg
Low-fat icecream	60g (2 Tbsp)	90mg
Salmon (with bones)	100g (small tin)	335mg
Sardines (oil drained)	100g (drained weight)	380mg
Oysters	100g	135mg
Almonds	50g	125mg
Tahini	20g (Tbsp)	190mg
Spinach (cooked)	145g (1 cup)	72mg
Soy milk	200ml (glass)	45mg
Fortified soy milks (e.g. So Good)	200ml (glass)	290mg
Tofu	100g	130mg

Source: NUTTAB 1991–92, Australian Department of Community Services and Health

Most of these claims can be dismissed for lack of evidence: for example, no relationship between milk intake and mucous production has been found. And although some babies suffer a cow's milk intolerance during their first months of life, most outgrow this in early childhood. Low-fat and reduced-fat dairy products have grown almost exponentially in both quality and range over the past 5 years, now offering athletes many ways to enjoy valuable protein and calcium with little or no fat content.

Lactose intolerance is a problem suffered by a small percentage of Caucasians, but in larger proportions by other racial groups such as Asians and Australian Aborigines. It is not an allergy to milk; rather, those who are lactose intolerant lack adequate amounts of the enzyme lactase, which aids the digestion of lactose, the principle carbohydrate in milk. Inadequate digestion of lactose can lead to gastric discomfort, flatulence and diarrhea. However, this problem does not prevent those affected from consuming dairy foods. For a start, products such as yoghurt and cheese do not contain large amounts of lactose, and it is now possible to buy special tablets which can be added to milk to 'predigest' the lactose before drinking it—you may even be able to buy milk already treated. Even so, lactose intolerance is rarely absolute: most people can tolerate small amounts of lactose-containing products, especially when they are consumed with other foods as part of a meal. All in all, dairy products can form a valuable part of the athlete's peak training diet. If you haven't drunk a glass of milk since you were in school, there are many other ways to enjoy low-fat dairy foods—the following guidelines show many meal and snack ideas that incorporate carbohydrate-rich and low-fat foods. Three or more choices such as these each day will help you to meet your calcium intake goals.

Those who can't or won't eat dairy products will need to make calcium-enriched soy milk an important dietary choice. Note that soy milk contains a similar amount of fat to whole milk, unless you choose a low-fat brand. Other foods can make a calcium contribution—for example, tofu and other soy products, and fish that is eaten bones and all—however, most of us will not eat these foods regularly enough to make them our most important calcium source. Some athletes will not be able to meet their calcium goals from diet alone and may be prescribed a calcium supplement. This should be done on the advice of a sports dietitian or doctor after making sure that dietary potential has been reached.

HINTS FOR A CALCIUM BOOST

The following meal and snack ideas feature calcium-rich eating for the peak training diet—high in carbohydrate and low in fat.

- Cereal and milk*
- Carton of low-fat fruit yoghurt with sliced fruit
- Low-fat soft serve yoghurt or specialised icecreams (e.g. Gise ice-dessert)
- Wholemeal sandwich with salmon and salad (eat the bones!)
- Sardines on toast—drain the oil or buy brands canned in tomato sauces or juice
- Homemade pizza topped with low-fat cheese slices or a sprinkle of reduced-fat mozzarella cheese
- Banana smoothie made with milk*, banana and low-fat icecream/yoghurt
- 'Skinny' hot chocolate* or cappuccino* plus toast or English muffin
- Macaroni cheese—white sauce made with milk* and low-fat cheese
- Tofu in a vegetable and rice stir-fry
- Stewed fruit with custard or rice pudding made with milk*
- Liquid meal supplement (e.g. Sustagen Sport, Gator-Pro or Exceed Sports Nutrition Meal)

* Choose a low-fat milk—especially brands that are calcium-enriched —or a calcium-fortified low-fat soy milk

2.7 *Timing of meals*

Being an athlete probably means having a hectic lifestyle. Your daily schedule may include work or school, training (or competition), perhaps some physio or a massage, adequate sleep—and who knows what other commitments. Somewhere among all these activities, food has to be squeezed in, and unfortunately it often becomes an afterthought.

Your optimal training diet needs to be planned rather than haphazard. This way you will be sure that you are achieving all your nutrition goals. In addition, the timing of food can be an important factor in making it all happen—matching your food intake to the times when your body most appreciates it.

Your daily timetable and your commitments will be unique. Write down how you organise your schedule of events each day, and then take note of the following factors to see how you can best plot in your food stops over the day.

HINTS FOR MEAL TIMING

- Spread the same food intake over five or six meals and snacks, rather than three large meals. The possible advantages are:

  — more even blood glucose levels rather than big peaks and troughs over the day. This may help to avoid 'flat spots' or afternoon fatigue.

  — lower blood fat levels and less likelihood of storing body fat for the same kilojoule load.

  — stimulation of your metabolic rate. Each time you eat a meal there is a small rise in your metabolic rate. More meals—better stimulation.

  — no need to 'stuff' yourself to eat lots of kilojoules. It is more comfortable to have a 'grazing' pattern—eat a little now and come back for more later.

  — avoids 'hunger spots' when you are on a reduced energy diet.

- Time your last meal before training (or competition) so that you can exercise comfortably. This may mean 1–2 hours for a light snack or a liquid meal (low-fat milk smoothie or Sustagen Sport etc.) and up to 3–4 hours for larger or heavier meals.

- Promote recovery after heavy exercise sessions (training or competition) by eating some carbohydrate as soon as possible. Your high-carbohydrate breakfast or tea might be waiting for you as soon as you finish. If not, start muscle glycogen storage straight

---

59

away with a carbohydrate drink or snack within 15–30 minutes of exercise, and continue to top up carbohydrate levels at your next meal. Don't neglect your fluid needs either. (Read Chapter 6 for more details on strategies to promote recovery.)

- Having access to food when you need it will be an important factor in achieving your nutrition goals. If you live your life on the run, you will need to plan ahead. Having a portable food supply with you will help you to eat on the go. Think of some suitable snacks to store at work, in your locker, in your sports bag or in your car.

3 Matters of physique—losing and gaining

You may have noticed while watching an Olympic Games opening ceremony, that athletes come in all shapes and sizes. You may also have tried to guess what type of sport was involved by examining the size and shape of a particular athlete. The issue at point is that various aspects of exercise performance are favoured by certain physical characteristics. Athletes, particularly at the highest level of play, will tend towards the physique that favours the demands of their sport.

Your physique will reflect both the basic structure you inherited from your parents, and the remoulding achieved by your training and diet. Hopefully you have chosen your parents well and selected the sport to which you are best suited! Physical characteristics that you may need to fine-tune are:

- your body-fat level
- your total muscle mass.

3.1 Desirable body-fat levels

We require a certain minimum level of body fat for good health. For men this is approximately 3–5 per cent of body weight, and for women about 12–15 per cent. Of course, most people carry considerably more body fat than this. In terms of sports performance, extra body fat can improve floatation, provide insulation against the cold, and protect body organs against damage during contact sports. However, these benefits must be weighed up against the extra weight of 'dead tissue' that must be carried. Extra body fat causes a decrease in your ratio of active to inactive body weight—often referred to as your 'power to weight' ratio.

Some sports will not be disadvantaged by a higher level of body fat, particularly those based on skill rather than aerobic fitness. Think of golf or archery perhaps. By contrast, a low level of body fat is crucial for athletes such as triathletes and marathon runners, who must carry their own body weight over long distances. Similarly, athletes who compete in weight divisions will be better off if muscle is at a maximum level, and body fat is sacrificed to reach a weight limit.

In another set of sports again, success is partly or solely based on the athlete's appearance. Body builders, gymnasts and even divers pursue a 'trim, taut and terrific' look to impress the judges in their sports.

Typical body-fat levels for various sports have been compiled by taking measurements from large groups of elite athletes. This work is not meant to provide compulsory body-fat targets for each type of athlete. Rather, it should be used to describe a range of body-fat levels that appear *acceptable* or *desirable* for the top participants in a sport.

Within this range, athletes can probably find their own ideal body-fat level, based on the following information:

- at what body-fat level do you seem to perform best?
- can you also maintain good health at this level?
- can you achieve and maintain this body-fat level without unreasonable effort, and without compromising other nutritional goals?

Be aware that some athletes will perform at a top level, or at their personal best, at body-fat levels that fall outside the acceptable ranges. But then some top athletes don't fit the expected moulds in lots of ways—you probably know of very tall marathon runners or very short basketball players. And before you pursue the lowest level of body fat possible, be aware that too little body fat has its problems also. Athletes who become too lean can experience early fatigue, an increased risk of infection, intolerance to cold, and for some females, the loss of regular periods. There may be other penalties to pay, directly resulting from the methods used to achieve such a low body-fat level, such as drastic dieting or excessive training. So be sensible with your body-fat goals.

3.2 Assessment of body fat

There are a number of high-tech methods of estimating an athlete's body fat. Underwater weighing is considered the golden standard, although like many methods it is expensive, belongs in a laboratory, and is generally only available to a few athletes. Even with the latest equipment and tightest techniques, no method is completely accurate. The results, usually given as the percentage of body fat in total body weight (% body fat), should always be interpreted with this in mind.

The ideal method would be portable, inexpensive and accessible to all athletes, without sacrificing its accuracy. The 'pinch test', using skinfold calipers to measure the amount of fat under the skin at various body sites, has long provided a simple alternative. Traditionally, subcutaneous fat has been measured at three to seven sites and a prediction equation used to convert the results into an estimation of total body-fat content. This conversion step has always been regarded with suspicion, however, since it is impossible to find an equation that perfectly measures the relationship between skinfold fat and total body fat.

Since the 1980s, the Australian Institute of Sport has taken another approach to the skinfold exercise by doing away with the conversion to percentage body fat. Instead they have set new standards in terms of the skinfold measurements themselves—or at least the sum of the readings from the series of body sites. Even as this book is being written, the protocol is being updated slightly, to standardise the sites and measurement techniques in line with international standards (ISAK standards). When the technique is standardised and practised all over the country (as well as overseas), we will be able to build up a huge data bank on the typical 'sum of skinfold' measurements for a variety of sports and at various times of the sporting season. This will help greatly in understanding the range of body types that suit performance in certain sports. But remember that the 'ideal' skinfold level for any specific athlete is individual and specific to that person.

The key points to the AIS skinfold protocol are:

- A larger number of sites have been chosen to better represent body-fat distribution over the whole body. (See Figure 3.1 for a description of the sites—eight for males and seven for women.)
- Skinfold measurements should be taken by an experienced caliper technician using a good set of calipers (for example, John Bull or Harpenden calipers). Readings should be made on the right-hand side of the body, and after each site has been measured once, the whole sequence should be repeated. Where the second reading differs by more than 0.5mm, a third measurement should be taken. The average of the two closest values is used.
- The sum of the eight or seven skinfold readings is then calculated. This can be compared to the 'sum of skinfold' standards for the particular sport, or, better still, to previous measurements made on the same athlete.
- If an athlete has skinfold measurements repeated over a period of time to monitor changes, it is preferable that the same technician takes the readings on each occasion.

Typical readings for the sum of skinfolds using this AIS protocol will be presented for various sports in Part II of this book. These readings

Figure 3.1 Sites for taking skinfold (fat) measurements for determination of skinfold sum

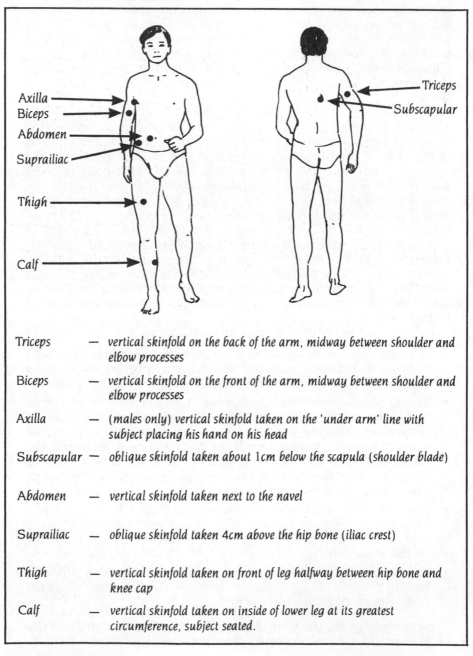

Triceps	—	vertical skinfold on the back of the arm, midway between shoulder and elbow processes
Biceps	—	vertical skinfold on the front of the arm, midway between shoulder and elbow processes
Axilla	—	(males only) vertical skinfold taken on the 'under arm' line with subject placing his hand on his head
Subscapular	—	oblique skinfold taken about 1cm below the scapula (shoulder blade)
Abdomen	—	vertical skinfold taken next to the navel
Suprailiac	—	oblique skinfold taken 4cm above the hip bone (iliac crest)
Thigh	—	vertical skinfold taken on front of leg halfway between hip bone and knee cap
Calf	—	vertical skinfold taken on inside of lower leg at its greatest circumference, subject seated.

will gradually be replaced over the next years by standards using the updated ISAK protocol.

3.3 Losing body fat

So your lycra outfit is showing bulges in the wrong places or perhaps you have come back from injury to find that your skinfold sum has jumped by 20mm. Maybe you need to lose 3kg to row in the light-weight crew. At some point in their lives or their sporting careers, most people try to lose weight. Typical situations are summarised in the following box.

The real aim is not to lose weight but to lose body fat, and this is achieved by consistently eating less kilojoules than your body expends, thus creating an energy loss situation. This might sound simple, but in actual practice, the weight loss attempts of most people end in failure. Instead of simple and consistent means, some athletes seek a magical program that will require no effort and produce results by last Thursday. Some turn to grapefruit diets, herbal powders or 'fat burning' supplements. Others take drastic measures such as severe food restriction, dehydration techniques, diuretics and laxatives.

TYPICAL REASONS FOR ATHLETES WANTING OR NEEDING TO LOSE BODY FAT

- *Athletes in skill-based sports such as golf or archery who do not burn many kilojoules during training to help with energy balance*: These athletes generally want to lose body fat to improve appearance and general health and fitness, rather than to achieve a direct effect on performance.

- *Athletes in 'appearance sports' such as gymnastics, figure skating, diving and ballet who need to look trim, taut and terrific to impress the judges as well as to assist their sports skills*: These athletes often want to achieve lower body-fat levels than is natural for their bodies. Although they spend many hours in training each day, this training is low-intensity (e.g. technique, strength and flexibility work) rather than 'kilojoule-burning' aerobic exercise.

- *Endurance athletes such as runners, road cyclists and triathletes who transport their own body weight over long distances, and sometimes up hills*: A low body-fat level will generally mean less 'dead weight' to carry; however some of these athletes (predominantly females) also want to achieve an unnaturally low body-fat level for their bodies. The intense and prolonged training sessions assist most

---

65

endurance athletes to 'naturally' achieve suitable low body-fat levels; however at times some assistance from diet is needed.

- *Athletes who are returning from a period of inactivity such as a break in the competitive year, retirement, or injury*: These athletes usually gain body fat during the lay-off—sometimes excessive amounts due to inappropriate eating (and drinking) patterns. An increase in training energy expenditure and a decrease in energy intake is required.

- *Athletes, particularly young males, who have moved away from a stable home situation where they have had all their meals prepared for them, to a new environment where they must look after their own cooking (for example, football players, basketball players)*: Lack of nutrition knowledge and cooking skills, or lack of time in a busy day often lead to poor food intake and reliance on high-fat take-away foods. This can be a time of body-fat gain and requires a new self-reliant eating plan.

- *Athletes living in an athletes' village, residential institute or boarding school where food is supplied at an 'all you can eat' cafeteria*: The change (and temptations) of a new food environment, the unlimited quantities of food and the example of others, can lead to increased food intake and gain of body fat. Learning to eat the right amount for you is the plan!

- *Athletes who are constantly on the circuit, travelling to train or compete (e.g. tennis players, cricketers)*: It is difficult to establish set eating patterns, and reliance on restaurants and take-away foods may lead to over-consumption and poor food choices. Loss of body fat will require an eating plan that can travel with you.

Since these methods fail to address either energy loss or long-term issues, they also fail to produce the desired fat loss. In addition, some attempts will actually depress the body's metabolic rate, making it even more difficult to create an energy loss situation. In the worst case scenario, there may be direct effects on your exercise performance or your health. While some people make a life-time career of being on (and off) diets, there is only one successful way to approach weight loss—and that's once and for all!

The first step is to forget the magic and miracles, and to be prepared to invest a little effort and sufficient time. The time element is essential. To lose 1kg of body fat, you must create an energy loss of almost 30 000 kilojoules (7000 Calories). Since most people can only afford to spare 2000–4000 kilojoules per day (500–1000 Calories), you will need 7–14 days to burn up one kg of body fat. On the bright side, once it is gone, it is gone—unless you revert back to your old food habits and put yourself into an energy gain situation.

KEYS TO A HEALTHY FAT-LOSS PLAN FOR ATHLETES

- *Goals* Set realistic weight and skinfold targets, including short-term targets and a long-term aim.

- *Time frame* Plan to lose about 0.5–1.0kg per week, or about 5–10mm from your skinfold measurements each fortnight. This may not happen in a consistent and consecutive way, but can still be used to set your overall time-line.

- *Energy intake* Plan to shed 2000–4000kJ (500–1000 Cals) daily from your present diet or energy requirements. More extreme energy deprivation may cause a metabolic adjustment. Athough these figures are arbitrary, do not go below daily energy intakes of 5000kJ (1200 Cals) for women and 6400–7600kJ (1500–1800 Cals) for men for prolonged periods. Further restrictions may promote metabolic and physiological adaptation, as well as make it difficult for you to find all your nutrient requirements.

- *Carbohydrate intake* Make sure that you are still eating enough carbohydrate to fuel your training sessions, otherwise you will quickly become fatigued. Slight cut-backs may be tolerated, but look after carbo needs during long training sessions and in the recovery phase. See Chapters 1.3, 2.2 and 5.

- *Protein intake* Make sure that your reduced-kilojoule diet still meets your protein requirements—e.g. 1.2–1.6g per kilogram of your weight each day. See Chapter 2.3.

- *Fat intake* Make the most of your energy cut-backs by eating less fats and oils. See Chapter 1.2. A low-fat intake is important in producing a low-fat body!

- *Vitamins and minerals* Your health and your performance will suffer if you become nutrient depleted. You will need to choose nutritious foods to ensure that you can meet your vitamin and mineral requirements from a smaller energy intake—that is, to choose foods with maximum nutrients for minimum kilojoules. A sports dietitian will advise you if it is useful to take a multivitamin/mineral supplement.

- *Flexibility* Make sure that your new eating plan fits in with your lifestyle and uses foods that are readily available. This is why most dietitians prefer to help you plan an eating program that is simply an improvement of your old, familiar ways. Most people fail when they 'follow a diet' from a book or magazine—even when the nutritional ideas are sensible—because generic diets are usually too strict to fit in with their own special requirements and lifestyle.

- *Long term view*   Can you see yourself maintaining these eating habits as long as you want to maintain your fat-loss goals? Be prepared to make permanent improvements to your eating program to maintain your achievements.

- *Enjoyment*   Every eating program should have room for treats! Make sure that your fat-loss program includes some of your favourite foods—perhaps in smaller amounts, or for special occasions.

What is the formula for the peak nutrition fat-loss diet? The box above summarises the key features that you should plan to incorporate, with realistic goals and adequate time being first on the list. It is best not to juggle weight loss and a competition schedule. Plan to tackle it early in training or even in the off-season. By protecting your intake of important nutrients, you should be able to continue training without fear of fatigue caused by dietary deficiencies.

Such an eating plan can come from a dietitian or a good sports nutrition book. Depending on your present energy requirements you may need a 8400kJ (2000 Cal), 10 500kJ (2500 Cal) or even 12 600kJ (3000 Cal) daily food plan.

Another approach to body-fat loss is to remodel your present diet, which hopefully already meets some of the goals of peak nutrition. For a start you probably enjoy what you eat and it fits your lifestyle. So take a good look at your present eating patterns and decide where some cost-cutting can be done to reduce total energy intake, while preserving your other nutritional goals. A dietitian is an expert at this exercise, but you may be able to plan some changes by yourself.

Of course, make sure that you work with a realistic picture of what you actually eat, rather than what you think you eat. A helpful way to sort this out is to keep a food record for a week, writing down everything that you eat or drink at the time it happens. Additional comments about why you ate (or drank) these items can help you to find the right strategies to make changes.

You may need to work on three basic issues of eating: the quantity you eat, the type of food you eat, and your reasons for eating. You will need to make permanent changes to your eating patterns along these

HINTS FOR SUCCESSFUL AND SUSTAINED LOSS OF BODY FAT

Quantity of food

- Decide exactly how much you *need* to eat, as distinct from what you would *like* to eat or what everyone else is eating. This may mean reducing your usual serve by a half or a third, and stopping yourself from going back for seconds.

- Avoid letting yourself get too hungry before you eat. A small but well-timed snack may prevent you from eating everything in sight later on.

- Eat slowly so that you enjoy your food and can stop before you overeat.

- Make your meals as filling as possible:

  — drink water (or a low-kilojoule drink) before and during your meal

  — enjoy high-fibre foods

- Eat fruit rather than drink juice. Take care with all high-energy fluids—it is easy to quaff litres of kilojoules, especially when you are thirsty after training!

- Enjoy your special or favourite foods, but in smaller quantities. For example, share a dessert in a restaurant, or have a chocolate frog rather than a family block.

Type of food

- Target fat, alcohol and sugar in your diet. These are high-energy nutrients that contribute little nutrient value to your diet (see Chapter 1 for more details, particularly 'Hints for Eating less Fats and Oils').

Eating behaviour

From your food record, take note of the reasons that you eat without being hungry or really needing the food. Stop the eating by changing your behaviour, for example:

- Eating when depressed or upset—tackle the problem that is causing you to be depressed or upset. Think up other activities to pamper yourself that don't involve food.

- Eating when bored—find a non-food activity, as above.

- Eating because the food is around—either remove yourself or remove the food. There is no such thing as willpower!

69

- Eating at social functions—at a restaurant, order exactly what you want and don't be afraid to make special requests. Eat just what you want and don't be afraid to say 'no thank you' to your hosts when eating at other people's homes. Better still, ring your hosts ahead of time and explain what you need. As a last option, don't eat at all (eat before you go, or when you get home).
- Find non-food ways of rewarding yourself for successful changes in your food habits.

lines and check periodically, by keeping another record, to see that the effort is sustained.

3.4 Low-energy consumers

Some athletes, particularly female athletes, seem to defy energy logic. Many claim that they can't lose weight, or need to drop to very low kilojoule intakes to reduce their body fat, despite 1–2 hours of intense training each day. Others claim that they need to exist on these low levels just to maintain their body fat levels. For years this phenomenon has puzzled scientists and athletes alike. Many dietary surveys of elite or intensely training female athletes—from swimmers, runners and basketball players to gymnasts and ballet dancers—have reported average energy intakes for the group below 8400kJ/day (2000 Cals), and below 5000kJ/day (1200 Cals) in the case of individual athletes. And every sports dietitian and coach has worked with athletes who complain that they can't seem to be able to eat 'what they deserve' in return for their hard work. It's frustrating to do the same training as the guys in the next lane, and then watch them eat twice as much food as you while remaining at least 20mm lower in sum of skinfold readings.

Of course, this problem is not exclusively a female one: some males also seem to draw the short 'energy requirement' stick. Of course, these female athletes are simply reflecting the complaints of a large percentage of the female population as a whole.

Does this energy discrepancy really exist? Can a female runner athlete run 100km per week and remain weight stable on less than 7500kJ (1800 Cals) per day? A number of recent studies have tried to examine the energy balance situation in various groups of female athletes. Remember from the beginning of this Chapter that we know it is not necessary to eat exactly the same number of kilojoules as we expend every day; however, over a period of a week or more the figures should begin to balance if our weight (body fat level) is stable. Accurately measuring either energy intake or energy expenditure is a hard task. Traditionally, scientists have relied on athletes to keep detailed records of everything they do and everything they eat and drink for a week. This is tedious for both the scientists and their victims! What's more there are numerous inaccuracies—both in arriving at the kilojoule amounts on both sides of the balance sheet, and in making sure that what is described during the study period truly reflects the real-life situation.

It is a well-known problem that many people under-report their food and drink intake when they are keeping a dietary record. Consciously or unconsciously, they forget to write down every morsel that they consume, or perhaps they consume less than normal durng the recording period. In fact, in some studies when athletes have been provided with a diet that matches the energy content they recorded in a previously kept food record, they lost weight!

Energy expenditure measurements have recently made a great leap forward with the development of the 'doubly-labelled water' technique. While it is a very expensive method (and at present only belongs in the hands of researchers), it has the benefits of being quite accurate and user-friendly for the athlete. In very simple terms, the athlete drinks some water that has been 'labelled' with charged particles called stable isotopes (it's only a tiny dose and it's quite safe!). Both the hydrogen and the oxygen components of this special water have been marked and it mixes in with the rest of the water in the body. After a period of days or weeks, a remeasurement of the amount of labelled hydrogen that has disappeared (through metabolism) compared to the rate of oxygen disappearance, will allow scientists to use a complicated formula to estimate the total energy expenditure during that period. All without discomfort or disruption to the athlete's program!

A recent study of elite female distance runners by scientists at Indiana University, measured the match between energy intake (estimated from 7-day food records) and energy expenditure recorded over the same period using the doubly-labelled water technique. The results showed that average daily energy intake (8530kJ/day) accounted for only 70 per cent of average daily energy expenditure (12 520kJ/day). However, the athletes did not lose body weight or change body composition during that time. Other careful studies of energy balance in female athletes, using different techniques to measure energy expenditure, have reported similar findings. In some cases, the energy balance oddity was particularly striking in amenorrheic athletes (those with interrupted menstrual cycles) compared to those who were menstruating regularly.

The laws of thermodynamics state that any independent system must be in energy balance—in other words, that unless these athletes were losing body fat then energy intake must equal expenditure. So there are two ways to interpret the energy discrepancy reported in these studies. First, these athletes may have become 'metabolically

71

efficient' and have adapted to their heavy training schedules in some way that reduces energy output. In other words, the energy expenditure figures in these studies are wrong and represent an overestimation of real energy requirements. Alternatively, we can suggest that the energy intake figures are wrong; that they are artificially low. Since weight has not been lost, the subjects must be under-reporting the food and fluid consumed—either by not writing down everything or by underestimating the size of the portions consumed.

It is probable that some individual athletes really are 'metabolically efficient'. However, at the present time those who have studied groups of athletes cannot find definite proof of this finding. The problem is that studies of groups of randomly-chosen athletes may hide the characteristics of individual subjects within the group, because the results are 'averaged' out. In other words, the average hides the 'extremes' or 'outliers'. To find support for 'metabolic efficiency' we may have to wait until studies are conducted on large numbers of these special athletes—those who have had low-energy requirements already confirmed in prior tests. This technique may allow the outliers to stand up and be counted (and be studied!). We need to know how and why these athletes became metabolically efficient. Is it a direct genetic effect? Or are these athletes being 'punished' for resorting to very low kilojoule intakes or for trying to reduce body fat levels or particular fat stores in conflict to their 'natural' body levels? And what part of energy expenditure adapts—is Basal Metabolic Rate reduced, or does the athlete become more efficient at their exercise so that it costs less energy? Stay tuned for the answers to these questions!

However, for the moment the consensus view is that at least some 'energy-conserving' athletes actually underestimate and/or underreport their true energy intake. In fact, in the study mentioned above, the authors also included a questionnaire on attitudes to food and body image. They reported an interesting result: there was a positive relationship between body size/weight and energy expenditure (as you would expect since heavier people require more kilojoules to keep themselves living and moving). However, there was an *inverse* relationship between body weight/size and energy balance—that is, the bigger you were, the less kilojoules you ate compared to your energy expenditure. As well as having the highest energy discrepancies, the bigger runners also had the poorest body images. The authors concluded that the more 'weight conscious' and dissatisfied with your body you were, the more you tended to underreport your food intake. In other words, you may create your 'energy discrepancy' in your own mind because you are stressed over your body weight/fat and what you eat.

It's easy to underestimate what you really eat—especially when you are thinking about it all the time. People tend to play down the size of the portions they eat, or forget about the little 'tastes' and 'nibbles' they have—especially when a series of these are substituted for a 'square meal' or a single plate of food. Also they like to remember the 'good' days and forget the 'binge' days. Some low-energy conservers exist for a number of days on very restricted energy intakes then splurge with high-fat foods. Since fat is so Calorie-dense, high-fat nibbles or splurges may not seem large in quantity, however they can significantly increase total energy intake. What's more, dietary fat splurges appear to be more fattening than previously realised.

But let's get back to the true low-energy consumer. We might describe this as any male athlete who chronically eats less than 8400 kJ (2000 Cals) per day, or any female athlete who chronically eats less than 6400kJ (1500 Cals) per day. (These figures are arbitrary and should be adjusted according to body size.) Likely candidates for this group are athletes who strive to be petite and lean against their natural body type and/or without the assistance of high-energy expenditure training. For example, athletes in 'appearance' sports such as ballet, gymnastics, diving and figure skating undertake skill-based rather than kilojoule-burning training yet demand very light and lean bodies. Even athletes who 'do the miles' such as runners, cyclists and swimmers may desire to be leaner and lower in body fat than seems natural for their bodies. Female athletes of all types, as well as athletes who 'make weight' constantly might be nominated in this group.

These athletes are set enormous challenges to meet their nutrient requirements and nutritional goals from such a small energy budget. The features of the peak nutrition fat-loss plan (see box pp. 67–8) are still important, but to these we might add the following ideas:

HINTS FOR LOW-ENERGY CONSUMERS

- Check to see if you are really a low-energy consumer by keeping a truthful food diary for a week.
  - See if you are really nibbling or consuming more than you realised (and see if those kilojoules can be better used to increase your intake of nutritious foods).
  - See if you are eating more fatty foods and high-fat splurges than you realised. Exchange for some lower-fat, higher-carbohydrate choices. This will help with extra energy for training and will make it harder to deposit body fat.
  - See if you lose weight while you are recording. Most people will consciously or unconsciously cut back when they are accounting for their food intake. This will not only tell you that your energy requirements are greater than you thought —but you may lose some unwanted body fat as well!

- Look at ways of increasing your energy requirements, either by increasing the cost of energy for exercise, or by increasing/preserving metabolic rate:

  — if your program consists of skill- or strength-training only it may be possible to add some aerobic activities to increase the total energy cost of your training. Talk to your coach about this.

  — Even on a fat-loss program, do not drop below a daily intake of about 5000kJ (1200 Cals) for a female and 7600kJ (1500–1800 Cals) for males. Further restrictions probably promote metabolic conservation and make nutrient intake goals almost impossible to achieve.

    Although these are arbitrary figures, the following guidelines may provide a minimum safe energy intake (that is, the level below which metabolic conservation or nutrient inadequacy are likely to occur):

Small female (<45kg)	3600kJ (860 Cals) + energy cost of daily training (see Table 2.3)
Average female	4320kJ (1030 Cals) + energy cost of daily training
Large female (>75kg)	5015kJ (1270 Cals) + energy cost of daily training
Small male (<60kg)	5000kJ (1260 Cals) + energy cost of daily training
Average male	5480kJ (1310 Cals) + energy cost of daily training
Large male (>85kg)	6190kJ (1480 Cals) + energy cost of daily training

  — Spread your energy intake over the day. Do not skip meals—especially breakfast—if you want to preserve your metabolic rate.

  — Experiment with a small increase in energy intake, using carbohydrate-rich foods to provide an extra 800–2000kJ a day (200–500 Cals).

    You may be surprised—not only will you *not* gain weight, but the extra training fuel will put more spring in your step and help you to perform better in all aspects of your life. What's more, a kick-start to training and to energy metabolism can often actually result in a loss of body fat.

- You will need to work hard to achieve maximum nutrient intake from minimum kilojoules:

— consult a dietitian to learn how to look after your special nutrient requirements and how to choose foods with 'maximum nutrients for minimum kilojoules'

— you will probably need to take a multivitamin/mineral supplement to add to your food intake. A dietitian can advise you on the best type and the right dose.

3.5 Making weight

Weight-matched sports include boxing, wrestling, judo, weight- and power-lifting, horse racing and lightweight rowing. There are two traditions in these sports that show an unfortunate side of athletic nutritional practices. The first is the desire to compete in a lower weight division than your normal training weight—theoretically gaining an advantage over a lighter, weaker opponent.

The second tradition is to shed the excess weight in a rapid fashion—often three to six kilos in as many days. This is when the drastic techniques come into play—such as dehydrating in saunas or plastic suits, fasting, or using diuretics and laxatives. These methods may effectively cause a loss of body weight, but the athlete loses body water, muscle and glycogen stores to achieve it. Are you prepared for the loss of performance and the health hazards involved? Even if you have time for a meal after the weigh-in, cramming yourself with food and drink cannot quickly reverse the damage.

Clearly, there needs to be a radical change of thinking and practice in these sports. The bottom line? You will compete best at the weight that corresponds to your lowest healthy body-fat level. Achieve this once and for all, and leave yourself only minor adjustments of one or two kg before an event. With pre-competition nerves and a few last minute tricks, you should be able to weigh-in confidently and in peak form.

HINTS FOR 'MAKING WEIGHT'

- Select a competition weight that is safe and sensible, by assessing your lowest healthy body-fat level. Use the fat-loss methods above to slowly and surely achieve this weight, well ahead of your competition.
- Stay within one or two kilos of your weight division during training.
- Final adjustments might be made over the last week to ten days

75

with a further slight reduction in energy intake—especially if you are in an exercise taper.

- Over the last week, reduce salt intake and stay away from high-salt foods to prevent fluid retention.
- To lose the final kilogram, make use of a low-residue diet over the last 12–24 hours. The easiest plan is to replace meals with liquid meal supplements. These products will supply carbohydrate for muscle stores and other nutrients, but leave your gut empty and light.
- Leave your pre-event meal until after the weigh-in. This doesn't need to be a huge feast, but should top up your energy and fluid levels before the event.

3.6 Bulking-up

Many athletes, even outside bodybuilding, dream of looking like Arnold Schwarzenegger. Often they try to buy these dreams with pills, potions, powders and three helpings at each meal. But it is not pure weight gain that is desired. Athletes in strength-based sports such as throwing events, power- and weight-lifting, and some football codes, really desired a gain in muscle mass. Despite all the magic and misconceptions, there are only a few real requirements for muscle gain, and these, in order of importance are:

- genetic potential—did you pick the right parents with the right body type?
- weight training—muscles only grow when given the right stimulation.
- a high-energy diet—you need more of everything, including, but not exclusively, a high protein intake. In fact, carbohydrate is still the most important energy source, since the muscle must be fuelled to do the work that will stimulate it to grow.

Set realistic goals based on the first two points in this list. You may need to seek expert advice—a strength coach to set a program of progressive muscle overload, and a dietitian to support this with a high-energy diet. Periodic measurement of body-fat levels and muscle circumferences will reassure you that any resulting gains in body weight are those that are desired. See the next section for advice on 'action-packed' eating.

3.7 The high-energy diet

Whether you are trying to gain muscle mass or simply maintain a strenuous training load, you may need to consume a large daily energy intake. To outsiders this may sound like paradise—and for some it *can* be enjoyable. But for other athletes it can range from a chore to an impossible task. Hurdles to chewing through all the necessary kilojoules include:

- lack of time, including time to buy and prepare food. Subtract your training time, your work, sleep and all the other commitments in your day, and this probably leaves you with three hours to consume 25 000 kilojoules (6000 Cals).
- the bulk of the food. A high-carbohydrate, high-fibre diet mean lots to chew and digest.
- fatigue and loss of appetite after training.
- lack of access to food (or suitable food) at possible eating times.
- need to limit food intake prior to training to avoid gastrointestinal discomfort during exercise.

If you are having trouble, a dietitian can help you to look over the day's schedule of activities. Keep a record like that suggested in the fat-loss section. This will help you look for opportunities to increase your energy intake.

HINTS FOR ACHIEVING A HIGH-ENERGY INTAKE

- Above all, be organised. You will need to apply the same dedication to your eating program that you apply to your training. A haphazard approach—eating what is available, when it is convenient—is no way to ensure the quality and quantity of food that you need.
- Increase the number of times you eat rather than the size of meals. A 'grazing' pattern of six to eight meals and snacks enables greater intake and circumvents gastric discomfort compared to the conventional pattern of three large meals. Build this into your day to suit your schedule.
- Plan to have food on hand for every eating opportunity. Portable snacks may be useful and an emergency food supply in your car, sports bag or locker is another good idea.
- Increase the energy content of high-carbohydrate foods by adding a little sugar or low-fat protein. For example, add jams and syrups to toast and pancakes, and make two or three layer fillings in sandwiches. This adds extra kilojoules to a nutritious meal, without adding bulk.
- Avoid excessive intake of fibre, and make use of some 'white' cereal foods with less bulk (e.g. white bread, Cornflakes and Rice Bubbles). You may find it impossible to chew your way through a diet that is solely based on wholegrain and high-fibre foods.

- • Drink high-energy fluids. Make low-fat milkshakes and fruit smoothies, or try liquid meal supplements such as Exceed Sports Meal, Sustagen Sport or Gator-Pro. These drinks provide low-bulk nutritious kilojoules and can be consumed with meals or as snacks between meals—even quite close to training.

4 Competition nutrition

Competition is your time to 'seize the day' and push yourself beyond your best. Your training and tapering should leave you well prepared for this. The final detail to consider is what could go wrong, to acknowledge the physiological issues that might hold you back, and then to plot nutritional strategies to keep these problems at bay. Each type of sport will have its own 'walls' to hit—whether it be hydrogen ion accumulation, muscle fuel exhaustion, or dehydration. Your nutritional strategies will involve issues of preparation over the last days as well as special practices during the competition itself.

4.1 A checklist of fatigue factors

The fatigue factors in a sport relate mostly to the type and duration of exercise involved. But the environment also can add to the problem list.

In brief, for explosive efforts such as jumps and lifts, fuel is supplied by high-energy phosphate compounds within the muscle cell— adenosine triphosphate (ATP) and creatine phosphate. These compounds can only supply several seconds of work but are quickly generated between efforts.

As events move from seconds to minutes, still at high workloads, metabolism continues anaerobically (without oxygen) with muscle glycogen now providing the main fuel source. If you start the event with extremely low levels you will suffer from inadequate fuel. But more likely, your normal muscle glycogen stores will see you through and it will be the build-up of acidity (hydrogen ions) and other by-products of muscle metabolism that cause the burning fatigue that slows you.

As the exercise duration becomes longer—and therefore at a lower intensity—aerobic metabolism becomes more important. Your muscles burn a fuel mixture of fat and carbohydrate, with the relative proportion of each depending on factors including the intensity of exercise (the carbohydrate contribution is greater at a higher work-load), your pre-event diet and your level of training.

Team sports usually involve a mixture of (anaerobic) high intensity bursts, interspersed with (aerobic) recovery periods. Meanwhile, athletes in relatively steady-state exercise, such as running or cycling, will gravitate to a predominantly aerobic workload just below the threshold where there is significant accumulation of blood lactate. Both groups should be able to continue activity until carbohydrate fuel stores become depleted.

The failure of carbohydrate stores to keep pace with the energy demands of the muscle occurs typically after 60–90 minutes of continuous exercise at maximal aerobic pace. Fatigue can be manifested in two ways, known by runners as 'hitting the wall' or in cyclists' and triathletes' terms, as 'bonking'. The 'wall' describes local muscle fatigue —heaviness or cramping in the exercising muscle—causing the athlete to slow down, and sometimes even stop completely. The likely cause is the exhaustion of muscle glycogen stores, leaving the muscle to rely on fat and the uptake of glucose from the blood stream to supply energy.

'Bonking' is caused primarily by the lowering of blood glucose levels, and occurs when the muscles take up blood glucose more quickly than it can be replaced by the liver (or by eating/drinking carbohydrate). This often happens in conjunction with muscle glycogen depletion, but in some sensitive individuals it may occur as an independent event. 'Bonking' produces a central nervous system fatigue— dizziness and mental confusion, and an overwhelming tiredness and desire to sleep. The smart athlete will try to avoid both consequences of carbohydrate depletion.

Recent work suggests that there are other aspects of central nervous system function that can cause fatigue, such as changes in brain chemicals like serotonin. Nutritional factors can alter these brain chemicals and future research will help to pinpoint strategies to minimise various causes of 'central fatigue'.

Dehydration is a fatigue factor in many sports, with as little as 2 per cent body fluid loss (1–2kg for a 50kg athlete and 1.5–3kg for a 75kg athlete) being shown to cause a reduction in aerobic exercise output. When fluid losses move into the range of 5–10 per cent of body weight, heat exhaustion may become a threat—although heat-related problems also present separately without dehydration.

Dehydration can occur in sport from two angles. Firstly some athletes purposely dehydrate themselves before an event to make a weight category. Talk about starting the event behind the eight ball! Secondly, dehydration can occur during exercise as athletes fail to replace the sweat losses that occur to cool their bodies. Just like a car, you produce heat as a by-product of work and this must be dissipated to keep your body at its preferred temperature. The harder you work and the heavier you are, the more sweat will be produced to cool you down. If the environmental temperature is hot and humid, your body will find it difficult to dissipate this heat.

The final nutritionally-based fatigue factor to be discussed is blood sodium imbalance. This is really only an issue for athletes who exercise at high intensities for very long periods—perhaps six hours or more—especially in the heat. Athletes such as ultradistance runners and Ironman triathletes actually do this! In recent years it has been found that many of these athletes finish with low blood-sodium levels, and a small percentage suffer severe effects as a result. Although the exact reason for diluted blood sodium levels is still debated, it is likely that problems arise when large amounts of sweat (water and sodium) are replaced with large amounts of low-sodium fluids such as water or cola drinks (e.g. Coke, Pepsi). There is a suggestion that a few athletes overdrink, but the choice of fluid replacement may be the major issue.

The message here is that you should drink to keep pace with your sweat rate—neither greatly underestimating nor drinking more than you are losing. While it is rare, it is possible for an athlete who is moving slowly—perhaps at the rear of the field—to spend too much time at the aid stations and outdrink small sweat losses. As for the choice of beverage, a sports drink containing electrolytes may better assist in maintaining blood volume and contents during situations of prolonged exercise.

CHECKLIST FOR COMPETITION PREPARATION DIET

Your checklist for competition preparation should include the following items:

- ensure that fuel stores (glycogen) are topped up in both your muscles and liver to meet the demands of your particular sport;
- in weight-class sports, achieve the required body weight without sacrificing performance;
- be well-hydrated;
- avoid gastrointestinal discomfort or problems;
- eat a pre-event meal that will continue to meet these goals.

4.2 General preparation for competition

Making weight to reach a competition weight class has already been discussed in Chapter 3.5. This leaves fuel and fluid needs as your preparation priorities on the day(s) leading up to the event. How hard you need to prepare depends on the challenges of your sport, the importance of the event and the frequency of competition. A long, intense event will probably throw out more fatigue factors to battle

HINTS FOR PREPARATION FOR GENERAL SPORTS
COMPETITION (events up to 80 minutes of continuous
exercise)

- In the absence of muscle damage, 24–36 hours of rest and a high carbohydrate diet will allow the storage of adequate muscle glycogen for your event. For some athletes the only change will be a well-earned rest from training.

- If you are competing frequently—once or twice a week for example, you may not always be able to organise the required rest from exercise. Try to taper exercise and achieve better preparation for your most important events.

- Schedule training so that the sessions which could potentially damage muscle fibres, (for example, those involving hard running, body contact or eccentric weight work) are early in the week, allowing more time for recovery.

- Your everyday training diet should already be high in carbohydrate. However, you may like to use the carbohydrate ready reckoner (Table 2.5) to check that your diet provides 8–10g of carbohydrate for every kilogram you weigh. For example, a 50kg athlete should aim to eat 400–500g of carbohydrate over the day preceding competition, while an 80kg athlete might aim for 600–800g of carbohydrate.

- If extra carbohydrate is needed over your everyday patterns, you might need to accentuate carbohydrate foods and reduce the protein component of meals. A little extra sugar and sugary foods can provide some compact carbohydrate—but don't make this an excuse to eat lots of fat.

- Drink plenty of fluids—especially if you anticipate that you will be competing in a hot environment.

- Top off with a good pre-event meal (see Chapter 4.4).

against, and if this is your major competition for the year then you will want to leave nothing to chance.

In preparing your fuel stores for competition, you can rest a little easier knowing that your training has given you an edge in this department. Aerobic endurance training teaches your muscles to store greater amounts of glycogen and to use it more sparingly during aerobic exercise, by increasing the contribution of fat to the fuel mixture. With your everyday (increased) muscle glycogen stores intact at the beginning of an event, you will have enough fuel on board to see you through all but the most prolonged sporting events.

To reach this everyday potential for muscle glycogen storage you require:

* 24–36 hours of rest or tapered exercise
* daily intake of 8–10g of carbohydrate per kilogram of your body weight
* absence of muscle damage.

For many athletes these conditions might be met simply by combining their everyday high-carbohydrate diet with a rest from training. Athletes in sports in which frequent competitions require more frequent preparation will need to plan carefully and prioritise their events. Notice in the hints on the previous page, that there is no need to cram yourself with food as if this is your last meal.

4.3 *Carbohydrate loading for endurance events*

Carbohydrate loading is probably the most talked about, yet least understood, nutrition topic in sport. For a start, all athletes, from darts players to ultramarathon runners think they need to do it. Secondly, many athletes use carbo-loading as a euphemism for gluttony— never mind the quality of the food, make up for it with quantity. And finally, the technique has been refined since its introduction in the 1960s, but many athletes have yet to catch up with the news.

To sort out the mysticism from what is a potentially valuable practice, you should firstly decide whether your sport requires you to have super-loaded muscle glycogen stores. If you are going to drive around the block, you don't need to have an extra petrol tank in your car—it would just be extra weight to carry. However, if you are driving in an endurance rally, then you will have an opportunity to use the additional fuel.

Typically, endurance sports which involve over 90 minutes of continuous high-intensity exercise, using the same muscle groups, will challenge the capacity of the athlete's normal fuel stores. Think about this definition carefully. Although your triathlon may take over two hours, it involves three separate sports and therefore different muscle groups. And while a team game may also play out this time, the actual duration of activity performed by any one player may be considerably shorter. You may need to think back to past events—did your pace or performance drop off late in the competition, accompanied by symptoms of muscle glycogen fatigue? If so, then you may be helped by super-loading muscle glycogen stores before you start. You won't run faster or work harder in the beginning, but it will prolong the time that you can exercise at your optimum pace. In the long run, you will come out on top.

Once you have decided that you compete in an endurance sport

Figure 4.1 The 'modified' carbo - loading program

Daily endurance training causes a daily cycle of depletion and loading of muscle glycogen stores. 72 hours of rest/taper and a high carbohydrate intake (10g/kg body weight per day) will cause an 'overloading' of glycogen in the trained muscles, enabling competition performance to continue for a longer period at an optimal pace.

and that carbohydrate loading could be useful, the next step is to forget everything you have read or heard about it—particularly about depletion phases and low carbohydrate diets. In its place try the following modified—and simplified—technique.

Without going into great detail, the original or classical carbohydrate loading program familiar to most athletes was developed using healthy but essentially non-elite subjects. We now know that well-trained endurance athletes are 'lean, mean glycogen-storing machines'. Every day in training they use up large amounts of glycogen, and every day their muscles rebuild the stores. In fact, this is a continuous mini-cycle of depleting and loading. With the storage techniques already well-rehearsed, all a well-trained athlete has to do to load up their muscle glycogen stores is to give their muscles the luxury of more time. In other words, it is no longer considered necessary (or useful) to undertake a severe depletion phase before the loading begins. In fact, it can be a disadvantage.

The same conditions needed for general competition preparation apply to modified carbohydrate loading, except that for a full glycogen storage effect you must extend the exercise taper and high-carbohydrate diet to a 72-hour period or more. Figure 4.1 illustrates how muscles become glycogen-loaded simply by extending the general preparation technique over a longer time. It is unlikely that you will compete in a true endurance event on a weekly basis, but if you do, save the full 72-hour preparation for important events only. As long as the taper doesn't interfere with your training schedule you can carbo-load, using this modified program, as often as necessary.

HINTS FOR A 'MODIFIED' CARBOHYDRATE LOADING PROGRAM

- Plan an exercise taper. This is not the time for last-minute training. As a suggestion, reduce your training load by 50 per cent going into the last week before the event, and reduce it by another 50 per cent over the last three days. The final day could be a day of rest or very light training—use it for stretching and mental preparation.

- Your daily diet over the 72-hour taper period should provide about 8–10g of carbohydrate per kg of body weight. Use the carbo-hydrate ready reckoner (Table 2.4) to check that you reach this daily target.

- Since the carbo-loading diet only lasts three days, you may take some liberties with your total nutritional goals and place carbo-hydrate intake at the top of the list. For example, don't worry about the protein foods at your meals—by de-emphasising the serve, you can leave yourself more room for large serves of the carbohydrate foods. In addition, sugar and sugary foods, including drinks such as sports drinks and soft drinks, can provide a compact carbohydrate source. Table 4.1 provides a typical carbo-loading menu.

- Be extra careful with your fat intake—save the kilojoules for carbo-hydrates. Don't get tricked with high-fat carbohydrate foods such as chocolate, icecream, rich desserts and takeaways. Although favourites with many carbo-loading athletes, these foods are a rich source of fat rather than carbohydrate.

- Enjoy the official carbo-loading functions before your event but don't let yourself get carried away. Leave your competitiveness for the event, not for food consumption races. Hopefully the event organisers have enlisted the aid of a dietitian in devising the menu, so that suitable food choices are available. Again, don't end up fat-loading instead of carbo-loading.

- Over the final 24 hours you may wish to reduce your gastric contents so that you race feeling 'light'. To do this, switch to low-fibre foods and make extra use of compact sugar foods. You may even like to use liquid meal supplements or high-carbohydrate 'carbo-loader' supplements to supply some or all of your carbohydrate needs over the last 12–24 hours. These are very low in residue and will leave you with an empty gut to race light.

> • Drink plenty of fluids. You will need to be well-hydrated for a long event, especially in hot weather. Perhaps carry a water bottle around with you over the last 24 hours as a reminder.
> • Finish up with a light pre-event meal two to three hours prior to the event (see Chapter 4.4)—and compete with action-packed muscles!

Table 4.1 A typical plan for carbohydrate loading

These meal plans provide about 600g of carbohydrate per day—suitable for a 60kg athlete to meet the 10g/kg recommendations. You may need to adapt the menus to eat more or less carbohydrate.
The menus are proposed for carbohydrate loading days only—while meeting carbohydrate requirements, they do not meet all nutritional goals for everyday eating.

Day 1: (602g CHO, 80 per cent of energy intake—12 200kJ)
Breakfast: 2 cups Weeties + 1 cup skim milk
            1 cup sweetened canned peaches
            250ml sweetened fruit juice
Snack: 2 slices thick toast + scrape marg + Tbsp honey
            250ml sports drink
Lunch: 2 large bread rolls with light salad
            375ml can soft drink
Snack: Large coffee scroll (unbuttered)
            250ml fruit juice
Dinner: 3 cups of boiled rice
            (made into light stir fry with small amount of lean ham, peas, corn and onion)
            250ml fruit juice
Snack: 2 crumpets + scrape marg + Tbsp jam
            Tea/coffee
Extra water during day

Day 2: (605g CHO, 77 per cent of energy, 12 700kJ)
Breakfast: 2 cups porridge + 1 cup skim milk
            1 banana
            250ml sweetened fruit juice
Snack: 2 muffins + scrape marg + Tbsp jam
Lunch: Stack of three pancakes + 60ml of maple syrup + small scoop icecream
            250ml fruit juice
Snack: 50g jelly beans
Dinner: 3 cups cooked pasta + 1 cup tomato puree
            2 slices bread
            250ml sports drink
Snack: 1 cup fresh fruit salad
            2 Tbsp non-fat flavoured yoghurt

Day 3:
same as Day 1 or 2, switching to white cereals, bread, etc.
OR: in place of lunch, dinner and afternoon/evening snacks:
            4 × 500ml liquid meal supplements or high carbohydrate supplement (carbo-loader) plus light snack if desired
Extra water during day

4.4 The pre-event meal

The pre-event meal is another nutritional practice that has attracted superstition and ceremony over the years. Its value to performance can vary from positive (in the case of an athlete who is still carbohydrate-depleted from a previous event), to neutral or cosmetic value (for the athlete who is already well-fuelled and hydrated) and finally to a negative or disastrous effect (for an athlete who chooses the wrong foods and suffers a gastric upset during the event). And even when the physiological effects of a pre-event meal are minor, the psychological factors can be of great importance. During the last hours before an important competition, athletes need to feel focused and prepared and most athletes and teams have a special eating ritual to suit their situation and needs.

The major goals of the pre-event meal are:

- to finish topping-up glycogen stores in muscles and the liver. Liver stores are important to consider if you are competing in morning events since they may be low after an overnight fast.
- to top-up fluid levels, especially if dehydration is likely to be a problem during the event
- to leave your gastrointestinal system feeling comfortable during the event—not too empty so that you feel hungry, but not over-filled or prone to gastrointestinal upsets
- to leave you feeling confident and ready to perform at your best!

Practical issues that must be considered are:

a. How well prepared is the athlete, or more specifically, has the athlete recovered from their last training or competition session?

The importance of the pre-event meal in topping-up fuel and fluid levels depends on the timing of the last major training or competition session, the degree of depletion caused by this session, and the amount of carbohydrate and fluid consumed since. For example, an athlete who has been preparing exclusively for an event may have tapered and eaten carefully in the day or days leading up to it. In this case, the role of the pre-event meal is a minor 'topping-up' since the major work has already been accomplished. On the other hand, if the athlete is competing in a tournament situation, or back-to-back in a weekly competition, and has recently completed a gruelling event, then the pre-event meal will be a crucial part of recovery and preparation. Similarly, an athlete who trains hard right up to the event, or restricts food and fluid intake to 'make weight', will look to the pre-event meal to repair suboptimal fluid and fuel levels.

b.   What time of day is the event scheduled?

Athletes who compete early in the morning will have to juggle the need for sleep against the need for adequate time to digest pre-event meals and snacks. While muscle glycogen levels can be prepared in the days leading up to the event, liver stores are more labile and need to be restocked after the night's fast. A moderate-sized carbohydrate meal on the morning of the event will be sufficient for this task. However if the event starts too early to allow 3–4 hours for a meal to digest, the athlete may choose a smaller carbohydrate meal 1–2 hours pre-event. To compensate for this, the athlete could pay more attention to carbohydrate intake during the event, thus supplementing the liver's ability to maintain blood glucose levels during prolonged competition events (see Chapter 4.7).

c.   Is the athlete at risk of gastrointestinal discomfort or upset?

Factors such as the timing, the amount and the content of pre-event meals (e.g. too much fibre or fat intake) can increase the risk of gastrointestinal upsets during exercise. Certain types of athletes are predisposed to such problems, and events involving running or 'bouncy' movements are also more likely to be associated with gut trouble. Manipulation of pre-event meals will be important for athletes at risk.

Thus the pre-event meal is rather a mixed bag in dealing with the various needs and timetables of different athletes—as well as their individual likes and dislikes. Some athletes prefer to keep to a meal plan that mimics their everyday eating patterns while others prefer to have a special plan to make competition day feel important. Others may need to manipulate some component of their normal diet—such as reducing the fibre intake—to ensure that the pre-event meal is 'spot on'.

In any case, high-carbohydrate eating is still the name of the game. Suitable meal and snack suggestions are found in 'Ideas for pre-event meals'. Since sport can be played at any time of the day, the pre-event meal schedule may vary considerably from one athlete to the next. When the event starts late in the day (e.g. a basketball game or a swimming final) the athlete may follow normal daily eating patterns early in the day, and then plan a special meal about four hours pre-event. Alternatively, they may like to eat their major meals earlier in the day and finish with a pre-event snack around 2 hours before the start of competition. In both cases, significant amounts of carbohydrate have been consumed during the day to assist glycogen stores.

Athletes competing in morning events may choose a breakfast according to the amount of food that can be comfortably eaten before the start of the competition. Early afternoon events might be tackled with a breakfast and a midday top-up, or a single larger brunch. All athletes should experiment with their pre-event meal plan so that they can come up with strategies that build confidence as well as fuel stores.

The psychological impact, and even superstition attached to favourite pre-event foods must also be considered. In many situations the pre-event meal is just a fine-tuning effect after all the important preparation work has been done. Even where pre-event meal practices don't exactly meet the scientific theories, some athletes will not be significantly disadvantaged. If the athlete is emotionally or psychologically boosted by a strategy, it is often best to leave well enough alone.

HINTS FOR THE PRE-EVENT MEAL

- Plan your day so that the final meal is eaten four hours before the event in the case of a larger meal, or one to two hours pre-event in the case of a snack.

- Choose high-carbohydrate, low-fat foods to ensure easy digestion and to top up carbohydrate fuel supplies. Many people find their normal breakfast choices are a great pre-event meal, even when it is not breakfast time. Other suggestions are found in 'Pre-event Meal Ideas'.

- Experiment with the type, timing and amount of food that works best for you. Practise in training or some minor competitions so that everything is right for important challenges. Learn which foods, if any, cause you discomfort or upsets and avoid these. High-fat foods are often a problem, but you might also find that you need to reduce your normal fibre intake in pre-event food choices.

- Drink plenty of fluids leading up to the event. If it is a hot day, or your sport provides little opportunity to drink during the competition, make sure that you are well-hydrated at the start of the event.

- In sports where you must weigh-in prior to the event to meet a weight division, you will probably choose to leave your pre-event food and fluid intake until after the weigh-in. Check-in times can be early in the morning on the day of the event, or an hour before it starts. Hopefully you have used sensible weight control measures to reach your weight target, so your pre-event meal will only need to top up fuel and fluid stores. There should never be a need for a last-minute panic to cram in food. It is too late in the day to correct the effects of dehydration and starvation practices.

- It is important to eat some carbohydrate before morning events, especially if you are competing in an endurance-length sport. If the liver's glycogen stores are low from an overnight fast, you may be less able to maintain blood glucose levels, especially late in the event. Experiment with a small snack or carbohydrate drink if time is short. In addition, compensate for low liver glycogen stores by consuming carbohydrate during the event (see Chapter 4.7).

• If you have a busy competition schedule (e.g. competing daily in a tournament or cycle tour), it may be difficult to recover food and fluid levels between events. Post-event eating, pre-event eating and during-event eating may all share an equal role in achieving carbohydrate and fluid goals. Even if you are becoming tired, don't neglect any of these eating opportunities.

• If you suffer from competition nerves or need to eat quite close to your event, you might find liquid meal supplements or a fruit smoothie a useful pre-event meal. These are high in carbohydrate and low in fat and bulk. Being easy to digest, you can probably drink them in comfort even up to an hour pre-event.

4.5 Sugar prior to the event?

In days past, some athletes thought that a last-minute intake of sugar might provide instant energy to boost their competition performance— hence the cramming of chocolate bars, glucose tablets and other foods thought of as quick energy. However, some of these foods are high-fat as well as high-carbohydrate. And in many cases, the most important carbohydrate source for muscle at the start of exercise is stored right inside it. That is why you carefully prepared your diet and taper over the day(s) leading up to this event.

One effect of a large dose of sugar or glucose in the 30–60 minutes prior to exercise is to increase your carbohydrate metabolism, by increasing blood glucose and insulin levels. This is a bit like pulling out the choke on a car to make it burn a richer fuel. Some researchers have found that the increased carbohydrate burning continues on into the exercise bout, increasing the ratio of carbohydrate that is burnt in aerobic exercise at the expense of fat-burning.

For an endurance athlete this was thought to pose a problem, since body carbohydrate fuel stores might now be depleted at a faster rate. Some athletes seem to be sensitive to another side-effect—the lowering of blood glucose levels.

However, most studies have shown that, despite pre-exercise carbohydrate intake, as soon as the exercise gets into full swing (e.g. after 10–30 mins), metabolism reverts back to its usual pattern and no problems occur. In fact, in many cases, any extra carbohydrate-burning was more than compensated by the carbohydrate consumed. In studies

PRE-EVENT MEAL IDEAS

- Breakfast cereal* + skim milk + fresh/canned fruit
- Muffins* or crumpets* + jam/honey
- Pancakes + syrup
- Toast* + baked beans* or canned spaghetti
- Baked potatoes with low-fat filling
- Creamed rice (made with skim milk)
- Pasta* with tomato-based or other low-fat sauces
- Rolls* or sandwiches* with banana filling
- Fruit salad plus low-fat yoghurt
- Liquid meal (supplements or homemade fruit smoothie)

* You may need to avoid high-fibre types if you are at risk of gut discomfort or problems during events.

where the athlete was not already fully 'fuelled-up' (e.g. muscle glycogen levels not maximised or liver glycogen levels depleted by an overnight fast), consuming carbohydrate an hour prior to the event actually improved the athlete's carbohydrate status—and improved endurance performance.

In the majority of other cases, there was a neutral effect on performance. Only a small group of subjects suffered problems—be it fatigue from faster carbohydrate depletion or problems with gastrointestinal side-effects. A suggestion for athletes who suffer the blood glucose roller-coaster after consuming pre-event carbohydrates, is to switch to low glycemic index carbohydrate-rich foods (see Chapter 2.2). Some studies have suggested that low-GI foods such as lentils and oatmeal can provide pre-event carbohydrate while maintaining more stable blood glucose and insulin levels. Be careful with this strategy however: many low-GI foods are high in fibre and may cause gastrointestinal problems when consumed close to intense exercise. Of course, in most situations the best strategy to overcome carbohydrate depletion during exercise is simply to consume carbohydrate during the event.

Athletes who compete in high-intensity anaerobic events lasting seconds to minutes are already big carbohydrate-burners. For these athletes, carbohydrate between and before events will be part of recovering between one heat or bout, and preparing for the next. Small carbohydrate snacks, including sugary foods, can be spread over the day of competition and will help to preserve blood glucose levels.

In summary, the question of sugar or carbohydrate intake in the hour prior to exercise has several answers. These vary according to the individual athlete, the success of their competition preparation, and the type of event they compete in. In many situations it is likely that additional carbohydrate intake is unnecessary—particularly if you are already 'fuelled-up' with a good competition preparation and a well-chosen pre-event meal. It can be a disadvantage to those who suffer blood glucose swings or gut problems as a result—particularly in the extra stress of competition. But it can be helpful for athletes who are still trying to refuel, especially from a series of hard training or competition sessions. Similarly, athletes who compete in very early morning events may need some pre-event carbohydrates but lack the opportunity to eat any earlier. Since performance is at stake, and the cost may be high, it makes sense to experiment to see which group you fall into. Practise in training sessions or in minor competitions before you introduce any new strategies into your competition routines.

4.6 Fluid intake during events

During any sport it makes sense to stay as well-hydrated as possible. Although it may go unnoticed in some sports, in hot weather and at a strenuous pace, athletes can lose in excess of a litre of sweat per hour. In fact Alberto Salazar was reported to sweat an astounding 3.7 litres/hour during the 1984 Olympic marathon in the hot Los Angeles conditions! Dehydration has a number of effects on performance, according to the type of sport involved. There has been a popular belief among athletes that performance is not significantly impaired until a 'critical' level of dehydration is reached—most commonly thought to be around 5 per cent of body weight (i.e. 2.5 litres for a 50kg athlete; 3.5 litres for a 70kg athlete).

However, more recent studies have established that there is no 'critical' point, but rather a gradual erosion of performance as the degree of dehydration increases. Heart rates are higher, you feel you are working harder and body temperature regulation becomes more difficult with every percentage of sweat loss. Because the effects creep up on you, just like your hair growing, you may not notice it happening.

The following comments summarise our current understanding of dehydration and performance:

- You cannot learn to adapt to chronic dehydration or 'toughen up' by repeated exposure.
- Any level of dehydration begins to exert an effect on prolonged aerobic performance, but the effects become significant when fluid losses exceed 2 per cent of body weight (e.g. 1kg for a 50kg athlete, 1.4kg for a 70kg athlete).
- The effects are more pronounced when exercising in hot conditions.

- The effects of dehydration vary according to the way you became dehydrated. Dehydration techniques used by some athletes to 'make weight', such as the use of diuretics, cause a different ratio of fluid loss from various parts of the body and may have a more pronounced effect on performance.

- Dehydration also affects mental functioning—decision-making, concentration and skill. Therefore dehydration may be more detrimental to a tennis player or football player whose performance relies on skill and judgement, than to a runner who just needs to keep putting one foot in front of another!

- Dehydration above 3–4 per cent of body weight greatly increases the risk of gastrointestinal discomfort and upsets. It appears that stomach-emptying rates are greatly reduced, so any fluids consumed may not effectively rehydrate the athlete. In the worst case scenario, bloating may stop the athlete from consuming more fluids, and vomiting may add to dehydration woes.

In general, any athlete undertaking an event with a duration in excess of 30–60 minutes of high-intensity exercise (particularly in hot conditions) may need to consider their fluid levels. In many sports the disadvantages of dehydration can be removed, or at least reduced, by the consumption of fluids by competitors during the event. While this is not necessarily practical in every sport, as the environmental conditions become hotter and the duration of the sport continues, fluid intake during the event becomes more critical. A healthy tradition in many sports is to have quarter or half-time breaks (with drink stops), aid stations along a race route, or trainers armed with water bottles waiting for a stop in play. Look at your sport to see whether the need arises and what opportunities can be provided for fluid intake.

Of course, there are some limits to the volume of fluid that can be consumed during an event. The amount of fluid that is actually delivered into your body depends on three factors: the volume that is consumed, the rate at which this empties from your stomach (which is basically a 'holding bay') and the rate at which it is then absorbed through the intestinal walls. To encourage you to consume it in sufficient quantities, an exercise drink must be palatable and available. Drinks that are very sweet or luke-warm are not very appealing, especially during hot conditions. Availability means not just having the drink on hand, but having adequate opportunity to consume it.

Sports which make fluid consumption difficult include those in which it must be done literally 'on the run'. This includes running, cycling, cross-country skiing and triathlon events. It is a skill to consume rather than spill fluids when you are moving; this must be practised well in training. There is always the risk that drinking during exercise will cause gastrointestinal problems—a stitch, indigestion, or bloating. This is usually more of a problem in sports which involve running or other 'bouncy' movements, and can occur even when the drink is consumed during a break. More importantly, grabbing and/or drinking the fluid on the move will necessitate a slowing of pace, or a change from your streamlined position. The athlete needs to know that the few seconds lost in drinking will be more than compensated by better performance later in the event, thanks to better hydration levels. More studies are needed to know just how great the trade-off is. At the present time, many elite athletes seem to take the conservative view and drink minimally when it disturbs their race pace. However, since they often can't tell that they are moving fractionally slower, or having to work fractionally harder to keep up performance, they may never really appreciate the detrimental effects of even moderate dehydration.

Once fluid has been drunk, the next stages are for it to be emptied (stomach) and absorbed (small intestine). Interestingly, even when you are just trying to replace body water levels, water may not be the most rapid way to achieve this. A dilute carbohydrate–electrolyte solution may actually achieve faster rehydration than water. Small amounts of sodium and glucose may increase the rate of intestinal absorption of water, and may help this fluid to be retained in the body instead of causing you to make a trip to the toilet! However there is a limit to how high these concentrations can go. High carbohydrate concentrations reduce the stomach-emptying side of the process and can become too sweet, while high sodium-concentrations, although of benefit to absorption processes, make the taste too salty.

In the next section, we will discuss situations that call for carbo-hydrate-replacement during exercise. However, at this point we will just consider those events which will benefit purely from fluid intake. Water will do the job in most cases, and is often the most available (and cheapest) fluid option. However, if you don't mind paying the extra cost, then flavoured drinks such as sports drinks, soft drinks and cordial can also be used. The carbohydrate content probably does not provide any physiological advantages in most non-endur-ance sports, but if you like the taste then you may be tempted to drink more, and therefore look after your fluid needs better. Sports drinks are formulated at a suitable concentration already (see next sections) but soft drinks, fruit juices and cordials should be diluted by 50–100 per cent to bring them into line with a good stomach-emptying concentration. See the Hints for Fluid Intake during General Sports Competition so that you can set up some good drinking strat-egies to suit your sport.

4.7 Endurance events—fluid and food intakes

An endurance event might be defined as one that will challenge the athlete's fuel and fluid reserves. Typically, we consider that sports

---

HINTS FOR FLUID INTAKE DURING GENERAL SPORTS COMPETITION

- Events typically lasting for 30–60 minutes of continuous exercise should provide opportunities for fluid intake during competition. Depending on the nature of the sport you may need to organise aid stations, scheduled drink breaks, or the use of trainers/water-carriers to bring out drinks.

- Athletes who compete in brief, intense sports lasting seconds to minutes should rehydrate fully after events, especially where they intend to compete or train again later in the day.

- Athletes who are slightly dehydrated before a competition weigh-in, should work hard after the weigh-in to fully restore fluid levels. If the competition involves further sweating, such as a wrestling match or a rowing event, then extra care should be taken with fluid levels. A sports drink or oral rehydration solution (e.g. Gastrolyte) may promote speedier rehydration than water.

- Water is a suitable drink during most events, though sports drinks, and diluted (de-fizzed) soft drinks or cordials offer no real disadvantages other than their cost. Above all, a drink must taste good and must be available.

- Cold drinks are more refreshing and palatable.

- Try to drink regularly rather than waiting until you become thirsty, and drink a comfortable amount on each occasion—for example, 150–250ml. If you have done some fluid balance measurements during previous competitions or similar training sessions (see box pp. 29–30) you may be aware of your likely fluid loss. In most cases a good fluid intake plan will keep total deficits below 2 per cent of body weight.

- In some sports these fluid intake guidelines might clash with tradition, attitudes and sometimes even sports rules. There may be a need for re-education of athletes and re-organisation of event practices to transform these ideas into action. Athletes should appreciate that the concern over fluid balance is not just to prevent severe dehydration, but to promote optimum performance at all times.

---

involving 90 minutes or more of continuous high-intensity exercise fit this description—for example, marathons in running and cross-country skiing, triathlons and long cycle races. Some sports can become endurance events on occasions—for example, a tennis match that is played out over 5 hours. Sometimes, the sport evolves into an endurance event because repeated performances are required with insufficient time to recover fully between. In such a case (e.g. a basketball tournament), a 40–60 minute event can become fatiguing for players because fluid and carbohydrate levels were not optimal at the onset of play.

The bottom line is that despite the best preparation possible, the athlete is likely to become fatigued during the event from carbohydrate depletion as well as possible dehydration. Studies have repeatedly shown that in these circumstances, additional carbohydrate consumed during the event can prevent, reduce or delay the symptoms of fatigue—and improve performance.

Once glycogen stores have become depleted, a well-trained muscle is able to take up glucose from the bloodstream at a rate sufficient to meet the fuel needs of continued exercise. A significant amount of carbohydrate is needed to keep pace with blood glucose uptake—on average about 50g of carbohydrate per hour, or 1g per minute. In addition to supplying the muscle's continuing fuel needs, carbohydrate intake can prevent blood glucose levels from falling into 'bonking' or hypoglycemic territory. Since lowered blood glucose levels can affect the brain and central nervous system, it is possible that reduced levels interfere with skill and concentration, even before significant fatigue becomes apparent. Therefore, carbohydrate supplementation may be a particular advantage during sports which rely on skill and response, and are played in lengthy sessions (e.g. certain positions in team sports, some racquet sports).

Theoretically, carbohydrate intake needs to start *before* the onset of fatigue, whether from depleted muscle glycogen levels or from low blood glucose levels. Ideally it should start well in advance of obvious performance impairment—both because there will be a delay while carbohydrate is ingested, digested and absorbed, and because there will be a period of gradual performance reduction before the athlete becomes obviously fatigued. For some sports, this may mean that extra carbohydrate intake starts in the middle or later stages of the event. Other athletes may choose to supply extra carbohydrate right from the start, perhaps starting with smaller amounts and gradually increasing the supply. In any case, once carbohydrate feedings start they should continue throughout the rest of the event. Supplementary carbohydrate is best consumed as a series of small feeds, rather than one giant load. However, sometimes the practical considerations in your sport will dictate how often you can manage this.

How much carbohydrate you need to consume will depend on your muscle fuel needs (how fast they are burning carbohydrate), and how well their own glycogen stores can meet this need. In lower intensity sports (e.g. hiking or bike touring at a recreational pace) or at the beginning of higher-intensity exercise when muscle glycogen levels are adequate, you may find that 20–30g of carbohydrate per hour will be sufficient to keep you performing well. However, at the 'business end' of a marathon or ironman triathlon (when stores are low and you want to go hard), you may need 50g/hr of carbohydrate or more. Studies show that there is wide variation in the supplementary carbohydrate needs of athletes—even when they have prepared similarly for an exercise session and are carrying out the same relative work load. You will need to experiment in your sport to identify if carbohydrate intake during the event helps you to perform, and how much you need to consume. You should also experiment to find practical opportunities to take your additional fuel on board.

Alongside the 'why', 'when' and 'how much' issues, you will also need to consider 'what'. In various sports there are different traditions of carbohydrate feeding during exercise. For example, cyclists have traditionally eaten chocolate bars, sandwiches and bananas, while triathletes probably started the market for specially manufactured 'sports bars'. In cross-country skiing, thick sugary syrups are often drunk, while runners might try jelly beans. Whatever carbohydrate choice is consumed during endurance exercise, the following conditions must be met:

- the carbohydrate choice should not delay stomach emptying, thus interfering with fluid delivery as well.
- the carbohydrate should not cause gastrointestinal problems such as diarrhea, bloating, vomiting or discomfort.

Again the individual athlete and the type of event will determine the importance of each of these considerations. We have already mentioned that some athletes are at greater risk of gut problems during exercise, and similarly have different rates of gastric emptying. Practice and training may be able to improve that. These disturbances are more likely to occur in sports which are very high in intensity or in which the gut contents are joggled around, compared to low-intensity exercise and sports like swimming, cycling or skiing where the movement is more horizontal or gliding. You may need to choose your competition menu according to the type of event.

Solid forms of carbohydrate generally take longer to empty from the stomach than fluids, particularly if they contain significant quantities of fat and fibre. These nutrients may increase the risk of gut upsets in some athletes. Athletes may also lose touch with their fluid needs if they are concentrating on solid foods—especially products like bread, dried fruit, confectionery and sports bars which have a low moisture content. However, many solid foods do offer the advantage of being a more compact and portable fuel form—which may be useful if you have to carry all your own supplies in a bike race or a cross-country ski event. And in very prolonged events, it can be a long time since breakfast, and some solid food may help to prevent or alleviate that hungry, empty feeling. Table 4.2 lists some popular food choices and comments about their use as competition fuel.

Table 4.2 Common food and fluid choices used in endurance sports

Food/fluid	Description	Amount needed for 50g CHO	Comments
Water			May be drunk in addition to solid foods or sports drinks to make up total fluid needs. Can be poured over athlete for additional cooling effect.
Sports drink	5–8% CHO + 10–25mmol/l sodium	600–1000ml	Theoretically the most efficient way to meet CHO and fluid needs simultaneously during exercise. Sodium has some useful roles. A powdered product will allow you to manipulate the CHO concentration within the 4–10% range, allowing you to promote fluid or carbohydrate intake according to your needs.
Cola drink (e.g. Coke, Pepsi)	11% CHO minimal sodium	500ml	CHO content may be a little high for most efficient stomach emptying —perhaps dilute a little with water or ice. Could provide a change of taste on occasions in a long event, and may give a caffeine 'buzz'. Beware that excessive intake (e.g. 10–15 cans) may exceed the IOC limit for caffeine. Defizz before drinking. Lacks sodium.
Fruit juice	8–12% CHO minimal sodium	500ml	CHO content as for cola drinks. See comments above. Lacks sodium.
Cordial	8–12% CHO	400–800ml	Concentration depends on how you mix it—dilute according to instructions on bottle for 8% strength, or more diluted in very hot conditions. Can be used as a more economical sports drink. Lacks sodium.
Bananas	Solid form of CHO + fibre	2–3 medium	Portable form of CHO. However, solid foods (theoretically) may cause gut discomfort if consumed in large quantities in high intensity sports—especially running. May be most useful as an adjunct to carbohydrate drinks, when the athlete becomes hungry, or needs to carry compact supplies. Don't neglect fluid needs.
Oranges	Solid CHO —CHO drink the juice only is consumed.	3 medium	Most athletes suck out the juice rather than eat the fruit—so you can often treat it as fruit juice. See comments above. May provide a refreshing change of taste in a long event.

Table 4.2 (Continued)

Food/fluid	Description	Amount needed for 50g CHO	Comments
Dried fruit (sultanas, figs etc.)	Solid CHO + fibre	65g	See comments for bananas.
Jelly beans	Solid CHO	60g pack	Compact carbos—but eating a large amount all at once may cause gut discomfort or diarrhea. Don't neglect fluid needs.
Jam sandwich	Solid CHO (+ fibre if wholemeal, + fat if buttered)	2 thick slices + 4 tsp jam	Commonly made with peanut butter or butter/marg. These high-fat foods are unnecessary. Fat or fibre content may cause gut problems in some athletes. See comments for bananas.
Chocolate bar	Solid CHO + fat	1.5 x 50–60g bar	High fat, solid CHO. This is theoretically not the best carbohydrate choice; however, many athletes have used chocolate successfully during endurance events or training. Don't forget fluid needs.
Choc-chip cookies	Solid CHO + fat	4–8 depending on size	See comments for chocolate.
Muesli bar	Solid CHO + low–moderate fibre	2	Choc-coated or choc-chip types may have higher fat levels. See comments for bananas.
Sports bar	Solid CHO	1–1.5 depending on size	Specially manufactured for use by athletes. Usually low in fat and fibre (check the label). Convenient and compact way to carry carbohydrate. Eating too many bars may cause gut upset or diarrhea in some athletes. Don't forget fluid needs.

Perhaps the most efficient way to provide carbohydrate while looking after fluid needs is to consume sugar-containing drinks. Although there are a number of everyday drink types to choose from (see Table 4.2), the most efficient and purpose-built product is the sports drink. As we will discuss in the section below, sports drinks allow the athlete to provide carbohydrate and fluid needs simultaneously, and encourage consumption by being flavoured to appeal to an exercising athlete.

However, to finish this section it is worth recalling that dehydration is another factor that has been shown to increase the chances of gastrointestinal disturbances during competition. This is especially relevant, because some athletes do not start to take in fluids or food during events until they are already dehydrated or carbohydrate-depleted. Many attribute the resulting stomach upset to the fluid they eventually drank, rather than recognising the problem that it was consumed too late. Similarly, food intake may be blamed for problems that are at least partly due to poor hydration strategies. It can be tempting not to stop or slow down for the first few aid stations in the effort to keep with the lead pack, or to keep going while your rhythm seems strong. But the risk is that you become dehydrated before you realise it—perhaps suffering minor losses of performance, but increasing the risk that it may be too late to turn the processes back. Your competition plan should be to prevent/delay dehydration and carbohydrate fatigue, not to try to deal with problems after they have already occurred.

Whatever your competition plan, it should be practised and fine-tuned in training—particularly under conditions that will mimic the Big Day. Often, practical issues will force you to adopt a plan that falls below (or even outside) the optimal guidelines. Do the best that you can—and follow what works for you. Many athletes have been observed to perform well on practices that look less than ideal on paper, but seem to work in real life!

HINTS FOR INTAKE OF CARBOHYDRATE AND FLUID DURING ENDURANCE EVENTS

- A combined fluid and carbohydrate intake plan may assist performance in prolonged aerobic sports (e.g. marathons, cycle races, triathlons) and in prolonged intermittent sports (e.g. team games, racquet sports). Effects may be greater in sports played in the heat, or in repeated performances where inadequate recovery occurs between events. Think back to previous performances and experiment to see if carbohydrate supplementation and better hydration can be of benefit.

- Form a strategy to meet your expected fluid and fuel needs during the event. Look both to past experience in competition and to the arrangements that are proposed by event organisers.

- Practise in training with the types and amounts of fluids (or food) that you intend to use so that you can become an expert. Make sure that you enjoy the taste of your exercise refreshments.

- Fluid needs during endurance events will vary according to environmental conditions, as well as the duration and intensity of the event. Use opportunities in training to estimate expected sweat losses using body weight changes (see box pp. 29–30). Ideally, you should aim to replace about 80 per cent of sweat losses as you go. However, the typical (comfortable) gastric emptying rate (600–1000ml/hr) may fall well behind fluid losses in extreme circumstances. Do the best you can to keep total fluid deficits below 2 per cent of body weight.

- Intake of fluid should begin early in the event and be taken at regular intervals as practical. An intake of 150–250ml of fluid every 15–20 minutes is a good benchmark but use the opportunities that exist in your event.
- Cold fluids are more refreshing and palatable and may add an additional cooling effect.
- Don't let yourself become dehydrated. A reduced stomach-emptying rate plus an increased risk of gastrointestinal complaints will put you further behind in your exercise intake.
- The stomach empties fastest when it is fullest. In extremely hot conditions you may need to maximise fluid intake to meet extreme sweat losses. Make use of the 'volume effect' by drinking the largest amount of fluid that can be comfortably tolerated just before starting the event (e.g. 300–600ml). Top this up each 15–20 minutes as it empties, thus maximising gastric emptying rate and fluid intake. With this technique and with practice you may be able to tolerate intakes of 800–1200ml/hr.
- Carbohydrate intake may start simultaneously with fluid intake or may start later in the event. In any case, begin a significant intake before you start feeling fatigued, and continue throughout the event. Often, a sports drink consumed to meet fluid intake needs will also supply adequate carbohydrate intake.
- Carbohydrate needs may vary from 30–60g/hr; experiment to see what works for you. You may find that a steady intake (small, frequent feedings) is beneficial; alternatively you may be able to increase carbohydrate quantities as the event continues.
- A sports drink may allow you to meet fluid and carbohydrate needs simultaneously. At the recommended concentration it provides about 30–70g of carbohydrate with an hourly intake of 600–1000ml. However, if you buy a powdered form you may be able to manipulate the carbohydrate content to increase fluid or carbohydrate delivery according to your needs.
- Although it is not necessary to use solid foods to provide carbohydrate requirements, many athletes will still enjoy the tradition or the convenience. If possible, avoid carbohydrate foods that are high in fat and fibre, since these nutrients may delay gastric emptying. Experiment in training. Table 4.2 provides a summary of common exercise foods and fluids with comments about their use.
- In events that last over 6–8 hours, it is possible that you will become 'hungry' and empty in the stomach. While you may de-

pend on carbohydrate drinks for fuel intake, a small amount of solid food can help to allay these feelings.

• A low level of electrolytes may be useful in an exercise fluid, especially during an ultra-endurance event. The sports drink is valuable for this reason.

Table 4.3   Analysis of some common sports drinks

Drink		Carbohydrate (% = g/100ml)	50g CHO	Electrolytes Sodium (mmol/l)	potassium (mmol/l)
Bodyfuel	7%	fructose glucose polymer	700ml	12	2
Exceed FER	7%	glucose polymers fructose	700ml	10	5
Gatorade	6%	sucrose glucose	850ml	23	3
Isostar	6%	glucose polymer sucrose	850ml	24	4
Maximum	7%	glucose polymers	700ml	10	5
Replace	8%	glucose glucose polymers fructose	650ml	10	5
Staminade	4%	glucose sucrose	1250ml	10	5
Suntory	6.5%	sucrose glucose	800ml	12	5
Isosport	7%	sucrose glucose polymers	700ml	20	5
Powerade	8%	glucose polymers glucose, fructose	650ml	10	4
Sportplus	7%	sucrose, glucose	700ml	17	7.5

4.8   Sports drinks—the rebirth

The first sports drink, Gatorade, was produced in the late 1960s as a special game drink for an American Gridiron team. It was formulated to 'replace what sweat takes out of you during exercise'—namely water and electrolytes such as sodium. The basic formula contained water plus electrolytes, with sugar added to make it palatable. Early sales were very promising.

However, in the mid 1970s the results of studies of stomach function during exercise suggested that sugar dissolved in fluid caused a reduction in the rates of stomach-emptying. Scientists felt that the first priority during exercise was to keep hydrated, and therefore suggested that it was wrong to consume carbohydrate at the expense of fluid replacement. The American College of Sports Medicine issued a position statement, saying that water was the best fluid for athletes to drink during exercise. Furthermore, it recommended that if sports drinks and other sugary drinks were used, the carbohydrate concentration should be kept below 2.5 per cent (2.5g per 100ml or 25g per litre). Sports drinks, not surprisingly, got a bad reputation—being labelled as 'too concentrated' and 'too salty'. It was also popularly said that sports drinks could 'dehydrate' rather than rehydrate an athlete during exercise.

The late 80s saw a rethink on the use of sports drinks. New scientific research produced the following findings:

- carbohydrate intake during endurance exercise can benefit performance, but significant amounts need to be consumed
- early concerns about gastric-emptying qualities of carbohydrate-containing drinks seem unwarranted—new techniques of measuring gastric-emptying show that most athletes can handle solutions of 4–8 per cent carbohydrate without impairing fluid delivery or hydration levels during exercise
- a small amount of sodium in an exercise drink can serve a number of useful functions.

The 90s has brought with it a mushrooming of the popularity and availability of sports drinks, with many new brands hitting the markets. Table 4.3 summarises the composition of a number of well-known sports drinks—or more precisely the composition of the 'ready-to-drink' forms or the suggested concentrations achieved when powdered forms are mixed according to the instructions. You will notice that the sports drinks generally fall within a narrow range; that is, 5–8 per cent carbohydrate and 10–25mmol/l sodium. This is the formula that would appear to meet the needs of most athletes during prolonged exercise, and achieves what is called a hypotonic to isotonic concentration (meaning it is lower than or equal to the concentration of blood).

Drinks with 5–8 per cent carbohydrate concentration have been shown to have favourable stomach-emptying characteristics—that is, they promote a reasonable rate of fluid delivery to the exercising athlete. At the same time, they deliver a significant amount of carbohydrate. A typical hour's intake of 600–1000ml of a 6 per cent drink would supply 36–60g of carbohydrate. Such a concentration is thought to be a common ground for the needs of most endurance exercise situations. Different drinks use a variety of types of sugars to make up the carbohydrate content. One of the more 'high-tech' carbohydrate forms is the glucose polymer—formed by the splitting of large starch molecules into glucose chains of usually 7–10 units. It was first thought that glucose polymers might empty from the stomach quicker than single glucose or sucrose molecules. However, studies have not shown

103

Figure 4.2 Concentration and volume of drink necessary to supply fluid and carbohydrate needs

Concentration in drink % (gram/100ml)	30 gm/hr	40 gm/hr	50 gm/hr	60 gm/hr	
2	1500 ml	2000 ml	2500 ml	3000 ml	Volume too large > 1250 ml/hr
4	750	1000	1250	1500	
6	500	667	833	1000	Adequate fluid replacement 600–1250 ml/hr
8	375	500	625	750	
10	300	400	300	600	
15	200	267	333	400	Low fluid replacement < 600 ml/hr
20	150	200	250	300	
25	120	160	200	240	
50	60	80	100	120	

Volume of fluid to ingest each hour to obtain
the noted amount of carbohydrate

Note: Gastric emptying does not usually exceed 1000–1200 ml per hour unless large volume consumed.

Source: E.F. Coyle and S.J. Montain, 'Medicine and Science in Sports and Exercise' *Official Journal of the American College of Sports Medicine* 24 (9 supp), SS.324-30.

the advantage to be as much as expected. Probably the major asset of glucose polymers is that they have a bland taste. When sugar concentrations get above 5–6 per cent they begin to taste too sweet—especially to an athlete who is working hard. Nevertheless all the mixtures probably have fairly similar physiological characteristics.

Of course, if you use the powdered forms of sports drinks, you can manipulate the final concentration yourself. In extreme conditions you may want to change the ratio of fluid to carbohydrate delivery, according to which has priority. For example, in very hot conditions you may want to maximise fluid delivery by lowering the concentration a little. A 4 per cent solution will probably achieve a slightly greater stomach-emptying rate—not important in most events, but of value in a very hot environment when your hourly sweat rates may be 1.5–2.0 litres and above. This means that you will have to drink more to achieve the same carbohydrate delivery—but that was your intent anyway! At the other end of the scale, if you were competing in very cool conditions and expecting a lower sweat rate (and lower fluid requirements), you might want to increase the concentration—say up to 10 per cent. This would allow you to achieve your desired carbohydrate intake without having fluid overload (leading to the need for a pit stop during the event). Some cross-country skiers, for example, drink very concentrated carbohydrate solutions. Figure 4.2 provides a graph that will help you to work out what drink concentration will supply particular fluid and carbohydrate amounts.

Some athletes who are able to look after their own provisions during an event mix up a variety of drink cocktails—often changing concentration during the event as nutritional needs change. For example, a marathon runner in warmish conditions might drink a 4 per cent carbohydrate mixture at the early aid stations (taking the opportunity to promote good fluid balance in the early stages while muscle glycogen stores are still the major fuel source), then, towards the end of the race when supplementary fuel needs are increased, the drink strength might increase gradually to 8 per cent. Because fluid levels have been well catered for along the way, the runner can now afford to focus on extra carbohydrate intake—being confident that gut problems resulting from dehydration won't interfere. Of course, experimentation is needed to develop such a specific plan as this, and it is only relevant where the athlete can plant their own race provisions at aid stations or with handlers. When you are part of a team competition, or participating in a big race field, it may not be possible to be so specific.

Sports drinks are specially flavoured to appeal to the taste preferences of exercising people. Their other purpose-designed feature is a small sodium level. This serves a number of important roles, in addition to adding to the flavour profile. Sodium replacement may be important in ultra-endurance events and may help to prevent the problem of hyponatremia (low sodium levels) that occurs in a small number of athletes who participate in such events (for example, Ironman triathlons, ultra-marathons). There is some belief that sodium helps to promote better intestinal absorption of the sports drink, but this may not be significant until the sodium level becomes much higher than is present in the current range of sports drinks, and higher than most people would consider palatable. However, sodium does have a role in rehydration—by helping your body retain the fluid that you have drunk and to quickly rebalance its fluid compartments (see Chapter 5). In the majority of cases, athletes whose exercise pursuits benefit from the use of a sports drink will benefit from this extra sodium intake. Therefore, when used correctly, sports drinks do not deserve the label of 'too high in salt' or cause any problems of high blood pressure.

Sports drinks will be discussed again in the recovery chapter and supplement chapter. We will see that they represent a practical way for the athlete to meet nutritional goals during and after exercise—and that this often justifies the cost. The most common question asked, after 'do they work?'—is 'which one is the best?' There is no single answer to that query either. Sports drinks 'work' when they are used by an athlete to meet a goal of sports nutrition—and most of the current sports drinks can be used in this way. Once you have established whether they are of benefit to you in your situation—and whether you can afford them—the choice is often based on side-issues. For example, you might choose the drink with the flavour that most appeals to you. If you are going to drink a 'swimming pool full' while training and competing for this year's Ironman triathlon, then you had better like it!

Alternatively, it may be sensible to go with the drink that is already being supplied in the race or competition. Perhaps you want to support a drink that sponsors your team or sport in some way. Or again, perhaps you are happy to support a sports drink company that sponsors various opportunities for sports nutrition education. After all, they are most likely to teach you how to use their product well. Whatever your choice, remember that competition success is the result of carrying out well-devised plans rather than grabbing a magic potion at the last minute.

5 Eating to recover

Being an athlete in the nineties means pushing yourself hard and long, striving to go beyond your best and hold it together until the finish. And then do it all over again tomorrow.

In many sports events, you may be required to compete more than once, with the interval between events being anything from 30 minutes to 24 hours. For example, you may be racing in an athletics carnival where you have to run in heats, semi-finals and even the final in the one day. In a basketball or tennis tournament you may be scheduled for one or two games each day. A cycle tour may be composed of one or two stages each day, lasting for a week or more. Indeed, the training schedules of many athletes pose a similar challenge to optimise recovery between sessions, particularly when two or even three hard sessions are planned each day. In all cases, performance is dependent on your ability to recover from one session and present yourself at your best for the next.

In the nineties, recovery should be regarded as an active part of training or competition. It is no longer passive, happening by itself, in its own good time. Rather, special strategies are employed to speed up recovery processes and promote the level of return. There are many components to this, including massage, relaxation and sleep. Nutritional recovery includes:

- replacing the fluid and electrolytes lost in sweat
- refuelling muscle glycogen stores
- repairing any damage caused by the exercise and building new structures to adapt to the workload.

The peak training diet includes active recovery in its checklist of goals. In the main, your eating patterns should now provide all the building blocks and the vitamins and minerals necessary to build and repair. These processes probably happen over a longer time frame than the acute challenges of rehydrating and refuelling. Recent scientific studies have focused on the acute situation to find special strategies to enhance these recovery issues—not just what to eat and drink, but when to do it!

5.1 Restoring fluid and electrolyte balance

Even where planned fluid intake has been carried out before and during an exercise session—either competition or training—it is likely that you will still finish the session with some degree of dehydration. This is particularly true for prolonged and intense sessions in a hot environment, where sweat losses exceed the usual intake of fluid. However, this may also be expected in short events where there is little or no opportunity for fluid intake during exercise. If you are required to compete or train again within a short period, whether hours later or the next day, it is important that fluid levels be restored.

Most athletes will not be fully aware of the degree of dehydration that has occurred during a session. Human beings have a poor in-built ability to gauge and repair this, so it is better to rely on an objective assessment and a definite plan of attack, rather than simply listening to thirst. The amount of fluid needed to restore fluid levels may vary from 500ml to three litres, depending on how much sweat you lost during the session, and how well you attempted to replace it during the exercise itself. A quick guide to dehydration state is to weigh yourself before and after the session—minus sweaty clothes, of course (see box pp. 29–30). A kilogram of lost weight is roughly equal to a litre of fluid that needs to be replaced—except in endurance events where you weighed in heavier than normal with loaded glycogen stores. If you carbo-loaded before the event, subtract 1–1.5kg from your pre-event weight to account for the extra glycogen and the water that is stored along with it, leaving you with true fluid losses. Alternatively, go by your usual training weight.

Restoring hydration requires attention to what, when and how much fluid is consumed.

a. Amount of fluid

Pre- to post-exercise weight changes may give you a rough estimate of your dehydration levels (see box pp. 29–30). But this is not the end of the story. For example, you may do some calculations at the end of your session to determine that you are roughly 2kg 'behind'. However, this does not mean that drinking 2kg or 2 litres of fluid will see your fluid levels fully restored. It will take more than that, because over the next few hours you will continue to lose fluid—by continuing to sweat a little, and by needing to urinate. You may actually have to drink 3 litres to regain the 2 litres you need! It will also take time for the fluid to equilibrate back into the various body compartments from which it was lost. Be prepared to drink at least what you have lost over the next couple of hours, and then keep topping up until fluid levels are fully restored.

b. Type of fluid

On the surface, any drink should help to restore fluid levels. However, at a more sophisticated level there are some fluids which are better than others—and in some situations, speed will be the name of the game. As we discussed in the 'during exercise' situation, a fluid has to be consumed before it starts to be useful, so post-exercise drinks need to be available and appealing. Some studies have shown that athletes will drink more of a flavoured drink than plain water when left to choose their own post-exercise fluid strategies. It helps if your recovery drink is enjoyable, but remember that if you have a reasonable degree of dehydration to overcome, you should be drinking to a plan rather than to desire.

One thing you may not know is that some fluids are better than others in being retained—in particular, by influencing urine production. Fluids containing a little sodium—for example a sports drink—are superior to plain water both for rebalancing the body fluid compartments and for promoting fluid retention. The sodium may also help to replace salt losses. If water is considered the standard fluid, and sports drinks can reduce urine production compared to this, then beware of other drinks that actually increase expected urine losses. Alcohol and caffeine both have a diuretic action—that is, they stimulate urine production. Alcohol has a number of other effects that make it a poor choice for rehydration fluid (see Chapter 1.6). But if you need to rehydrate quickly and efficiently after a hot, sweaty session, then caffeine-containing drinks (e.g. Coke and other cola drinks, strong tea and coffee) are also not the best choice.

A recent study from the laboratories of Professor Ed Coyle in Texas, illustrates the significance of the retention rates of various post-exercise drinks. Subjects exercised in a hot environment until they had lost 2 kg of sweat (approximately 2.5 per cent of body weight) on a number of occasions. For the two hours after each trial they sat quietly at a comfortable temperature and replaced the missing two litres of fluid. Drinks were consumed in two sittings, immediately after exercise and 45 minutes later. Over the course of the study each subject got to drink each of the following beverages: water, diet-cola, and a sports drink. The order of each trial changed for each subject to avoid bias. The volume of fluid that was retained after two hours was as follows:

Diet cola	54%
Water	65%
Sports drink	73%

Urine production was greater with the diet cola than the other drinks. The gassiness of the cola was also reported to be a problem—many of the subjects felt uncomfortably full after drinking the required amount of this drink when compared to the other fluids. While the total differences in fluid balance may seem small (e.g. 200–400ml), this could make a major difference if dehydration was severe and the next session was looming. This situation is frequently faced by heavily-training athletes, or athletes competing in tournaments. (It's also worth noting that another study has reported greater fluid retention when athletes eat some solid food at the same time, than when they drink alone.)

The benefits of a carbohydrate boost provide another issue in the choice of a post-exercise beverage. Sports drinks, cordials, soft drinks and fruit juices will all provide carbohydrate intake to assist restoration of glycogen levels, while simultaneously looking after fluid recovery. As discussed in Chapter 4, the sports drink comes out slightly ahead when you need to balance efficient fluid delivery with carbohydrate delivery, since you can count on it to be rapidly absorbed. So when the situation calls for quick replacement of moderate to large amounts of fluid and carbohydrate, consider the sports drink as a well-rounded choice. Other fluids will also do an adequate job, although alcohol and caffeine-containing drinks should not be consumed in large amounts.

c. When to drink and other factors

Obviously you should start to rehydrate as soon as possible after you have finished an exercise session. Drink frequently and drink as much as you can comfortably manage, so that you maximise the rate of stomach emptying. Depending on the size of your losses you may need 4–24 hours to completely replace and rebalance your body fluid losses. Some organisation will be needed to have suitable drinks on hand.

Plan ahead for your post-exercise requirements—and for the rest of the day if necessary. You may need to bring some drinks down to your training session or competition venue. A jug of drink on your desk at work or in front of the fridge can be a good reminder of the task at hand. Similarly, carry your water bottle around with you for the day.

Lastly, don't forget that other post-exercise practices may work against your hydration plans. Staying in a hot environment will continue to make you sweat. Avoid sitting in the sun to get a tan or to watch how other competitors are faring in an event. Don't spend long hours in a hot tub or spa, unless this is part of your recovery and extra fluids have been planned.

5.2 Replacing glycogen stores

Depending on the length and intensity of your training session or competition event, it is likely that your muscle glycogen stores will need topping up before the next session. Active recovery strategies will be important if you have depleted most of these stores and/or your next session is less than 24 hours away.

Figure 5.1 Daily recovery from prolonged exercise

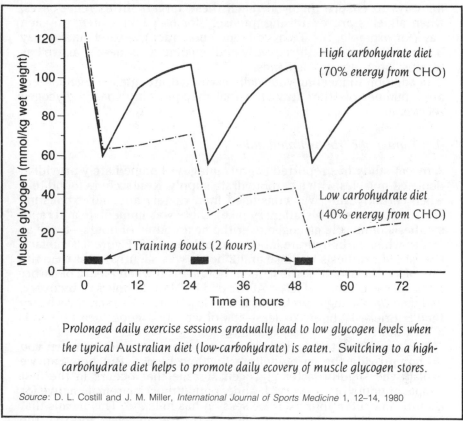

Prolonged daily exercise sessions gradually lead to low glycogen levels when the typical Australian diet (low-carbohydrate) is eaten. Switching to a high-carbohydrate diet helps to promote daily ecovery of muscle glycogen stores.

Source: D. L. Costill and J. M. Miller, *International Journal of Sports Medicine* 1, 12–14, 1980

Optimising glycogen storage can be a daily challenge for many athletes. Figure 5.1 illustrates the benefits of good refuelling strategies, compared with the bad news facing athletes who do not efficiently recover. This now famous graph compares the success of muscle glycogen recovery with two different strategies—the typical Western diet, and a high-carbohydrate eating plan. It illustrates clearly that athletes with heavy daily commitments to training or competition need a special dietary program. Failure to follow such a program may impede recovery and prevent good performance on subsequent days. The effect can be quite dramatic—or creep up on you gradually—but nevertheless it's the Wall!

Daily intakes of 8–10g of carbohydrate for each kilogram of your body weight are needed to restore maximum amounts of glycogen.

This equates to 500–800g of carbohydrate per day—see Chapter 2.2 for ways to ensure that you reach these targets. In extreme cases, when athletes are exercising intensely for 6–8 hours or more each day (for example, the Tour de France bike race), greater intake may be needed to cope with recovery and ongoing daily needs, as well as to meet huge energy demands.

In addition to meeting your daily carbohydrate intake targets, there are a number of other strategies that may promote speedy glycogen recovery.

a. Timing of carbohydrate intake

A recent study has reported the advantages of immediately providing depleted muscles with a carbohydrate supply. Researchers found that when carbohydrate was consumed immediately after an exhausting session (2 hours on a stationary bike), there was immediate and rapid synthesis of muscle glycogen over the next couple of hours—twice as fast as when carbohydrate intake was delayed (see Figure 5.2). In fact, the rate of synthesis in those first 2 hours was slightly faster than the rate of synthesis in the subsequent hours, even when plenty of carbohydrate was consumed later. At the end of 24 or 48 hours of recovery, you may have caught up from such a slow start, however, if recovery time is brief—10 hours or less—it's obviously a good idea to give it a 'kick start'.

It makes sense that muscle glycogen recovery is slower when you do not provide the carbohydrate building blocks. But how can we explain the slightly faster glycogen storage that occurs in the first couple of hours of recovery? It appears that muscles remain active for a short time after your exercise session has finished. This means that blood flow will continue to be diverted to the muscles, and that the muscle cell will continue to be able to take up glucose across its walls at an accelerated rate. Since depleted muscles enjoy an enhanced glycogen synthase enzyme activity, all the conditions are there to stimulate a fast synthesis rate. However, this window of opportunity seems to close after about two hours, and glycogen storage drops back to a more typical rate.

To take advantage of the enhanced storage rate, or even just to ensure the rapid restoration of muscle fuel stores, an athlete should consume about 1g of carbohydrate per kilogram of body weight as soon as possible after the finish of the session (i.e. within 15–30 minutes). Such a snack—50–100g of carbohydrate for a typical athlete—should be repeated every two hours until the athlete is back into their normal meal schedule. See Table 5.1 for some examples of high carbohydrate snacks and mini-meals. Over a day of recovery it doesn't appear to matter whether the muscle receives its carbohydrate supply in big meals or as a number of small snacks—at least from the

Figure 5.2 Short-term recovery after prolonged exercise

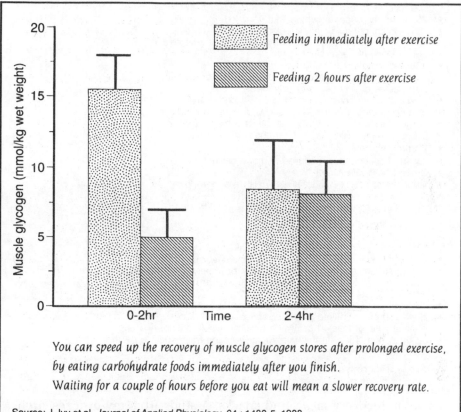

You can speed up the recovery of muscle glycogen stores after prolonged exercise, by eating carbohydrate foods immediately after you finish.
Waiting for a couple of hours before you eat will mean a slower recovery rate.

Source: J. Ivy et al, *Journal of Applied Physiology*, 64 : 1480-5, 1988

glycogen synthesis point of view. As long as you can eat your way through your total carbohydrate needs each day, the timing details are up to you once an early start has been made. For some people, a 'grazing' pattern is less filling and more fun. However, other athletes do not have access to food or the opportunities to eat it all day and for them a routine of larger meals may be more suitable.

b.   Types of carbohydrate foods

Glycogen storage is influenced by the type of carbohydrate that is consumed. Fructose, a sugar found in many fruits, fruit juices and some sports drinks, is not very effective in restoring muscle glycogen stores. However it enhances liver glycogen storage, and is therefore

Table 5.1 Examples of 50g carbohydrate snacks

Light and easy to eat:
- 250ml of carbo-loader supplement
- *250–350ml of liquid meal supplement
- *250–350ml home-made low-fat milk shake/fruit smoothie
- 800–1000ml of sports drink
- 800ml of cordial
- 500ml of fruit juice, soft drink or flavoured mineral water
- 50g packet of jelly beans or jelly lollies
- 1 round of jam sandwiches (thick-sliced bread and lots of jam!)
- 3 medium pieces of fruit (e.g. apple, orange and banana)
- Large Mars Bar (70g)—note that this is a high-fat choice
- 3 Muesli bars—also high in fat if choc-coated
- 2 breakfast bars
- *sports bar (note that * applies to many but not all)
- 3 rice cakes with jam or honey
- large bread roll (or two small rolls) with a banana
- *2 × 200g cartons of low-fat fruit yoghurt
- *1 × 200g carton of fromage frais plus a breakfast bar

Quick, low-fat and nutritious:
- *250–350ml of liquid meal supplement
- *250–350ml home-made low-fat milk shake/fruit smoothie
- Cup of thick vegetable soup with a wholemeal roll
- *Salad sandwich with slice of lean meat or cheese and a piece of fruit
- *Carton of low-fat fruit yoghurt and a muesli bar (not chocolate)
- *Bowl of cereal with low-fat milk
- *Bowl of fruit salad with 1/2 carton of low-fat fruit yoghurt
- *220–250g tin of baked beans or spaghetti on 2 slices toast
- banana jaffle or toasted sandwich (using a whole banana)
- *200g carton of low-fat fruit yoghurt or fromage frais, sprinkled with
  1 cup breakfast cereal

* denotes snack contains 10g or more of protein

useful in recovery meals and snacks. A study from my own research group has shown that carbohydrate-rich foods with a low Glycemic Index are less effective than those with a high Glycemic Index in restoring muscle glycogen levels (see Chapter 1.3 for a description and identification of low Glycemic Index carbohydrate foods). For this reason, some nutrition experts have recommended that such foods should not make up more than 1/3 of the carbohydrate provided in recovery meals and snacks. However, because these foods tend to be filling and fibrous—for example, lentils, porridge, baked beans—it is unlikely that you would choose to eat a meal exclusively based on low Glycemic Index foods anyway. All in all, enjoying a variety of carbohydrate foods will probably ensure that both muscle and liver glycogen stores are looked after.

c. Muscle damage

Muscle damage, either through direct body contact and bruising, or through eccentric exercise (the type that makes you sore a day later), causes a delay in the recovery of muscle glycogen. In fact, some studies of runners who have completed a marathon show that muscle fuel stores are still below par nearly a week later. Running involves eccentric muscle contractions, and a single hard or lengthy running session may cause significant muscle damage. This damage causes a disruption of the muscle fibres and physically interferes with their glycogen-storing capabilities. Furthermore, the white blood cells which rush to the area as part of the immune system's 'mopping-up' brigade, use up glucose for their own fuel needs. The major effect on muscle fuel stores appears to occur in the second 24 hour period of recovery—that is, 24–48 hours after the session.

Some studies have shown that problems with glycogen storage following muscle damage can be at least partly overcome by increasing carbohydrate intake even further, and by capitalising on the first 24 hour period before the main effects take over. Therefore, athletes who have completed a hard race, contact sports, or other events in which bruising or other muscle damage has occurred, should pay extra attention to their eating strategies during the first 24 hours of recovery and remember that additional high-carbohydrate eating may help to compensate for the storage delays.

5.3 Other recovery issues

There are many processes in recovery and adaptation that occur after and between exercise sessions. Many involve the 'cleaning-up' of damage, or the building/rebuilding of new cells. Nutrients such as proteins, vitamins and minerals are involved in these processes, accounting for some of the increased nutritional demands of the athlete. It is important that your everyday diet be based on wholesome foods that can meet increased requirements for various nutrients. And while these issues are not yet clear, there may be some benefit in supplying at least some of these nutrients in immediate post-exercise meals and snacks.

There are some indications that eating protein straight after a hard exercise session might help with various recovery aspects. Some studies have reported that a carbohydrate–protein combination may assist the restoration of muscle glycogen, and may reduce muscle damage or speed the repair process. There are still many questions to be studied—such as why and how much. However if your training or competition schedule is punishing, and you need help to recover from long intense sessions, then try a carbohydrate—protein combination. Look back to Table 5.1 for nutritious carbohydrate snacks that also provide a protein boost. Items that are marked with an asterisk provide 10g or more of protein with a rich supply of essential amino acids, along with the 50g carbohydrate serve. Alternatively, you may be able to schedule your next meal soon after the exercise session for an even larger carbohydrate and protein supply.

There may be other reasons to choose carbohydrate recovery foods with more than just carbohydrate and fluid in mind. For some athletes these recovery carbohydrate snacks and meals make up a significant proportion of the total eating plan—for example, an athlete with low energy requirements who is trying to make every kilojoule 'count', or an athlete competing in a 3-week bike tour who is eating for recovery day in, day out. In these circumstances, recovery carbohydrates also need to be able to provide a significant contribution towards total nutrient needs. Wholesome carbohydrate-rich foods should therefore be chosen, and perhaps supplemented with other low-fat nutrient-dense foods.

5.4 Putting it all together—practical considerations

A summary of hints which draw all this information together is found below. In this chapter we have seen that speed and timing in delivery of recovery nutrients can be important in promoting the efficiency of recovery. The period immediately after a hard exercise session is a crucial time to supply fluid, carbohydrate and perhaps other nutrients to a fatigued body and depleted muscle. This might sound great in theory, but in the real life of an athlete this important time is usually when you have the least desire or opportunity to consume foods or fluid.

HINTS FOR RECOVERY AFTER PROLONGED STRENUOUS EXERCISE

- Previous training and competition experiences should give you a rough idea of your expected level of dehydration after an exercise session. If you are confident that this is a litre or less, then a general fluid plan should be sufficient to see you well rehydrated before the next session.
- If you are likely to be moderately to severely dehydrated after an exercise session (despite your best attempts to look after fluid needs before and during the session), then check body weight changes pre- to post-event to get an estimate of your overall fluid deficit. This will give you a rehydration target.
- You will need to drink more than your estimated fluid deficit to regain fluid balance. Be aware of continued sweating and urine production to get an idea of how much of your rehydration fluid is being retained.

- Use other tactics to reduce ongoing sweat losses. Keep cool by staying out of the sun, avoiding excessive time in saunas and hot tubs, and wearing appropriate clothing.
- Avoid alcohol and caffeine-containing drinks when you are re-hydrating. These drinks, particularly in excessive amounts, stimulate urine production and are therefore inefficient rehydration fluids.
- Eat or drink a carbohydrate snack within 15–30 minutes of the end of your session. A carbohydrate boost of 50–100g (about 1g per kilogram of your weight) will start the recovery process. Choose carbohydrate foods and/or fluids that are practical to your location or appetite (see Table 5.1).
- Continue to replenish carbohydrate stores with more 50–100g carbohydrate snacks every 2 hours until you can get back into the swing of your usual high-carbohydrate meal plan. Your total daily target should reach 8–10g of carbohydrate for each kilogram you weigh—500–600g for a typical athlete (see Chapters 1.3 and 2.2).
- If you have suffered muscle damage and are likely to experience soreness—whether through direct injury or eccentric-type exercise—take extra care with your early carbohydrate recovery. The first 24 hours are the most important for efficient refuelling. Even after that, extra carbohydrate intake may help to overcome the effect of the damage on glycogen recovery rates. Any alcohol within the first 24 hours after an injury may cause problems with repair and recovery.
- Plan ahead to have your recovery snacks, drinks and meals accessible and suited to your appetite and eating opportunities. Even if you have to juggle a number of activities after your training or competition sessions, use a little creativity to find refuelling and rehydration supplies that can travel with you while you attend to your commitments.

There are many factors that stand in the way of good recovery nutrition:

- There may not be any food or fluid available at the track, pool, field or velodrome, or perhaps the catering facilities only serve high-fat rather than high-carbohydrate choices.
- You may have other commitments and distractions—e.g. your stretching and warm-down program, coach's meetings, collecting or cleaning your equipment, post-competition officialdom, press conferences, driving to your next appointment, etc. This may tie up your time making it difficult to find or eat a recovery snack.

- You may have no appetite. Many athletes feel nauseous or disinterested in food after a hard exercise session. Or perhaps you are too tired to chew anything, let alone go home and prepare a meal. After a game or match you may be in celebration mode, and figure you can party tonight and have a rest from good eating—then pick it up again at the beginning of the week.

This is where good planning and organisation comes into play. You need to think ahead to recognise the obstacles, and plan a strategy to overcome these hurdles. Bringing your own food and drink to a training session or event may help both with the lack of catering at the venue, and with the demands on your time and attention. Many carbohydrate-rich snacks and drinks are portable and non-perishable—check the list in Table 5.1. At worst, some choices need minimal preparation time and a little help with storage—an esky can be a great investment if there are no fridges or lockers around. With a few minutes to grab your drink bottle, your package or your bowl, you may be able to attend to your next commitment while munching on your recovery supplies.

For those who finish the session feeling hot, tired and a bit queasy, a drink may be more suitable than solid food. Carbohydrate drinks include sports drinks, fruit juices, soft drinks and cordial, and when served cold will appeal to even the tiredest athlete. For additional nutrients, try a fruit smoothie or a commercial liquid meal supplement. Some of these can be bought in ready-to-go cans or tetra packs. Next up the rung are high-fluid foods that don't take much chewing: yoghurts, fromage frais and fruit pieces can be appetising to hot, sweaty athletes, while hot soup or hot chocolate (boosted with extra skim milk powder or powdered liquid meal supplement) can grab your attention when you come in wet and freezing. In general, bite size or finger foods can be most practical. When you're too tired to chew, sandwich quarters or a slice of pineapple look far more manageable than a triple-decker super roll or a huge plate of pasta.

It's understandable when you've finished a hard match or event that you want to celebrate or commiserate by taking some time out. This may not create any problems if this is the end of the season or a one-off competition. However, for those playing in a weekly competition, or in a tournament situation, you need to live to fight another day. And the next hours are crucial in the recovery process, especially if you are severely dehydrated, fatigued or suffering injury and damage. Put first things first and get the recovery thing happening. Refuel and rehydrate aggressively—a well-organised team will have suitable post-event recovery snacks and drinks waiting in the change rooms or club house. This makes it easy to get the right things happening quickly and automatically. Perhaps, once you have the recovery processes under way, there will be time to have some fun. Take care with alcohol intake—excessive intake is not a good recovery plan (see Chapter 1.6).

Finally, when you get home after training or competition you may be looking to boost your fuel intake again. When it's late and you're tired, or the clock has been ticking away since your session finished, you need to be organised to be able to prepare a quick meal. Breakfast-type meals are easy since breakfast cereal and toast are quick to prepare and require minimal culinary skill. Sandwiches and toasted sandwiches/jaffles are also speedy—provided you have shopped to have some tasty and nutritious fillings available. It's usually the evening meal that takes time to prepare if you're in charge of your own cooking, however there are many quick recipe ideas and convenience ingredients that can see a meal on the table in 20–40 minutes. Many organised athletes cook ahead, so that on busy nights after late training or competition they only need time for reheating. Or why not have a snack as soon as you walk in the door, to keep you going until the meal is cooked. It doesn't have to be extra kilojoules if your total intake is a concern. You can always start with your dessert first—have some yoghurt or fruit immediately, and then eat your main course later when it's ready.

5.5 Multi-event competitions

There are a great variety of competition situations and schedules that require an athlete to compete over and over. Between events you will need to consider recovery from the first session, and then specific preparation for the second. In some ways, good recovery leaves you well-prepared. The fine-tuning is to add the pre-event meal strategies covered in Chapter 4. Your overall strategies will vary according to the following features:

- The physiological requirements of the event—the length, intensity and type of exercise will decide both the level and type of depletion or fatigue that must be recovered from the initial event, as well as the limiting factors that must be prevented or postponed in the next event.

- The interval between events—this will decide how much recovery time you have, and whether you need to juggle solid food and drinks to avoid gut discomfort.

- The significance of total nutritional goals—if an athlete competes periodically in events over a couple of days, then it may be sufficient to concentrate on immediate fluid and carbohydrate issues. However, if competition extends over weeks, or makes up a significant proportion of the athlete's training life, then total nutritional

119

Table 5.2 Nutritional practices for various competition schedules

Description	Strategies
Short intense events repeated in the same day (swimming meet, weightlifting competition, etc.)	Replace mild to moderate fluid losses between events, and top up body carbohydrate stores over the day with a schedule of carbohydrate drinks or foods. Drinks will be handy when there is only a short interval between events, and where solid food may lead to gut discomfort. When you have more time between events (e.g. heats and finals) a carbohydrate snack or meal may be suitable. Liquid meal supplements can provide a half-way point, being more substantial than other drinks, but less upsetting than solids. Take extra care if you have dehydrated slightly to meet a weigh-in target, and be prepared to bring your own food and fluid supplies to the competition. Not all venues will cater adequately for your nutritional needs.
Moderate length events repeated in the same day (e.g. badminton or basketball 'lightning' championship)	The same principles apply as above, but you may need to work harder to replace both fluid and carbohydrate stores. Make sure that you start your plan straight after the event. Carbohydrate and fluid intake during the event may become more important if full recovery is not possible.
Moderate length events over successive days (e.g. basketball or waterpolo tournament)	During the day you may follow the same schedule as above. Once competition is over for the day you can turn your attention to preparing for the next day. Again, plan a post-event carbohydrate top-up, and make sure that all sweat losses are replaced. Meal schedules may need to be flexible if your events are held at different times each day. Pay attention to including nutritious food choices as well as using convenient carbohydrate and fluid forms. Carbohydrate and fluid intake during the event may become more important if full recovery is not possible.
Prolonged events over successive days (e.g. cycle tour, tennis tournament)	It will be a challenge to meet fluid and fuel needs both during events and between events. Sports supplements may be useful in many situations—e.g. carbohydrate drinks during competition, and low bulk 'carbo-loader' and liquid meal supplements as a boost to food intake when the day is over. Be aggressive with pre-event, during event and post-event nutrition—every opportunity must be used.

goals, such as vitamin, protein and mineral needs, will have to be taken into account.

Look at your competition schedule to plot out the times of your events and the intervals in between. Table 5.2 lists some common event time-tables and the typical nutrition issues that arise. Juggling these issues is often a challenging business. There is probably no single perfect system, but there are two overriding rules:

1 Experiment until you find the system that works for you and your sport. Practise in training to be sure.

2 Be prepared to organise your own supplies to make it happen on the day. Don't leave anything to chance or to the event organisers. Be in control.

6 Pills and potions

It is hard to open a sports magazine without being bombarded with advertisements for nutritional supplements—all promising to make you bigger, stronger, leaner, faster or whatever it takes to be a better athlete in your sport. How can you refuse such a tempting offer? Or, better still, how can you afford to let your competitor get an edge that you don't have?

In 1983, a survey of over 4000 Australian athletes reported that 47 per cent were regular users of nutritional supplements. Each year billions of dollars are spent in search of a bottle of the 'Winning Edge', and each decade a new set of wonder substances replaces the last set. Do they work? That is the question of the nineties.

6.1 Why do athletes use supplements?

There are three basic reasons why athletes turn to supplements and these need to be considered separately:

1 They consider that they eat poorly or perhaps they have an inadequate lifestyle. Wrong! How can some extra vitamins make up for late nights, too much alcohol or too much fat in your diet? There is only one solution to these problems—face the real issue and fix up your act properly!

2 They consider that their nutritional requirements for sport are too great, or their food supply is too low in nutritional value to meet their needs. Occasionally perhaps. But has a dietitian helped you to make best use of the food supply before you turn to supplements? And have you been advised about the right supplement for any remaining shortcomings?

3 They consider that some supplements can directly enhance sport performance. Maybe. But when, which ones and how much?

To sort out the answers, it helps to divide the large variety of supplements on the market into two categories: dietary supplements and nutritional ergogenic aids.

6.2 Dietary supplements in sport

A dietary supplement can be described by the following features:

- most commonly, it contains nutrients in amounts similar to the Recommended Dietary Intakes (RDIs) and to the amounts found in food, and provides these nutrients in a form that is practical or convenient for a sports situation;
- alternatively, it contains large amounts of a nutrient, specifically for the rapid treatment of a nutritional deficiency;
- rather than being 'magic', it is seen as being a means to an end, by being used to respond to a nutritional need or challenge that arises in sport—and by doing so, helps the athlete to achieve peak performance;
- it is supported by scientific trials and studies, and has the interest and approval of mainstream science.

Examples of dietary supplements are found in Table 6.1, with the situations in which they may contribute to sports performance. Some can be used to directly enhance exercise performance—for example, the sports drink—while others are used to contribute to the athlete's overall nutritional status and, therefore, indirectly contribute to peak performance.

Note that in all cases it is not the supplement that 'works', but rather the success of the athlete in understanding their nutritional goals and matching the supplement to the situation. The right supplement must be used at the right place at the right time, and in the right amounts. For example, an iron supplement will only benefit an athlete who is truly iron deficient, and can only reverse the deficiency when used in the correct dose for an appropriate time. A sports drink will not improve performance in a 100m sprint event, where the nutritional requirements for fluid and carbohydrate replacement have not been created. Some of these supplements and their application to particular sports will be discussed in Part II of this book. Talk to a sports dietitian if you are not sure how to make best use of these supplements in your situation.

Dietary supplements deal with well-known and well-studied nutritional and physiological challenges in sport. Scientific trials are continually being conducted to develop and support supplements and their strategies of use. Many of the supplements are produced by large pharmaceutical companies who contribute towards the research and provide nutrition education for athletes. This shows a good balance between the needs of the company, the athlete and the exercise scientist.

Of course, dietary supplements cost money. Even those of a simple nature—for example sports drinks—are more expensive than food items of similar nutritional value. It may be cheaper to use bananas and water, or cordial at the right concentration, to refuel and rehydrate during a lengthy exercise session, but because the sports drink will precisely meet your nutritional needs, and because it is practical and

Table 6.1 Some dietary supplements and their uses in sport

Supplement	Form	Composition	Uses
Sports drinks (see Table 4.3 for examples)	1 Powder (mix with water) 2 Ready to drink	5–7% carbohydrate (note % = g/100ml); 10–25mmol/1 sodium	• All exercise—fluid intake. • Endurance exercise—fluid and carbohydrate intake. • Post-exercise refuelling and rehydrating.
High carbohydrate supplements (e.g. Gatorlode Relode, Ultrafuel, Exceed High Carbohydrate Drink Source)	1 Powder (mix with water—or mix into food if unflavoured) 2 Ready to drink 3 Sachets of thick syrup	When made up, usually 20–25% carbohydrate. Some have B-vitamins added.	• Carbohydrate loading. • Post-exercise refuelling. • Carbohydrate intake during some endurance sports—make sure that fluid needs are not neglected. May need to 'dilute' by adding or drinking extra water.
Liquid meal supplements (e.g. Sustagen Sport, GatorPro, Exceed Sports Meal)	1 Powder (mix with water or milk) 2 Ready to drink	1–1.5 Cals per ml. Energy breakdown: 50–70% carbohydrate 15–20% protein low–moderate fat. 500–1000ml provides RDI levels of most vitamins and minerals.	• Training diet—a compact way to meet high energy and carbohydrate needs. • Competition preparation—low-residue meal for empty gut. • Pre-competition meal. • Post-exercise recovery—carbohydrate and protein. • Travelling—nutrition on the run.
Sports bar (e.g. Power Bar, Gatorbar, Exceed Sports Bar)	Chewy or slice-type bar	40–50g carbohydrate; 5–10g protein. Usually low in fat. Often with 50–100% of some vitamins and minerals.	• Training diet—a compact way to boost carbohydrate and energy intake. • Carbohydrate intake during some endurance sports —take care with fluid needs and with gut upsets. • Post-exercise refuelling. • Travelling—nutrition on the run.

124

Table 6.1 (Continued)

Supplement	Form	Composition	Uses
Vitamin/mineral supplement	Capsule or tablet	100–300% of RDI for broad range of vitamins and minerals	• Supplement dietary intake in low-energy or weight loss diet. • Supplement dietary intake in a restricted variety diet (e.g. vegetarian). • Travelling—supplement dietary intake when food supply is unreliable.
Iron supplement	Capsule or tablet	30–125mg iron per supplement (ferrous sulphate or gluconate)	• Supervised management or prevention of iron deficiency.
Calcium supplement	Tablet	500–1000mg calcium (calcium carbonate/phosphate/lactate)	• Calcium supplementation in low-energy or low-dairy food diet. • Treatment/prevention of osteoporosis?

tastes just right, you may think that this is money well spent during your marathon. However, it would be unnecessary and even a trifle extravagant to serve it at a family barbeque: there are lots of less expensive beverages to choose from when the situation simply calls for something that is wet and palatable.

If expense is a problem you may be able to fashion a 'home-made' version of some popular dietary supplements. Adding a little salt to cordial will give you the basics of a sports drink, and you can make your own liquid meal supplements with a blender and some milk, skim milk powder, fruit and optional yoghurt or icecream. Many athletes however, are glad to use the convenience of the 'ready to go' products, especially when they are 'on the move'—either through travel or living a busy day. Remember too, that part of the cost of the dietary supplement often sponsors the research that produces the state-of-the-art nutrition knowledge, as well as the education opportunities that brought it to your attention.

6.3 Nutritional ergogenic aids

By definition, an ergogenic aid is something that directly improves work output, or exercise performance. A nutritional ergogenic aid is a supplement containing a nutrient or food-related substance, eaten in the hope of an immediate boost to performance. It is these supplements that have captured the imagination (and wallets) of the athletic world. A general description includes many of the following features:

- it contains nutrients or other substances in much larger quantities than the RDIs or the amounts normally found in food;
- it aims to produce a pharmacological or (legal) drug-like action to improve performance. In other words, the action is outside the known physiological role of the substance;
- it is backed by a proposed mechanism that may sound scientific but is often untested. Where trials have been undertaken, most fail to detect an ergogenic effect. In fact by strict definition, 'proposed ergogenic aid' might be a better title for many supplements, since there is no certainty of their effectiveness.
- it is generally not supported by mainstream science except where sound evidence exists;
- it is often manufactured by small companies who have no pharmaceutical expertise and who fail to support research;
- it comes and goes in fashion;
- it can be expensive.

A quick guide to some popular nutritional ergogenic aids and the available scientific evidence is presented in Tables 6.2–6.4. You will see that there is good reason to think that some aids, such as caffeine and bicarbonate, may work for some athletes in specific situations. However, there's a lot more work to be done before the jury comes back with a result on the latest ideas about vitamin E, creatine and certain amino acids. The vast majority of nutritional ergogenic aids are either untested or have failed to impress in tests that have been done.

It's important to factor cost into the discussion since many of the currently fashionable nutritional ergogenic aids come with a hefty price tag—especially if they are taken in large amounts and with a large assortment of other products. Sometimes the expense reflects the cost of manufacture. Sometimes, however, it simply reflects the popularity and the promises of the product—in other words, what the athlete is prepared to pay for something they think they need. In the case of some nutritional ergogenic aids, food sources can provide a similar amount of the product in question at a fraction of the price. (see Figures 6.1 and 6.2)—it is always worth checking out this possibility. There may be some occasions when you need the most practical way of consuming certain nutrients, and on these occasions a 'designer-product' for athletes is worth the extra cost, but it is not always apparent from product advertising that a nutritional ergogenic aid might

Table 6.2   Some popular nutritional ergogenic aids for which there is some scientific support

Caffeine	Caffeine is probably the most widely-used drug in the world, and is found naturally in the leaves, nuts and seeds of a number of plants. Major dietary sources of caffeine—such as tea, coffee and cola soft drinks—typically provide 30–100mg of caffeine per serve, while caffeine is also found in some over-the-counter stimulant tablets (e.g. No-Doz) in 100–200mg doses. Caffeine has a number of effects on the body including stimulation of the central nervous system, adrenalin and muscle. It has been used by athletes for at least 100 years to improve sports performance, but since the 1970s it has received publicity and scientific attention for its effect on endurance exercise. Although scientists have debated the results of various studies, the general view is that a 300–500mg dose of caffeine (about 5–6g per kilogram of your weight) consumed in the hour prior to an event may improve the performance of prolonged aerobic exercise. The most popular theory to explain this effect is that caffeine stimulates fat metabolism during aerobic exercise, 'sparing' body glycogen stores and thus delaying fatigue. However other studies have indicated additional effects that also help performance—including effects on the nervous system which may give the athlete a 'buzz' and mask fatigue. However, caffeine-loading is not good for all endurance athletes. Like most drugs, caffeine elicits a variety of responses in different individuals. Some athletes receive a pronounced performance boost, others are actually disadvantaged by side-effects and some receive no effect at all. There are many factors involved, including your usual caffeine intake. People who drink strong coffee by the mugful every day may not get the same buzz as someone who rarely consumes any caffeine. Whether you are a caffeine 'responder' can only be determined by experimentation, and may be specific to you and your event. However, remember that large amounts of caffeine are banned by sporting organisations such as the International Olympic Committee. Urinary levels above 12μg/ml are considered to be 'doping', and will result in disqualification and bans. Drug education for athletes advises that such a level will only be achieved if 500mg or more of caffeine is consumed over a short period (e.g. 4–5 strong cups of brewed coffee or 10 cans of Coke). This probably exceeds the everyday use of most athletes but may be the level required to produce ergogenic effects in some athletes. So, even if you feel that it may be useful to your performance, make sure that caffeine doping is not banned in your competitive event or that you are below the legal limit.
Bicarbonate	In the competition chapter we identified one limiting factor during high intensity (anaerobic) exercise as the build-up of acidity or excess hydrogen ions. This causes a 'burning' sensation as well as an inability to maintain the exercise intensity. Sports which fit this description are those of 1–7 minutes of high intensity exercise and include 200–400m swims, 800–1500m runs and rowing or kayaking events. It has been proposed that extra muscle buffering capacity could improve performance in such sports—by mopping up more of the excess hydrogen ion than the body's present capacity will handle. Bicarbonate is such a buffer. Many studies have shown that a dose of 300mg of bicarbonate per kilogram of an athlete's weight (or about 20g for a typical 70kg athlete) will increase the blood buffer capacity. Furthermore, in many though not all of these studies, this was shown to delay fatigue when anaerobic exercise was undertaken. Again, the positive effects seem to be specific to individuals and to the event. You will need to experiment to see if you and your sport fit the bill. Some

Table 6.2   (Continued)

athletes already have such a well-developed buffering system that extra bicarbonate does not appear to be useful, and some events are not limited by hydrogen ion excess. While bicarbonate-loading is not considered illegal by sporting organisations, there are some side-effects. The bicarbonate dose is usually taken 1–2 hours prior to the event and can be taken either as common household bicarbonate of soda, or in the form of special pharmaceutical products known as urinary alkanisers (such as 'Ural'). Some people suffer gastrointestinal cramping and diarrhea as a side-effect, although it appears that this risk can be reduced by drinking a litre or more of fluid with the bicarbonate. In addition, alkaline urine is thought to mask the presence of a number of illegal substances, so if you are chosen for a drug test after your event you may have to wait a while until your urine reverts to a more acidic level that is considered OK for testing.

Creatine

Creatine phosphate plays a number of important roles in the provision of fuel to exercising muscles. It is probably best known as one of the high-energy phosphate compounds that supply fuel for rapid and 'flat out' exercise tasks lasting 1–10 seconds (for example, sprints or bursts of play in team sports). Stores can be quickly exhausted and then restored during the recovery period. However it also plays a role in anaerobic lactate-generating exercise (acting as a buffer inside the muscle cell), and during aerobic exercise (carrying the ATP energy produced inside one part of the muscle cell to the site where it can do its work). If creatine is a limiting factor in an exercise, and levels of creatine in muscle could be raised, then there could be a multitude of possibilities for performance enhancement. Shortly after the Barcelona Olympics, a study appeared in a European journal reporting that muscle creatine phosphate levels could be boosted by 3–6 days of a high creatine intake. Levels were increased by 25–50% by the intake of 5g supplements of creatine four to six times a day over this short period. This is a significantly greater intake than is provided by dietary sources (raw meats, eggs, fish, etc.) which normally contribute about 1–2g per day to the average adult. Following this exciting report, testimonials started appearing from a variety of sources—including successful British track and field athletes—claiming that their winning performances had been produced by creatine supplementation. Supplements hit the street, at great expense to the athlete, particularly because daily recommended doses were so high. Despite the enthusiastic start, there is still much to be studied before creatine supplements can be recommended to athletes with clear guidelines. Initial reports of effects on exercise performance are conflicting. Some studies have reported reduced fatigue and improved performance in repeated trials; others, however, have not. Effects on a single intense workout or a prolonged aerobic event are also unclear. It appears that individuals have different responses to creatine supplementation, with the most dramatic responses perhaps being seen in those whose initial muscle creatine phosphate levels were lowest. Vegetarian diets, low-energy diets and very high-carbohydrate diets are generally low in creatine. Athletes who follow such diets may be the ones to profit most by a creatine boost. However, it appears that there is a creatine threshold level in the muscle, and once this is reached extra creatine intake will not translate into greater benefits. Athletes who already have maximised muscle creatine stores are therefore unlikely to respond to creatine supplementation. It's a bit like the carbohydrate-loading effect. Like all effective ergogenic aids, creatine will only be useful when we know the answers to the following questions: what is the optimal dose

Table 6.2 (Continued)

(perhaps divided into an initial larger 'loading' dose followed by a reduced 'maintenance' dose)?; what types of sports events might it help?; are some athletes less able to take advantage of its effects?; are there any side-effects? Creatine has the potential to provide a useful performance edge to specific athletes in specific events—or it may fail to live up to its expectations. Stay tuned!

Table 6.3 Some popular nutritional ergogenic aids that are currently under review

Vitamin E

Vitamin E refers to a group of related compounds—the tocopherols. Back in the 1970s a number of studies of vitamin E supplementation were undertaken with athletes, usually swimmers. No effects on performance were reported and interest declined. However, more recently, the case has been reopened in recognition of the role of vitamin E (and Vitamin C) as anti-oxidants. The production of damage-producing 'free oxygen radicals' has been linked with the increased risk of cancers, heart disease and the general 'wear and tear' of ageing. It is believed that exercise increases the production of free oxygen radical species, and that recovery from an exercise session could be enhanced by a more efficient mopping-up of these potentially damaging compounds. Some studies have reported that supplementation with vitamin E (often together with vitamin C) reduces the markers of damage that follow a heavy exercise session; other studies have shown that repeated exercise sessions (that is, a training program) causes the body's own anti-oxidant systems to adapt to the new level of oxidative stress. This might mean that vitamin E supplementation may no longer be necessary or effective. Further work is needed to determine if extra anti-oxidant support is needed by heavily training athletes, and whether this is a long-term need or only necessary at the start of increased oxidant stress until the athlete's own body can catch up. Situations of increased oxidant stress might include the beginning of a new training program or an increase in training load, and training at high altitude or in a polluted environment.

Amino acids

Amino acids might be described as the sports marketing success story of this decade. But despite the hype and their undoubted popularity among athletes, the answer to whether they 'work' remains unclear. Just as the letters of the alphabet make up words, there are about twenty or so amino acids which are arranged in different combinations to form various body proteins. While protein is composed of amino acids joined in long chains, amino acid supplements provide 'free-form' or single amino acids. These are produced through special microbial fermentation processes, and are therefore much more expensive than food sources of protein or protein powders (see Figure 6.1). Manufacturers claim that free-form amino acids provide the benefit of more rapid absorption, although whether this does occur and whether it is a useful feature in healthy athletes has not yet been studied.

The major interest in amino acids lies in the claims that individual amino acids cause special metabolic responses. You may have noticed that amino acid manufacturers often market individual preparations making certain promises—for example, 'recovery' amino acids, 'anabolic or weight gain' amino acids and 'body fat loss' preparations. The list goes on. Unfortunately the research to support these claims does not. One theory that has been reasonably well tested is that the amino acids ornithine and arginine stimulate the release of growth

Table 6.3   (Continued)

hormone, and might therefore provide a 'natural' or 'legal' alternative to anabolic steroids, but a number of well-conducted studies have failed to find any increases in growth hormone release or body mass/strength following oral intake of these amino acids. However, there still appears to be some promise in the theory that branched-chain amino acids (valine, leucine and isoleucine) may have a role in exercise. These branched-chain amino acids (BCAAs) can be broken down, producing another amino acid, alanine, as a side-effect. Alanine, in turn, can be converted by the liver to provide another source of carbohydrate for exercising muscles. During prolonged endurance exercise events, blood BCAA levels may drop as a result of their use as a carbohydrate fuel producer. There has been recent interest in the theory that this may cause a complicated chain of events which affect the brain, via the increased production of a brain chemical called serotonin. Serotonin produces feelings of tiredness and may explain the 'central fatigue' that often overwhelms some athletes (in contrast to muscle tiredness). Some studies have shown that supplementation with BCAAs during prolonged exercise can stop the BCAA decrease and reduce this 'central' fatigue. However, carbohydrate supplementation will also produce this effect since BCAA levels will remain stable when no longer needed to produce a carbohydrate skeleton. Furthermore, carbohydrate supplementation will also address 'muscle fatigue' due to lack of carbohydrate fuel, thus taking care of a number of causes of performance impairment. In fact, moderate to large doses of BCAA supplements during exercise may actually be counterproductive. There is evidence that it may cause an increase in muscle ammonia production—yet another suspected cause of exercise fatigue. So the exercise story remains complicated.

The recovery situation is also full of unresolved theories—including the role of BCAAs in preserving blood glutamine levels. Glutamine is another amino acid that is important in immune system operations that mop up exercise-produced damage. BCAAs immediately after exercise may help to promote recovery and enhance immune system function.

Clearly, amino acids deserve more work. In the meantime, it is disappointing that promising theories are distorted by some amino acid supplement manufacturers and presented as extravagant 'facts'. The issue of safety and side-effects must also be explored. A grim reminder of the potential for tragedy can be found in the 'tryptophan' scare of the late 1980s when a number of deaths resulted from contaminated preparations containing the amino acid, tryptophan.

Probably the most neglected issue in the whole amino acid story however, is the potential for food to provide the same desired amino acid doses. Amino acid manufacturers have been clever in labelling their products in milligram quantities. A dose of 2000mg of branched-chain amino acids sounds impressive. Remember though, that 2000mg is merely 2g, and that the typical athlete probably consumes 60–160g of protein each day (a lot in the form of BCAAs). In fact, quite small amounts of everyday foods can provide 2000mg of BCAAs—and usually at a lower cost (see Figure 6.2). The problem is that food composition tables do not make this information available, and food manufacturers are not as skillful in their marketing. There may be some situations in which a designer-made amino acid supplement may prove to be the most practical form of intake—for example, if the value of amino acids *during* exercise is ever proved. However, in most situations it should be simple and inexpensive to boost your amino acid intake with food.

Table 6.4 Other popular nutritional ergogenic aids that have not yet passed the 'proof' test

Vitamins—megadoses	The most popular and enduring of the ergogenic aids. The role of vitamins at RDI levels has been well established. Following the 'if a little is good, more is better' rule, almost all of the vitamins have been tried in large doses in the hope of an extra boost to performance. To date, the evidence fails to support an ergogenic effect on performance.
Protein powders	Promoted to boost muscle mass. In Chapter 3, the principles of muscle gain were outlined: the right genetic potential, a strength training program, and a high-energy, high-nutrient diet. If you need a supplement to boost dietary intake, go for a complete nutrition aid (liquid meal supplements) rather than the more expensive protein-only supplements. Skim milk powder is the least expensive protein/carbohydrate booster (see Figure 6.1).
Bee pollen	Bee pollen offers a glamorous and exotic approach to performance enhancement. However, there is doubt over the real composition of some supplements. This might explain why the controlled trials have failed to find any improvement after taking bee pollen. However, the balance of studies suggest that there is no effect.
Carnitine	Carnitine is a carrier molecule which transports fat into the cell's energy chambers to be metabolised. Your body manufactures its own supply. A popular theory of weight-losers is that extra carnitine might speed up the delivery of fat, and the fat-burning process itself. It might also help the endurance athlete to burn more fat during prolonged exercise, again saving precious glycogen. Too good to be true? The studies that have been conducted show conflicting results. It seems too early to make a decision about the value of carnitine.
Coenzyme Q10, ATP	ATP is the final product in the cell's metabolic pathway to energy. Wouldn't it be good if you could jump the queue and get straight to the business end of energy production! There are a number of 'metabolic enhancer' products containing ATP or substances such as Coenzyme Q10 which are involved in the last steps of energy liberation. To date there is little evidence to support any ergogenic effect.
Inosine	Inosine is another proclaimed energy enhancer, because of its links with ATP production and the red blood cell lifecycle. Studies have not been able to transform this theory into a substantiated performance-enhancing practice. In addition, there are some questions about the safety of inosine, because of possible connections with gout.
Ginseng	There is a long list of wonders attributed to this herb, and a number of 'active ingredients' have been identified. However, studies have generally failed to detect any performance changes in athletes using ginseng. Problems with standardising the composition of supplements makes the study process difficult. Check that your preparation doesn't contain any other additives that are banned.
'Vitamin' B15	Despite the well-known name, this substance is not a real vitamin. It has not proved successful in scientific trials with athletes.

Table 6.4 (Continued)

Gamma-oryzanol and Frac (ferulic acid	These are related compounds, found particularly in rice bran oil. They are most popular in the 'building' world, where they are claimed to increase body mass and strength while reducing body fat levels. The research to support these claims is scanty, and contradictory. Some experts question whether these and similar compounds are well absorbed. Further research is awaited. Meanwhile both products continue to sell well.
Chromium picolinate	Chromium has a role in insulin activity that is still poorly understood. It has also been of recent interest in the 'muscle building' industries due to claims of anabolic characteristics. Chromium picolinate is claimed to be a well-absorbed form of this trace element due to positive chelating properties. Athletes who have an inadequate dietary intake of chromium might be expected to show performance improvements following chromium supplementation. Some studies reported by the 'inventor' of chromium picolinate claim increased lean body mass following supplementation with his product. Other studies have failed to repeat these effects. More work is needed to understand chromium balance in athletes. Meanwhile clear evidence of beneficial effects from chromium picolinate is not available.

be available from Mother Nature as well as from Super Sports Products Pty Ltd. And Mother Nature doesn't go in for amazing claims on her labels!

Because there is no regulation of the nutritional supplement industry, at least at present, there is no legal requirement for a company to provide proof of its claims. Until the law—or the athlete—demands proof, there will be no clear answer to the question 'does it work?' To be fair, we still don't know that ergogenic aids do *not* work, but nor do we know if they are harmful or have side-effects. In an ideal world, supplement manufacturers would co-operate with scientists and athletes to carefully study the supplements and hunt for the answers.

What, then, is the basis of proof?

6.4 How do you prove something works?

The scientific theory

The mode of action of an ergogenic aid must be explainable—there must be some sort of scientific rationale to support how or why the supplement works. In the case of the dietary supplements this is easier, since they operate in the realms of exercise physiology that we already understand. However, many of the nutritional ergogenic aids are based on quite complicated manipulations of biochemical reactions. Many of the substances are found as coenzymes, cofactors and other products of the metabolic pathways of exercise. The basis of many of these 'scientific theories' is that if you provide much larger doses of

Figure 6.1 Cost of protein—supplements versus food

	50g of protein:	
Lean steak	250g raw weight approx 175g cooked weight	$8.99/kg = $2.25
'Super' body building protein powder (90% protein by weight)	60g powder	$32.95 per 750g tin = $2.64
'Weight Gain' formula body building powder (25% protein by weight)	200g powder	$22.00 per 750g tin = $5.86
Pharmaceutical liquid meal supplements (25% protein by weight)	200g powder	$16.00 per 900g tin = $3.55
Skim milk powder	150g powder	$8.80 per 2kg = $0.66
Amino acid supplements	50g bottle of powder or 100 capsules containing 500mg of aminos	$25.00

some compounds to the cells, metabolism will proceed faster and longer, thus improving performance. Sounds good on paper doesn't it?

Therein lies the problem. A little science can be a dangerous thing when it is extrapolated by someone who can't look at all sides of the situation properly. The full scientific perspective may require the input of a range of specialists trained in human physiology and digestion, exercise physiology, enzyme kinetics and biochemistry. The human body is a complex unit, and many steps occur between popping a tablet into your mouth and having something happen in your muscle cells. Even if a substance might enhance metabolism from *inside* the cell, the experts may tell you that this substance won't be able to pass through your digestive system intact, or that the molecule is too big to pass across the cell membrane to get inside. In other words, eating

Figure 6.2 Cost of amino acids—supplements versus food

		2000 *mg* BCAAs (*valine, leucine and isoleucine*)
Typical amino acid supplement	4 capsules (500mg) or 1/2 tsp powder	85 cents
Liquid meal supplement	45g powder	80 cents
Lean grilled steak	40g (cooked weight)	52 cents
Eggs	75g (= 1.5 eggs)	22 cents
Skim milk	260ml	31 cents
Low-fat fruit yoghurt	170g (2/3 carton)	51 cents
Almonds	65g	130 cents ($1.30)
Wholemeal bread	145g (5 slices)	54 cents

Note that the food souce is usually cheaper—and think of all the other nutrients that you get at the same time!

large amounts of the substance is not necessarily going to work as you first thought.

A theory is just that—a theory. It is the first line of enquiry, but should never stand alone as proof. When experts have judged it from all angles, and found it to hold some possibilities, then the next stage is to put it under the scrutiny of the scientific trial.

Personal endorsements and anecdotal stories

In the eyes of the athlete, the most powerful proof that a supplement works is the endorsement of another athlete—particularly an elite athlete. If your hero swears that 'Product X' helped him to win the world championship, you will at least be interested, if not sold on the supplement. If you don't believe how emotive this is, just look at how the ergogenic aid companies advertise.

Not all the personal endorsements for ergogenic aids are paid for or appear in glossy full-page ads. Athletes are continually searching for the winning edge, and many conduct their own supplement trials—with a study population of one! The results are rapidly spread by word-of-mouth. How does this stand up as proof? What does it mean if you, or the world's greatest swimmer, or the school's football team performed well while taking 'Product X'? Unfortunately, under the scientific microscope it means little. It is equally possible that you would have performed as well without Product X. In some cases, where there were negative effects, you may have performed well in spite of it.

For a start, performance is multifactorial. It is affected by your equipment, your diet, training methods, natural ability, mental attitude, sleep, and the environment. It is almost impossible in real life to control all these factors so that the effect of the supplement can be judged on its own. You might have ridden a faster time in the triathlon this year, but how much of this is due to Product X, and how much is due to the extra year of training, your new aerodynamic handle bars, and the tail wind?

Secondly, there is the placebo effect. This describes the ability of your mind, when you really believe in something, to make it come true—even for a short period of time. It has been well-documented that when a group of people are given a tablet, and sold on the story of how it will work, a large number of that group will report that the effect actually happened, even when the tablet only contains sugar. Sometimes they can create the effect themselves, sometimes they just believe that it has occurred. Just like a rabbit's foot, or your 'lucky underwear', a supplement can provoke a psychologically-powered improvement even without a physiologically-based reason.

So personal experiences can create the next level of interest in an ergogenic aid—but however impressive they sound, there is no real seal of approval until scientific trials have been done.

The scientific trial

A well-conducted scientific trial remains our best hope of substantiating the claims about supplements—whether dietary supplements or the ergogenic-aid type. However, such trials must be carried out with extreme care and strict guidelines. They should involve a large number of subjects, and be designed to mimic a real sports situation with relevant physiological and performance changes.

A dummy supplement should be used in a scientific trial to counter the placebo effect. The subjects should be divided into two groups with one receiving the real supplement and the other the dummy. Neither the subjects nor the testers should know which is which until the end—in this way no-one can bias the experiment and its results.

Sometimes the trial is conducted twice in each group, switching the tablets over so that each group has one period on the real substance and one on the dummy. With this cross-over, each subject acts as their own comparison or control, thus cancelling out some of the individual factors that affect performance. In all scientific studies, much effort should be aimed at controlling other performance variables. Lastly, for a fair trial, the scientist should be sure to test the supplement in a dose, a duration, and with the type of subjects in which changes are most likely to occur.

These criteria obviously mean that a good study is time consuming, expensive to run and requires a great deal of co-operation from subjects. It is not hard to see why so few studies have been done, or why questions are not fully answered when a study has a few flaws. Until the ideal world is created—with scientists, athletes and supplement companies joining forces to provide the scientific answers—the decision about using nutritional ergogenic aids rests with you.

6.5 *Making your own decision about ergogenic aids*

The positive side about the large array of nutritional ergogenic aids is the chance that one or more, might actually improve your performance, whether by real action or by the placebo effect.

What are the costs of being a human guinea pig? Firstly, there may be side-effects from the long-term and heavy use of some products. If they are as powerful as they are reported to be, then how do you know that all the effects will be in your favour? All nutritional ergogenic aids, including vitamins, are chemicals—too much of any chemical can cause problems. Ergogenic aids will certainly affect your wallet, as many are extremely expensive and many athletes use a number of products.

By strict definition, an ergogenic aid causes a pharmacological or a 'legal drug' effect. There is always the possibility that any substances that are found to directly improve performance will then be judged as unfair in competition and subsequently banned. Already, many sports bodies have deemed that large doses of caffeine constitute 'doping'.

Finally, don't pin your hopes on the ergogenic aid and overlook factors that definitely affect performance. There is no pill or potion that can replace good training, an optimal training diet, a strong mental attitude, and adequate sleep and recovery.

II Sports nutrition in action

Introduction

In this section we will turn theory into practice, by looking inside a number of sports to see the nutritional challenges faced by athletes. Typical nutrition issues arising from the physiological requirements of training and competition as well as the lifestyle of the athlete will be identified.

These sports were chosen to represent a variety of different nutrition issues. If your sport has not been specifically covered, you will probably find that you can identify with another sport, or with various issues that arise in a combination of sports. Think about the features of your sport—both the characteristics of competition and the way that you train. By reading the brief description at the beginning of each chapter you may be able to identify another sport (or group of sports) that makes similar demands to yours. Alternatively, you may already know some of the nutrition issues that interest and concern you. Use the lists at the front of this book to look up a case history or a relevant checklist. For example, loss of body fat is a goal shared by athletes in many sports, and even if you are a lacrosse player you may be able to identify with the weight loss efforts of Vicki the netballer. Similarly, if you are vegetarian or thinking of becoming one, you will find Maureen's experiences of interest in the gymnastics chapter, and the hints for the travelling athlete in the tennis chapter will be valuable no matter what your sport is.

Finally, appreciate that each chapter covers *typical* issues, and is by no means complete or exclusive. Your nutrition goals and interests may be a little different to those in the chapter on your sport. Hopefully, however, you will find something that addresses you personally and individually. Above all, enjoy this section for the chance to think about the practical and human aspects of nutrition for sport. It should help you to convert science into food choices and eating habits, and thus help you to take your sport as far as your ambitions reach.

Triathlon

Triathlon, described as the boom sport of the 1980s awaits its Olympic debut in Sydney at the 2000 games. In this multi-sport event, competitors complete a swim, cycle and run in immediate succession, with races broadly categorised as follows:

Short course: 500m swim/20km cycle/5km run

Olympic distance: 1.5km swim/40km cycle/10km run

Long course: 2km swim/80km cycle/20km run

Ultra distance/Ironman: 3.9km swim/180km cycle/42.2km run.

At present men dominate the race numbers, with women making up 10–15 per cent of the field. In most triathlons, all competitors race alongside each other, with a prize structure that recognises males and females, elite and recreational, as well as different age groups. There are not too many sports that allow everyday athletes to toe the starting line with their heroes!

Training

It is not surprising with three sports to master that triathlon training can be time-consuming. Even recreational triathletes can spend more that ten hours each week in training, and top competitors may spend 20–40 hours—a full-time job! Typical weekly totals for a serious Olympic-distance triathlete are 10km swimming, 200–300km cycling and 40–60km running. A triathlete specialising in longer events may more than double this load.

The bulk of triathlon training is aerobic, with interval training being included in some sessions. Many triathletes include transition training in their schedules, with one sport being immediately followed by another (usually a cycle followed by a run). Weight training is sometimes included when time and facilities permit.

The most important fuel for training is muscle glycogen, and intense daily training will challenge the recovery of stores in the various muscle groups involved in each sport.

Competition

The official triathlon season extends from late spring to early autumn. Events are held on weekends (usually Sundays) and are typically held early in the morning to avoid the heat. During winter, when open water swims are impractical, triathletes may compete in run-ride-run races (duathlons). Elite triathletes may compete internationally in an almost year-round circuit.

Triathletes vary with their competition schedules. Some triathletes specialise in a set distance (either short or long course) while others compete over all race distances. Some athletes compete most weekends during the competition season, up to 20 times a year, but select a handful of key races to taper for. Others choose to spread their races over the season. Juggling competition and training schedules can present a great challenge to many athletes.

Triathlons are predominantly an aerobic event, with short course races taking as little as 45 minutes to complete, while ultra distance events take eight hours at best—and considerably longer for most competitors. A triathlon can be conducted at a higher intensity than a single sport of the same time duration and is less likely to be limited by the depletion of fuel stores, since the work is spread over a larger number of muscle groups. However, in longer triathlons the individual distances in each sport will challenge the fuel stores in the muscles involved, as well as the body's ability to maintain blood glucose levels.

The duration and environment of triathlons are important factors in terms of fluid loss and temperature regulation. While some triathlons threaten competitors with possible cold exposure and hypothermia, in most triathlons the problems of dehydration and heat distress are a greater risk. The famous Ironman race held in Hawaii each year challenges athletes not only with the long distances, but with strong winds and ground temperatures of over 40 degrees Celsius.

Physical characteristics

The only spare tyres that elite triathletes carry are under their bike seats in case of a puncture! Like distance running, triathlon performance is advantaged by a low level of body fat, so elite triathletes have similarly low skinfold levels to elite marathon runners. However, because swimming makes active use of upper body muscle mass, the total muscle mass and body weight of a triathlete will be greater than that of the marathon runner, with the greater muscle mass being found around the chest, arms and shoulders.

Typical physique (state level triathlete)

	Male	Female
Height	180–186cm	NA
Weight	70–76kg	51–63kg
Skinfolds	44–60mm	61–85mm

Common nutrition issues

Dietary extremism

Triathletes are renowned for their enthusiasm and self-discipline. They don't do things by half measures, and that includes diet. Many triathletes read widely about nutrition, including alternative diets such as vegetarianism and Pritikin. Some become skilled headhunters of 'bad foods' which are then single-mindedly eliminated from their diets. The result of this excessiveness is a restricted dietary range, causing a number of problems and missed opportunities (see the account of Victor at the end of this chapter). The most important rule of the peak training diet is to enjoy a variety of foods. Read Chapter 1 to see how this can be achieved while meeting all other nutritional goals for training.

Excessively low body-fat levels

Also along the lines of 'too much of a good thing', a current fashion in triathlon is to strive for the lowest level of body fat possible. This sometimes happens as a consequence of dietary extremism, but is often pursued as a goal in itself.

Triathletes should recognise firstly that optimum body-fat levels are individual, and that it is not necessarily an advantage to have the body-fat levels of Mark Allen or Dave Scott—unless you are Mark Allen or Dave Scott. Secondly, for *all* triathletes, optimum body-fat level includes the issue of good health. If your body fat drops to a level that causes problems with cold intolerance, loss of immune function, irregular menstruation (in women) and loss of strength/muscle mass, then this is *not* your optimum body-fat level—even if it does mean less 'dead weight' to carry over the course (see Chapter 3.1).

High energy requirements

The intense training program of a triathlete, especially the full-time or elite athlete, can chalk up massive energy requirements. This is how most triathletes naturally achieve their low body-fat levels. However, sometimes when a triathlete begins a training program, or increases the training load, body weight can drop below a desirable level. There are a number of reasons why food intake does not automatically adjust itself to meet the increased requirements of training. Being too extreme with food range has already been nominated; other factors include being too tired after training to cook, or even to eat. The bulk of the high-carbohydrate, high-fibre diet often becomes self limiting, especially when the athlete has to juggle eating times around work and training schedules. (See Chapter 3.7 for smart ways to increase energy intake by eating 'compact' kilojoules and by increasing the number of meals rather than their size.)

Loss of body fat

Sometimes, despite heavy training, a triathlete will need additional help to reduce body-fat levels. For some, this is a constant struggle. Females in particular, seem to need to eat less kilojoules than their training loads would predict. If you are a lower-than-expected energy consumer, you may find it frustrating when fellow athletes eat twice as much as you, or enjoy the feeding frenzies otherwise known as carbo-loading banquets, without gaining a gram. Chapter 3.3 will show you how to concentrate your efforts on a weight loss program and an energy intake level that is suitable for you.

Iron status

Triathletes, especially females, are in the high risk group for iron deficiency problems. The early stages of iron deficiency may reduce the ability to recover between training sessions, even before full-blown anemia causes a definite reduction in exercise performance. As discussed in Chapter 2.5, hard-training triathletes may experience increased iron requirements, perhaps due to increased iron losses from gut bleeding and red blood cell loss. However, the factor most likely to contribute to iron deficiency problems is the low intake of well-absorbed iron in the typical triathlete's diet. Read Chapter 2.5 to make sure that you are not overlooking iron in your nutritional goals, and have your iron status checked periodically to pick up low iron levels at an early stage.

Amenorrhea, low bone density, and stress fractures

An irregular menstrual cycle is a frequent result of the heavy training and committed lifestyle of the female triathlete, and perhaps low

143

body-fat levels and an inadequate diet are also involved. Whatever the cause, the effects should not be ignored. Studies show that low bone density can be a result of menstrual irregularity and its associated factors and there is also an increased risk of stress fractures. These problems, either singly or together, are complex in nature and treatment. See your sports medicine doctor early in the picture—and for more information read Chapters 2.6 and 3.4, and the profile of Sharon in the distance running chapter.

Daily recovery

With a twice daily training program, it is not surprising that recovery is regarded as a magic word in triathlon circles. The faster the recovery, the sooner or harder the next session can be. Triathletes often tread precariously along the fine line between hard training and overtraining. During the competitive season, recovery is important for those who want to race each weekend, or to pick up their training straight after each event.

Your peak training diet should supply all the nutrients required for recovery between sessions, with emphasis on fluid strategies (Chapter 1.5) and carbohydrate intake (Chapters 1.3 and 2.2). Chapter 6 has special notes for rapid replacement of fluid and carbohydrate stores after prolonged exercise sessions.

In planning your training schedule, organise the order of sessions to allow maximum recovery time for the specific muscle groups involved in each sport. Also note that hard running causes some muscle fibre damage and you will require a longer time to refill muscle glycogen stores. Plan the week accordingly, giving yourself adequate time and extra carbohydrate following intense running sessions or races.

Preparation for an event

Race preparation depends on the length of the race, the training state of the athlete, and race aspirations. Pre-race strategies are covered in Chapter 4 and should involve preparation of adequate fuel and fluid stores. You may also try to manipulate an empty gut to leave you racing 'light'.

For short events, a well-trained triathlete is able to store sufficient muscle glycogen with a 24–36 hour preparation of rest/taper and a high-carbohydrate diet. If it's your big race for the year, you might like to take a longer taper. Others who are training for longer events later in the season may not want to sacrifice even one day of exercise. Plan your preparation according to your short-term and long-term priorities.

Long course and ultra-distance events challenge muscle glycogen stores and therefore deserve a modified carbohydrate loading preparation. In this situation the last 72 hours, pre-race, should be devoted to glycogen storage, with a rest from exercise and a high-carbohydrate diet. With most races starting early in the morning, the typical pre-race meal is small and light, and eaten on rising about two to three hours pre-event.

Food and fluid intake during the race

For sprint races and events up to the Olympic distance, fluid needs are of greatest importance to competitors, and water is probably the most widely used fluid. Race rules generally insist that competitors carry a full bidon (water bottle) on their bikes, and race organisers provide additional fluids at aid stations in the transition areas, and sometimes on the run leg. While those who are out for long hours in the heat of the day are reminded about the need to take in fluids, even top athletes should be warned about the dangers of failing to drink on the bike or run. Chapter 4 explains that moderate fluid loss can reduce performance, and on hot days severe dehydration is a real threat to life and limb. Drinking pouches consisting of a pressurised sack with a plastic tube fitting along the bike frame to the triathlete's mouth (e.g. the 'Bike Stream') can provide easy access to fluid for those who worry about wasting precious seconds and losing their stream-lined riding position by reaching down to the bidon cage.

As events become longer, the advantages of consuming carbohydrate during the race become more obvious. Carbohydrate intake will improve performance in long-course distance and ultra-distance events, by supplying additional fuel sources for trained muscles once glycogen stores have been exhausted. You might like to experiment with carbohydrate drinks in Olympic distance races also, particularly for races in which your 'fuelling-up' may not have been optimal. In ultra-distance races, there is usually a well-organised network of aid stations at which athletes are offered a range of carbohydrate-rich food and fluids including sports drinks. See the account of the Ironman race below, and read Chapter 4.7 for guidelines to a well-organised feeding schedule. Most importantly, practise your intended strategies in training.

Ergogenic aids and dietary supplements

The past few triathlon seasons have seen a proliferation of supplements and ergogenic aids on the market, many bearing the endorsement of top triathletes. Read Chapter 6 to see which supplements can have an important and useful role in your training and competition, and which products are still awaiting scientific study. Make up your own mind once you have the facts in hand.

PROFILE: VICTOR
Variety is the spice!

Victor's friends complained that they never saw him any more—not since triathlon came into his life. Either he was out training or he was in bed early to recover for the next morning's session. There was little point inviting Victor over for dinner—he had become so fussy about his diet that there was little that you could serve him.

From the moment he bought his bike, Victor was hooked on triathlon and searched for any factor to improve his performance. One day while watching *Wide World of Sports* he saw an interview with Dave Scott. When he saw Dave wash his cottage cheese under the tap to remove the last bit of fat, Victor decided it was time for him to clean up his dietary act.

Once a chocolate fiend, he set about eliminating all sources of fat, sugar, salt and alcohol from his diet. He read Pritikin and decided to go one better by becoming a complete vegetarian. The key word, as in training, was discipline. He found that it was amazing how much he could give up, once he put his mind to it. Learning to read food labels was important in case there was some added sugar, fat, or worse still, chemicals. It soon became easier to go without manufactured food, and to cook up a plate of steamed vegetables instead.

Within a month the results were obvious. Gone were those stubborn four kilograms, and Victor felt trim and terrific in training. But by the end of six months another five kilograms was lost, and even Victor agreed that he was looking a bit too thin. Not that it mattered what he looked like—he felt it was how he rode the bike that was important. However, even that was becoming a problem. Victor found that his endurance and his recovery were beginning to waver, and that it was hard to do two solid training days back-to-back. The more he trained, the worse his times became. It was impossible to ride the wind trainer for more than an hour—without a comfortable layer of fat, he found his rear end became too numb on the hard bike seat. And had the pool forgotten to pay its electricity bill? The water had become so cold that Victor was shivering between sets of intervals. He thought of wearing his wet-suit to early morning training sessions to try and ward off another of the colds that seemed to plague him lately.

It was a delicate problem that finally prompted Victor to seek nutritional advice. Gradually over a period of time, he had developed gastrointestinal problems. His training partners were complaining about the 'sound-effects' and the constant pit-stops during runs. And nobody wanted to sit on his wheel when riding, no matter how strong the head wind was. He had become a one-man environmental hazard!

Victor wrote out a day's menu to show the sports dietitian (see below) and said, 'It's obviously something wrong that I'm eating. What else should I cut out of my diet?'

Victor describes his daily diet to the dietitian

Before swimming: 2 plain rice cakes (plain—jam and honey are as bad as sugar)

Breakfast: Large bowl of rolled oats, unprocessed bran, and water (I heard that milk gives you 'mucous' problems. I used to eat packaged cereals but I'm suspicious of what they put into them these days)
Pritikin bread + Pritikin jam (when I can get it)
Herbal tea

Morning tea: Rice cakes—plain
Occasionally Pritikin fruit bread

Lunch: Large container of salad
Rice cakes
4–5 pieces of fruit
(Sometimes I have a fruit-only lunch: 6–10 pieces)
Plain mineral water
(Are there any fruit juices that are *really* sugar-free?)

Afternoon tea: I've cut this out to help stop my diarrhea during after-work running sessions

Tea: Big plate of steamed vegetables or wholemeal rice with steamed vegetables or wholemeal pasta with tomato puree sauce (I have cut out all meats, fish and chicken to eliminate fat totally)
Fruit salad or another bowl of porridge

Supper: Toasted Pritikin bread with Pritikin sugar-free jam

During long rides: Water, rice cakes, bananas, dried fruit.

The answer that had eluded Victor, jumped out at the dietitian. There was no need to eliminate more foods—in fact the process of elimination was the cause of his present problem. While Victor was to be congratulated for his interest in his diet, his enthusiasm to curb his intake of salt, fat, sugar and food additives had gone too far. The advantages of a varied diet—flexibility, enjoyment and moderation with all nutrients—were lost.

Such a restricted diet was causing a number of problems. For a start, there were too few kilojoules due to the lack of food choices and the bulkiness of meals. Body weight had dropped, probably at the expense of muscle mass and strength, but also to a level of body fat that was no longer healthy.

By eliminating certain foods, Victor had been successful in drastically reducing his fat intake, but had also sacrificed other important nutrients from the same foods—protein from dairy foods and meats, iron and zinc from red meats, and calcium from dairy products. Since he had failed to explore alternative sources of these nutrients from plant food sources, in time it was likely that a nutrient deficiency would occur and further reduce performance.

As for Victor's fear about the chemicals in food, he had overlooked the most sensible approach—a widely varied diet will reduce the risk of overexposure to *any* one food component. The dietitian explained that all substances in food were technically chemicals, and that Victor's diarrhea and flatulence were due to overeating fibre. Clearly, Victor needed to learn about good uses of food—mixing and matching a variety of foods to maximise their valuable features while reducing any less-desirable aspects.

It took a while for Victor to overcome the fear and misconceptions that he had built up about food. But impressed with the arguments in favour of a varied diet, he gradually introduced or re-introduced himself to the great food range around him. He learned how he could still eat many of his favourite foods, but by modifying the type and amount eaten, he could still keep his diet low in fat. He was happy to incorporate animal foods back into his food plans.

Victor became intrigued with clever mixing and matching of foods at meals, and took delight in seeing how many different foods he could combine on his plate. Armed with recipes from the dietitian, he explored different pastas, grains and vegetables, even beans and other legumes. With wholemeal grains and cereals, and plenty of fresh fruit and vegetables, he realised that the fibre content of his diet was already high, so out went the unprocessed bran.

As he became more relaxed with his ability to choose foods well, he became confident about eating out at restaurants and with friends. There were usually a couple of choices on the menu that were suitable, even if he did have to ask the waiter to make some modifications to his order—such as leaving the butter off the bread, or making his cappuccino with low-fat milk. He was also delighted to find that the occasional Mars Bar didn't kill him—in fact it tasted terrific!

Gradually, his gut problems disappeared and his weight and training stamina returned. Most importantly, his friends and training partners no longer needed to avoid him.

PROFILE: GRACE
A 226-kilometre picnic

Grace stood on the pier at Kailua-Kona and thought of the race before her. This day had been the focus of her attention for the past six months. Since few people qualify for the Hawaii Ironman World Championship Triathlon she was determined to give her all to the gruelling event: a 3.9km swim, 180km cycle and 42km run. Just to finish would be enough, but Grace also set herself the goal of completing the race with a smile on her face.

Her preparation had left nothing to chance. Once her entry had been confirmed, she began to pick the brains of other triathletes who had competed the Ironman race in previous years. She asked about the food availability in Hawaii—would she be able to follow her usual food plan in the days leading up to the event? How were the aid stations organised at the race itself? What would they be providing to help her meet the massive nutritional challenges on the day?

Her friends assured her that the town of Kailua-Kona would provide her with similar food variety to that in Australia, and that in the days leading up to the event she could look forward to many 'all-you-can-eat' carbo-loading parties. Her race instruction booklet outlined the following aid station plan:

Aid stations:

Bike leg: aid station every 5 miles (8km)

Run leg: aid station every mile (1.6km)

Additional stations at race start and transition areas

Menu:

Water, Coke, Gatorade sports drink, oranges, bananas, jam sandwiches, chocolate-chip cookies

Although there was an opportunity to collect a special provision bag with her own food choices at the half-way mark, Grace decided to stick with the Ironman menu. She read plenty of sports nutrition articles and learned that her priorities would be firstly to keep as well-hydrated as possible, and then to supply herself with a constant intake of carbohydrate—about 50g of carbohydrate per hour was the amount recommended by sports scientists.

The carbohydrate drinks, particularly the sports drinks, seemed the best choice since they could supply both needs simultaneously. Theoretically at least, the drinks should be rapidly emptied from her stomach and quickly transported to her working muscles. Although the solid foods could supply carbohydrate, Grace remembered a couple of occasions when she had eaten during a long run, and had felt uncomfortable with the food sloshing around in her stomach. However, she realised this was personal, since many of her training partners could consume bananas and muesli bars without problems.

Grace bought some Gatorade and started using it in training. She read that on race day she should start drinking this early in the race, and then continue with small amounts at regular intervals. She calculated that an intake of about 800ml per hour would supply her baseline carbohydrate target (50g). Knowing that she should reach an aid station in the bike leg at about 15 minute spacings, this would mean an intake of about 200ml of drink between each. For her, the aid stations in the run leg would be about ten minutes apart, meaning that she should drink perhaps 125–150ml at each. Of course, this would not look after her fluid needs entirely. In the extreme heat in Hawaii she anticipated that she might lose over a litre of sweat per hour. She decided that she would take extra water at each station and drink additional fluid as needed.

The last thing she learned from other triathletes was to be flexible in her plan. What if she got to an aid station and missed the right drink? What if she got hungry? What if she got sick of the taste of the Gatorade? With commonsense, Grace realised that her plan might need to be altered as she went. She might need to drink extra fluid, or as her pace and the day's heat subsided her fluid losses might drop. If she got hungry a small amount of solid food should allay the discomfort. A drink of Coke could give her a 'change of scenery' at times. There was plenty of time over the six months of training to think and experiment.

Grace arrived in Kailua-Kona ten days before the race to acclimatise—to the weather, to the race atmosphere, and to the course itself. The last three days were spent carbo-loading, resting, and drinking plenty of fluid. A light breakfast on rising at 4.30am, and then she found herself at the race start with the other 1199 competitors who shared her own excitement and anticipation.

The race was all that she thought it would be. It was tough—but you don't earn the title of Ironman for nothing! After the swim she stopped briefly in the transition area for a drink, then departed on the bike. With two bidon cages mounted on the frame she was able to keep one bidon of Gatorade and another of water, replacing them alternately at each aid station. She judged her intake to be about 800–900ml per hour, mostly from Gatorade, and was glad of the extra water to throw over her head at times.

During the run, she alternated her drinks at each aid station—iced water, Gatorade and then Coke. A few orange segments were a refreshing change at times, and at one station she was grateful for a sandwich.

When the finish line loomed ahead, her weary legs felt as if they were running a four-minute mile over the last flood-lit stretch. But from the smile on her face, there was little need to ask if it was all worthwhile. She didn't feel like drinking a Gatorade cocktail to celebrate, but Grace would remember this race for the rest of her life— long after the Texta colour numbers 'sunburned' into her arms faded.

Swimming

Preparation for elite level swimming begins at an early age, usually around 10–12 years. Typically, the careers of elite swimmers also used to finish early, at around 20 years for women and 25 for males. There is now reason to see this as mental or lifestyle burnout rather than physiological burnout since in the '90s some elite swimmers have continued to compete until their 30s. In recent years there have also been some noted swimmers who have returned from retirement to swim again in open or Masters level swimming. Many have been able to improve or duplicate their earlier performances.

At the Olympic level, swimming events are held in a number of strokes (freestyle, breast stroke, backstroke, butterfly and medley), over distances ranging from 50m to 1500m. Long-distance swimming, in which a swimmer may complete an individual time-trial or group race in open water, has a much smaller following but was included in the World Swimming Championships for the first time in 1991. Long distance swimming races may involve distances from five to 50km, and are often held in the waterways between two famous landpoints— for example the English Channel. This chapter will be devoted to Olympic-event swimming.

Training

By the time they are 12 or 13, many swimmers have already taken on a serious commitment to training. Typically, training sessions are held in the early morning (e.g. 5–7am) and then in the late afternoon (e.g.

4–6pm) to fit around school or work commitments. The number of training sessions undertaken by a swimmer will vary, depending on their age, the events for which they are preparing, and the stage of the season. Typically, six to twelve sessions can be undertaken each week, with the distance covered in each session ranging from 1000–2000 metres of quality work for a sprinter in a taper phase, to ten kilometres for a distance swimmer in the base phase of training. The heaviest workloads can chalk up 100km of swimming each week, with two or three daily sessions adding up to six hours of training per day. At the club or school level, training commitments are considerably smaller than this, and swimmers may not train all year round.

Swimming training varies with the phase of the season, to include an initial aerobic endurance base, followed by various anaerobic training sessions where single or multi-effort intervals are swum at different percentages of maximal work output. Heart rate and blood lactate levels are measured to monitor the various types of work-outs. In addition to these sessions, swimmers commonly include weight training, typically three sessions per week. Some swimmers also undertake aerobic land training, such as running or cycling, to help reduce body-fat levels. Such a program calls heavily on muscle glycogen stores, and swimmers who fail to replenish their stores on a daily basis may be unable to complete such high-intensity sessions.

Peaking for competition involves a period of tapering with a reduced training load. Swimmers who compete in a number of competitions over the year may not fully prepare for them all, and may concentrate on peaking for one or two major competitions.

Competition

It takes about 25 seconds for an elite swimmer to race over 50 metres and about 15 minutes to complete 1500m—making swimming a highly anaerobic sport, with aerobic metabolism becoming more important as the race distance increases. Muscle fuel stores may not be depleted even over a 1500m swim, with the main source of fatigue being a build-up of the accompanying products of anaerobic metabolism such as hydrogen ions.

Swim meets are usually held over three to seven days, with swimmers typically competing in heats in the mornings and the final of that event in the evening. However, some Grand Prix meets may be held over one day, sometimes with timed finals. In minor carnivals, swimmers may enter a large number of events and be required to swim two or three times in one day, with 20 minutes to several hours between events. At major competitions, only exceptional swimmers will enter more than three events. Light warm-ups are completed prior to each competition session with the swim-down after each event being an important recovery strategy. Training is often scheduled on non-competition days.

Physical characteristics

Swimmers are noted for their upper body muscle development—back, chest, arms and shoulders. They are also usually tall, particularly in the case of sprinters. Since swimmers are required to move their own body mass through water, low body fat is an advantage. However, the buoyancy of water makes body fat less of a disadvantage than it is on dry land. In fact, some body fat in the right distribution can enhance floatation. Swimmers specialising in the longer events often have higher body-fat levels than the sprinters. Open water long-distance swimmers often carry large amounts of body fat to provide buoyancy, and insulation against the cold.

Typical physique (elite Australian Olympic swimmers)

	Male	Female
Height	181–193cm	168–177cm
Weight	72–86kg	57–67kg
Skinfolds	43–57mm	53–77mm

Other comments

Many top swimmers are in their teens, and the physical changes experienced with puberty may help to explain an interesting observation—male swimmers are more likely to have trouble eating enough kilojoules to meet energy needs, while female swimmers struggle to lose body fat. This is because male adolescence is a period of heavy growth and muscular development, requiring high energy support, while females undergo hormonal changes which promote an increase in body fat. For males then, the addition of an intense training program means that total energy needs can reach an almost unbelievable level, while the female swimmer, despite equally strenuous training, works uphill against the hormonal messages to lay down fat.

The long hours of training place a heavy restriction on a swimmer's lifestyle, limiting the social and recreational activities typical of teenagers. This can either reduce the opportunities to eat in a busy daily schedule, or conversely, raise the importance of eating for comfort or entertainment value. Thus, both underweight and overweight problems are common in swimming.

Access to food can also be an issue at swimming carnivals and meets, with many swimmers travelling away from home to compete. Hotels and 'athlete villages' may provide unsuitable food choices and the lack of supervision may further encourage poor eating patterns.

Common nutrition issues

Daily recovery

Strenuous daily training calls for a high-energy, high-carbohydrate diet. American physiologist Professor Dave Costill conducted a study on a squad of male swimmers who suddenly doubled their training load. While some of the squad adapted to this increase, the other swimmers experienced difficulty—complaining of fatigue and muscle soreness. Analysis of their diets showed that the first group had automatically increased their carbohydrate intake to match the increased cost of training, while the other group had not made this adaptation. Muscle glycogen levels of the second group were significantly lower.

This observation is explained in Chapter 5 on recovery, and is illustrated in Figure 5.1. Chapters 1.3 and 2.2 also provide information about good habits with carbohydrate foods to promote daily recovery in training. In Grant's story below, help was needed to make carbohydrate intake compact. A bulky diet requires more time to chew than most busy athletes can afford.

The Barry Sears diet—will it sink or swim?

In 1993 a new sports diet hit the streets—or rather the lanes of the pool. The Barry Sears diet (also known as the Eicotec diet), although promoted as the key to 'all athletic performance for the 21st century', first came to prominence because of alleged accolades from the Stanford Swim Team. 1992 was a year of amazing success for this team and its swimmers (winning both men's and women's NCAA titles and 7 Olympic gold medals in the US total), and it was claimed that the improvement was due to the special dietary program adopted by the team.

The diet, developed by Dr Barry Sears and team, claimed to be 'revolutionary' in promoting a special blend of macronutrients (40 per cent carbohydrate, 30 per cent fat and 30 per cent protein). It was claimed that this special (and unusual) ratio achieves a favourable partnership between the hormones insulin and glucagon—a partnership that favours loss of body fat, increases in lean body mass and other numerous performance benefits. Descriptions of the actual diet are a bit confused, but it does seem controversial in contradicting the scientifically proven high-carbohydrate training diet. Sometimes it is promoted as a 'high-fat' or 'fat-loading' diet; other times it looks simply like a low-kilojoule diet, reduced at the expense of carbohydrate. The dietary ratio it promotes is an unusual one, requiring unusual combinations of foods at meals and snacks. Of course, the athlete can be assisted to get the proportions right through the use of special 'Eicotec' bars which come at a hefty price (surprise!).

The Eicotec/Barry Sears diet is not the only program to promote a lower carbohydrate/higher fat (and protein) story at the moment. And while you can think up some fancy theories involving biochemistry and hormones to support the advantages of adapting the athlete to 'burn on fat' rather than carbohydrate, at this moment there are no real runs on the board for this idea. (See the skiing chapter for a full analysis of the fat-loading story.) Barry Sears has used the time-old advertising stunt favoured by travelling salesmen—tell your clients a plausible story and then amaze them with tales of satisfied customers. Of course he has given it a twentieth-century twist, by describing it as a scientific breakthrough. The proof can only come through scientific trials—and to date neither he nor other researchers have put his diet to a rigorous test.

But where does that leave the Stanford Swimming Team? Well, we don't actually have proof that any or all of the team used the Sears diet. Many athletes and teams dabble in nutritional supplements or programs without really taking them on board. And even if they did, how do we know that the Sears diet was responsible for their success? In the case of many of the swimmers concerned, good parents (in the genetic sense), hard training over many years, and a commitment to excellence are definitely involved. Maybe it was a coincidence that some of these swimmers tried a new dietary program. Maybe they even did well in spite of it (it was suggested by a leading American dietitian that some of the famous swimmers involved could probably eat sawdust and still be champions!). The Barry Sears diet, on paper at least, sounds too low in carbohydrate and, in some cases, too low in kilojoules to support the training needs of swimmers. In fact, swimmers probably have obligatory carbohydrate needs that are greater than many other athletes since they train for long periods at very high (carbohydrate-requiring) intensities. On competition day, swimming events of 200m and down are so heavily anaerobic that it makes sense to maintain swimmers as efficient carbohydrate-burning machines. While future research may let us reassess the fat-loading theory, for the moment the focus on carbohydrate seems a sensible and proven party line.

Fluid needs in training

Swimmers can churn up and down the pool for hours—often in the steamy environment of a heated indoor pool, and occasionally outdoors in the late afternoon heat. This can lead to reasonable sweat losses, which are not obvious when you are already wet. Hopping out of the pool to get a drink is not always possible. Smart swimming coaches now insist that swimmers bring their own water bottles to the pool deck. Drinking during rest periods or between sets will help you to train better. Sports drink or cordial will provide an additional fuel supply that may be welcome during a long training session, particularly when you're in heavy training.

High energy requirements

The energy cost of training, particularly when added to energy needs for growth, can mean a very high total energy requirement. This is typically an issue for male swimmers, and can be compounded by the lack of the time in the day to eat. Chapter 3.7 deals with hints to help a swimmer achieve a high energy intake, by increasing the number of meals and snacks in the day and making use of energy-dense foods. Planning ahead to have a portable and compact food supply can win the battle for you. See Grant's story, below.

Weight loss and the typical female swimmer

Female swimmers fight a notorious battle to keep body-fat measurements down at their desired levels. Despite heavy training they often complain that they do not seem to burn the expected kilojoules. Not only can this become frustrating, but the constant focus on diet and weight loss can mean that thinking about food almost takes over the day. Everything revolves around food—entertainment, comfort when upset or depressed, celebration or commiseration. It can become a vicious circle. You eat because you are upset. Your skinfolds go up, making you more upset, so you have something to eat to make you feel better. And so on.

While it may seem unfair that male swimmers can eat twice as much as you, or that some girls in your squad can eat what they like without dreading the mirror or the skinfold tests, if you concentrate on yourself instead of comparing yourself to others, you will probably find that you *can* improve your situation. Read Chapter 3, about setting a body-fat target that is realistic for *you*, and then committing yourself to a long-term fat-loss program that is right for *your* situation. Above all, set yourself the goal to become comfortable with your body shape and your enjoyment of food.

Eating disorders

There are many reports that female swimmers are at high risk of developing eating disorders—or more likely, that many swimmers resort to unhealthy techniques such as self-induced vomiting (bulimia), and the use of diuretics and laxatives. Most often these practices are used as a short-term solution to weight-loss problems. The problem is that they do not solve, or even attack, the real problem. In most cases the issue is overconcern about body fat and food, and a poor self-image. The body-fat problem itself is usually secondary, and in some cases wildly exaggerated. However, the unhealthy eating behaviour can add to your woes by directly impairing performance and health.

Read Chapter 3 for a sensible approach to goal-setting, with body-fat targets and fat-loss program. The best help may come from talking things over with professionals—a sports psychologist who can help you to restore your self-confidence, and a dietitian who can support you to get back into healthy training nutrition.

Iron status

Strenuous daily training places a stress on body iron stores. While swimming doesn't cause the same physical trauma as running, one study of swimmers reported that red blood cells were damaged by the continual impact of turbulent water. However, as in most cases of iron imbalance, a low iron intake is the major cause of poor iron status, and female swimmers on weight-loss diets are particularly at risk. Read Chapter 2.5 to learn about good sources of iron. Have your iron status checked regularly when you are in heavy training.

Competition nutrition

Muscle glycogen stores can be filled by 24 hours of a high-carbohydrate diet and exercise taper (see Chapter 4). Be aware, if you are doing a longer taper, that you may need to reduce your total energy intake to match the reduced workload, otherwise you may suddenly gain body fat.

Since events can be held at various times of the day, careful planning of the pre-event meal may be needed (see Chapter 4). This may be a challenge if you are away from home, and it often helps to bring some food supplies of your own.

Between events and between heats and finals you should replenish fluid levels and top up carbohydrate stores. If you have more than three hours between heats and finals a light carbohydrate meal might be eaten in comfort. During your swim-down, or when there is only a short interval between races, drink a carbohydrate-containing fluid such as a sports drink, fruit juice or soft drink. Carbohydrate-rich snacks such as yoghurt, fruit, sports bars, sandwiches or rice cakes can be brought to the pool and are suitable for longer gaps between races, or for a recovery snack at the end of a session. Don't forget fruit smoothies or commercial liquid meal supplements if your stomach or timetable calls for a 'lighter' snack.

Communal eating—the athlete's dining hall

A communal dining hall can be a culture shock to young swimmers, especially when being away from home is a new experience. This situation may be faced on swimming camps, at the athletes' village during big competitions, or by residents of the Australian Institute of Sport. For many, the change from the family meal table can provide a huge challenge, and bad decisions may be made with food. This can result in both short-term consequences (perhaps upsetting competition performance) and long-term problems (upsetting training nutrition goals). The dining hall story below illustrates that special tactics can be used to ensure that food is well chosen.

PROFILE: GRANT
Chewing through the carbos

A lot of Grant's day was spent staring at the black line on the bottom of the pool, especially since his squad had increased their training to twelve sessions a week. At first he had coped with the extra training load, but by the end of the second month he was feeling fatigued. Not only were his times beginning to drop off, but his school work had started to get on top of him as well. To cap it all off, his weight seemed to be going down and he could not really afford to lose any more body fat. Grant's mother encouraged him to eat a larger serve of meat at the evening meal, but by this time of the night he was often too tired to do more than pick at it.

A sports dietitian listened to Grant's story and examined his diet. She advised him that additional kilojoules were needed to cover the extra training, but that carbohydrate foods were the most important source of the energy for training. Chronic depletion of muscle glycogen stores were the likely cause of his current fatigue problems. At 80kg, a daily intake of 600–800g of carbohydrate was a reasonable target, and his present diet lagged considerably behind that.

They examined a list of carbohydrate foods together, and Grant found that they were all foods he liked to eat—bread, breakfast cereals, fruit, potatoes, rice and pasta. However, the problem was how to fit more of them into his day. He already left the meal table feeling too tired or too full to eat another mouthful. Listening to Grant's typical daily meal plan, the dietitian pointed out that he relied on only three meals per day—breakfast, hastily eaten in the car on the way from the pool to school, lunch, juggled between school activities, and a late evening meal at home.

The solution lay in increasing the *number* of meals rather than the *size*, and in choosing carbohydrate foods which were portable and easy to eat. Planning and preparation would be needed to have the right food on hand at school and during travelling times. Liquid meals, both homemade 'smoothies' and the commercial preparations such as Sustagen Sport, Gator-Pro, or Exceed Sports Meal, would come in handy, supplying kilojoules and carbohydrates with little bulk. These could be drunk in addition to meals, or as a snack between meals, without making him feel uncomfortable at training. The following plan was suggested:

Sample high carbohydrate (high-energy) eating plan for Grant (swimmer)

Breakfast: Brought from home and eaten at the pool after training:
2 large bowls of mixed cereals (untoasted muesli, Weetbix, Sustain etc) plus milk, chopped banana or other fresh fruit.
Fruit juice—500ml

Recess: 2 × 250ml tetra packs of Sustagen
Large piece of muesli slice or wholemeal scones
Grab-pack of mixed dried fruits and nuts

Lunch: 3 rolls, with salad and meat/egg/chicken/cheese
2 small cartons of fruit-flavoured yoghurt
Fruit juice

After school (on way to training):
250ml can of Exceed Sports Meal

After training (on the way home in the car):
Fruit juice or sports drink plus 1–2 Sports bars

Dinner (waiting for him when he got home):
Large serve of rice/pasta/potatoes
Lean fish/chicken/lean meat
Vegetables or salad
Bread or bread rolls
Fruit juice

Before bed: Milkshake or fruit smoothie with skim milk, fruit (banana, strawberries, etc.), icecream and extra skim milk powder.

Other snacks (weekends): Fruit or fresh fruit salad, crumpets, muffins, pancakes

This eating plan would increase Grant's intake to 800–900g of carbohydrate each day, and 21 000–23 000 kilojoules (5000–5500 Cals). The dietitian also pointed out that this pattern allowed Grant to begin eating wholesome carbohydrate-rich foods or drinks as soon as training was over. This way muscle glycogen storage would be activated as quickly as possible.

Within three weeks Grant reported a new feeling of energy at training, and a weight gain of a kilogram. This eating program certainly requires some planning and organisation, but with his new lease of life, Grant has plenty of enthusiasm.

PROFILE: ANGELA
Eating in a communal dining hall—special tactics for a special situation

By the time Angela had returned from the Commonwealth Games she had gained over two kilograms. Her coach at home was half expecting it. He had heard of other swimmers going to the Institute of Sport and gaining four kilograms in the first two months, mostly from increased body fat. His own daughters at boarding school seemed to have gained weight each time they came home for term holidays, although his son complained that at his University college there was never enough to eat.

159

Most people who eat in institutions, whether it be a boarding school, a hospital or the Olympic Athletes' Village, have definite views about the food. Common themes are: 'there's no variety'; 'all the goodness is cooked out of it'; 'it's fattening—you'll put on weight'; 'there's never enough to eat—weight just drops off'.

Dining rooms specially set up for athletes, such as the dining hall at the Australian Institute of Sport, or the cafeterias at Games' villages, are definitely not guilty of these charges. In addition to serving massive volumes of food, and staying open for long hours to cater for the various schedules of the athletes, these dining rooms pay particular attention to the nutritional needs of athletes. It is the athlete who is ultimately responsible for what goes into their mouths. In most cases when a situation of poor nutrition is closely examined, the real problem is found to be what the athlete is choosing—not the food opportunities themselves.

Most people are accustomed to a family meal environment, or to cooking for themselves. In these situations they get used to having one food choice at a time, and despite the fact that they think they eat a variety of meals, they probably stick to a handful of favourite recipes, with only an occasional change. In any case, it is all very familiar and under control.

The sudden switch to a communal cafeteria-style dining hall is a culture shock to most athletes. The following new features and challenges are thrown at you:

- Great quantities and many different choices of food. You can serve yourself as much as you like from a never-ending supply, and there are so many nice things to try. Many athletes find that under these circumstances, it is easy to eat more than usual, and more than they need.

- Limited access to food outside designated eating times. If the dining hall is only open at certain times, athletes with enormous energy needs may not be able to consume sufficient food at the customary three sittings. This may lead to weight loss in these athletes.

- Different and unusual foods. It can be challenging to find a new set of foods and meals awaiting you. You may be reluctant to experiment when it comes to trying new foods, or maybe you are unsure of their nutritional value. This can lead to weight loss or failure to meet nutritional goals.

- Lack of supervision. Many athletes come unstuck when they first move to the dining hall and find that Mum is no longer around to make them eat their vegetables.

- Distraction from other athletes. Surrounded by the eating habits of a large group of people, you may find it hard to concentrate on your own nutritional goals. And, given the competitive nature of athletes, it isn't surprising that official and unofficial 'eating competitions' can take place.

- Eating for entertainment. An athlete may not have much time and scope for leisure activities during the day. If the dining hall becomes the meeting place, a lot of extra food can be demolished in the name of relaxation and recreation.

Faced with these challenges, the athlete must develop special skills and tactics to use the dining hall to its optimum potential. The following hints will help you make good decisions:

HINTS FOR EATING WELL IN A CAFETERIA-STYLE
EATING HALL

- Develop the right attitude. The food is not 'fattening' or 'bad for you'. How you select from the food choices will determine whether you meet your nutritional goals.

- Treat the dining room like a restaurant. If there is no written menu, take the time to survey the choices before you commit yourself to a queue. Make a decision about what you will choose for that meal and then serve yourself. (Don't get into the line and keep adding more food to your plate as you pass by each dish.) Make certain that you meet your nutritional goals, rather than stumble on them by accident.

- Don't be distracted by the other foods you have not chosen for this meal. There will be other opportunities to try the things you missed today.

- Although the food choices available may generally reflect the guidelines for peak training nutrition, you may still have to exercise restraint or modify food choices to fully meet your goals. You may have the option of reduced-fat milk rather than full cream, or to cut the remaining fat from the meat. Make the best of these opportunities.

- Allow yourself some flexibility for special foods—but choose treats well, with your nutritional goals in mind.

- Don't concern yourself with the amount and types of foods that other athletes consume. Stick to what is right for you and realise that athletes vary with their nutritional needs.

- Remove yourself from the food environment once you have finished eating. Don't leave yourself exposed to boredom eating.

- If your energy needs go beyond the meal opportunities offered at

---

the dining hall, take a snack for later on—a sandwich, some fruit or flavoured yoghurt are good choices.

- If needed, make use of any opportunities to seek expert dietary advice or to have special services arranged for you. There is often a dietitian who can help with any queries or problems. They may also be able to arrange extra food or nutritional supplements to boost inadequate energy intake.

Cycling

Competitive cycling includes the separate sports of track and road cycling, both with distinct amateur and professional divisions, and the growing sport of mountain bike racing. This chapter will deal with track and road cycling events.

Cycle races range from sprint races lasting about ten seconds to stage races, such as the Tour de France, covering around 4000km over three weeks. They include individual events and team events and involve not only physiological demands, but a mastery of technique and tactics, as well as great courage. The variety of distances and types of races has resulted in the specialisation of cyclists into events which have similar demands.

Track cycling is undertaken on a sloped track at a velodrome, and ranges from the sprint event to the 50km point score race (basically a distance event). Other events include team and individual pursuits, the kilometre time trial and the Keiren. Track events rely on a range of capabilities from sprint power to speed endurance, and anaerobic energy production plays a vital role in most races.

Road races may be held over a number of stages (days), or as single day events. Other events include time trials (both team and individual) and the criterium (a race of varying numbers of laps around a circuit of roads). Races vary in distance from a couple of kilometres for some criteriums, to individual stages of 250km or more, and thousands of kilometres in multi-day events. Road cycling is primarily concerned with strength endurance and endurance, although anaerobic capacity may be called upon in breakaways, hill climbing and all-out sprints to the line.

163

In some countries, the road and track seasons are held at different times of the year, making it possible for cyclists to compete in both sports. However, the specialist nature of the different events means that very few cyclists excel in both areas.

Training

In the off-season, training consists primarily of road cycling to build up aerobic fitness, and weight training to develop strength. For cyclists who concentrate solely on track events, strength training is of considerable importance in building up power. Leading up to and during the competitive season, road work and weight training are reduced in favour of specific track training, with the emphasis on quality rather than quantity. During these sessions both anaerobic power and endurance are developed. Weight training may be continued throughout the season, but sessions are less frequent.

Road cyclists do most of their training on the road, and training distances vary with the time of the year. At the elite level, training involves at least daily sessions, with weekly distances tallying 400–1000km. At the height of the season in Europe, cyclists may do little training since they are continually racing—thanks to a packed race calendar and a selection of stage races.

Competition

Track cycling competitions, depending on their size, may vary from single-day to multi-day meets. Time trials and handicap races are one-off events, while the points score, the sprints and pursuits involve heats and finals. In the latter case, a competitor may be required to race more than once on the same day. Since most events are sprint-based, the depletion of fuel stores is generally not an issue.

Road cycling races are run as one-off events, and become more physiologically and nutritionally challenging as the duration of the race increases. In general, races of 80km or more require attention to fluid and carbohydrate intake during the event—a practical consideration for both competitors and race organisers. Races vary with their rules and support for intake during the event itself. Some organisers provide feed station(s) at intervals along the route, others require competitors to carry their own race food and drinks or to organise their own support crew. In stage races, accommodation and meals are often part of the race package, although many teams will provide their own or additional back-up.

Physical characteristics

Physical characteristics vary between cyclists specialising in different types of races. In general, cyclists are muscular and lean, with

increasing muscularity amongst track sprinters and increasing leanness amongst the distance competitors. Body-fat levels of cyclists are
low, particularly in the case of road cyclists where hill-climbing requires a high power-to-weight ratio.

Typical physique (elite track cyclists)

	Male	Female
Height	176–183cm	162–170cm
Weight	69–79kg	54–62kg
Skinfold sum	41–67mm	58–92mm

Typical physique (elite road cyclists)

	Male	Female
Height	174–187cm	162–172cm
Weight	67–80kg	52–60kg
Skinfold sum	35–57mm	50–74mm

Common nutrition issues

Training nutrition

Training for cycling, particularly distance road events, can be time
and energy-consuming. The long kilometres and hours of training
undertaken by elite cyclists call for a high energy diet—high in protein, vitamins and minerals, and high in carbohydrate for muscle fuel
stores (read Chapters 1 and 2 for a discussion of the optimum training
diet). Daily recovery between heavy training sessions requires a high
total carbohydrate intake, but also clever timing of meals and snacks
to enhance muscle glycogen restoration. Chapter 5 explains that a
carbohydrate snack immediately following a long training session,
will kick-start muscle glycogen synthesis and prepare fuel stores for
tomorrow's (or this afternoon's) training session.

A pattern of frequent meals and snacks may also be handy for
making sure that total energy and carbohydrate needs are met (Chapters 2.7 and 3.7). With the magnitude and bulkiness of food requirements, it can be hard to live on three meals a day. A dietary study of
elite cyclists estimated their average daily energy intake at over 26 000
kilojoules (6200 Cals). This was only made possible by a pattern of
constant 'grazing' over the day. Imagine trying to eat this as three
8000 kilojoule feasts every day—it would be the equivalent of three
Christmas dinners.

Iron status may be an issue for female cyclists—read Chapter 2.5
and see how a high iron intake can be compatible with a high carbohydrate diet. Female cyclists also need to take a sensible approach to

issues of body fat, a healthy menstrual cycle and a comfortable feeling about food. For more information, read Chapters 2.5 and 3.4 and the story of Sharon in the distance running section.

Body-fat levels

Most endurance cyclists take care of their body-fat levels through heavy training. In some situations, particularly in the case of female athletes or athletes coming back after a break, there may be an additional effort needed to help shed the 'spare tyres'. See Chapter 3 for a discussion of sensible and successful methods of weight loss.

Food and fluid needs during long rides

Whether in training or in competition, cyclists ride over distances that challenge their fluid and fuel levels. In hot weather and when working hard, sweat losses can be high. Of course you may not notice this since the sweat evaporates quickly in the wind. Nevertheless, moderate to severe dehydration will result in performance losses—obviously critical on race day, but also a disadvantage to good training.

Endurance performance is also affected by the depletion of body carbohydrate stores—through the depletion of muscle glycogen stores and/or low blood glucose levels. The heavy 'dead' legs that some cyclists experience are probably due to low muscle glycogen levels in the quads. Meanwhile, 'the bonk' or 'hunger flat' are more likely to be the result of blood sugar decline—notice how quickly you can pick up after eating some carbohydrate. Cyclists seem more susceptible to low blood sugar levels than other distance athletes such as runners. Some individuals are particularly susceptible—you may have observed that other riders can go all day on very little food, while more than 50km without a banana will see you falling off the bike.

Clearly, good performance will mean looking after fluid and carbohydrate intake during exercise. A cyclist can be more self-reliant than other athletes, in that food and drinks can be carried on the bike—food in the pockets of a cycling jersey or in a 'bum bag', and fluid in bidons (bottles) carried in cages mounted on the bike frame. Because of this, road races are less organised in providing aid stations to competitors than a running marathon would be. Depending on the history and tradition of the race, or the traffic safety rules under which it operates, a cycle race may provide little or no outside aid to competitors. Some races allow riders to have individual handlers to supply food and drinks during the race, but other events place competitors behind the nutritional eight-ball by allowing only what can be carried by the rider themselves. Some of these races can be over distances up to 260km.

Clearly, both cyclists and race organisers need to update their sports nutrition knowledge. Read Chapter 4.7 for the principles of endurance exercise intake. As a rule of thumb, carbohydrate intake should be organised for rides over 80km, and fluid needs will vary both with the distance and the weather conditions. Be prepared, according to the race rules, to take your own supplies, and to supplement these where allowable from aid stations (official or individual). Carbohydrate intake needs to start *before* you hit a hunger flat. Again, a rule of thumb is to start to eat by 40km into the race. As outlined in Chapter 4.7, an aggressive intake of about 50g of carbohydrate per hour is needed—perhaps even more in the last stages of a race when body carbohydrate stores are very low.

Amazing as it seems, in stage races such as the Tour de France, an added benefit of consuming carbohydrate during the race is that it can help to increase muscle glycogen stores as the cyclists are riding. It defies scientific logic that cyclists can continue to perform at such high levels for 2–3 weeks, with each day's stage lasting 4–8 hours often at an average speed of over 30km/hr. Not only do the cyclists back up from one day to the next, but they still have the energy and muscle fuel to sprint to the line at the end of each day's stage.

However, a couple of studies have shown that when cyclists ride at relatively low intensities (e.g. 40–50 per cent of VO_2 max.) while ingesting large amounts of carbohydrate, there may actually be a nett gain in glycogen stores in non-active muscle fibres while they are riding. In other words, cyclists who are breezing along in the relative ease of the peloton (or other packs sharing the workload) may benefit from consuming quite large amounts of carbohydrate. This carbohydrate may not only support the fuel needs of the slow twitch fibres that are supporting most of the present work load, but may promote glycogen storage in the fast twitch fibres which will come into demand during hill climbs, breakaways and the final sprint to the line.

On the bike, a range of solid and liquid forms of sustenance are possible, and indeed a wide range of foods have been successfully used during long races. While sports drinks provide state-of-the-art exercise intake, it may be difficult to transport sufficient liquid on the bike for the whole race unless you have a team of handlers. Two bidon cages should be mounted for long races in hot weather, particularly when no outside aid is allowed. A one-litre bidon in each can then provide a reasonable intake of fluid and carbohydrate (two litres of fluid and 140g of carbohydrate from a sports drink with a 7 per cent carbohydrate concentration). Extra fluid may be needed on very hot days and for very long races. If required, extra carbohydrate food can also be carried in your jersey—bananas, dried fruit, sports bars and muesli bars are popular choices. As discussed in Chapter 4.7, practise in training so that your competition plans are fool-proof.

A final word on training—good fluid and fuel practices will not only prepare you for your competition strategies, but they will also improve your training form. It is tempting to go out on four-hour training rides with a single bidon of fluid, and not want to interrupt your rhythm by stopping to refill the bottle. While you may not always 'blow up', you may spend the rest of the day with a headache and fail to bounce back for your next training session. Try not to let dehydration go beyond one or two kilograms of your body weight.

Competition nutrition and the pre-event meal

For most racing, especially track racing, a well-trained athlete should be capable of taking in adequate fuel stores with 24–36 hours of preparation. See Chapter 4.2 for details.

The pre-event meal is important for topping up stores and for making the athlete feel comfortable during the race. Choose a light meal or snack according to the guidelines in Chapter 4.4. Most people consider cyclists are not worried by a stomach of food to the same extent as a runner—after all, the food doesn't get 'joggled' around so much. However, if you are crouched over your bars in a streamlined position, then a full stomach can be uncomfortable and can interfere with your breathing. If this is a problem for you, try a liquid meal supplement such as Sustagen Sport, Gator-Pro or Exceed Sports Meal. This is a good way of taking in low-bulk sustenance.

Endurance competition—carbohydrate loading

Distance races should be tackled with full muscle glycogen stores. Where a weekly program of road racing is underway, it is not possible to undertake a carbohydrate loading schedule 3 days prior to each race. Good recovery nutrition will help to replenish carbohydrate stores throughout the training week, but there may not be adequate time to fully store muscle glycogen before the race. This will place more emphasis on carbohydrate intake practices during the race.

Of course, for very important races, you may like to reorganise your training and racing schedule to allow for a longer race preparation. See Chapter 4.3 for details of a full carbohydrate loading schedule.

Multi-stage races—the challenge of recovery

Whether in recreational bike tours or in important professional stage races, many cyclists undertake a schedule of successive-day riding, with individual stages up to 200km and events lasting up to three weeks. These events place enormous stress on the fuel and fluid reserves of the athlete, with the carry-over effect from each day's riding being important. As well as looking after needs during each day's stage, a successful athlete should undertake strategies to assist recovery between days. The main factor of success is not being the best on any one day, but being able to do it again tomorrow. This was highlighted by the feat of Greg LeMond, who in the 1990 Tour de France race became the first rider to win the Tour without having won a single stage along the way.

Recovery nutrition is covered in Chapter 5, with discussion of fluid and carbohydrate replenishment, and in the case of long tours, the need for adequate total nutrient intake. From a practical point of view, nutritional arrangements for multi-day events may be left up to individual competitors or teams, or they may be included in the overall organisation of the event. Often, accommodation and meals are included in the race or tour package and can vary from camp sites and army cooking, to hotel hospitality.

The disadvantages of relying on event organisation include unsuitable food, reliance on the event time-table rather than a time-table that provides for your needs or strategies, and the business of competing with lots of people for the same food. You may be safer to cater partly or fully for your needs—especially if the race organisation is unfamiliar to you, or if your nutritional needs are crucial to good performance. It doesn't hurt to bring some of your own supplies, especially the specific foods and drinks that are part of your race and post-race eating strategies.

Professional teams in important races will often come with a full back-up team and an aggressive nutrition plan. The Tour de France is perhaps the best known multi-stage cycle race, providing riders with an enormous challenge to their riding skills and nutritional knowledge. See the account below to see how the champions survive.

PROFILE
The Tour de France

The Tour de France is no picnic—4000km in 20-odd days over some of the most rugged mountain terrain in Europe. Yet eating and drinking, especially on the bike, plays a crucial role in allowing the cyclists to perform well, and for that matter, even to finish the race.

Recently some Dutch physiologists, led by Professor Wim Saris, conducted an extensive study of this race, following the fortunes of five male cyclists from one of the leading professional teams. Daily energy expenditure was estimated, with the cost of each day's cycling being taken from the detailed descriptions of each stage. Body weight and body fat was checked over the period, and cyclists kept a record of all food and fluid intake over the race.

The first and most remarkable result was the total energy expenditure estimated for the race—with an average daily energy expenditure of 25 400 kilojoules (6060 Cals). The heaviest day of exercise was estimated to cost 32 700kJ (7800 Cals), and on the one rest day, energy expenditure was estimated to drop below 13 000kJ (3100 Cals). Despite this energy output, there were only minor changes reported in body weight and body fat over the three-week period. And indeed the estimated energy intake from food, drinks and supplements was reported at a daily average of 24 700kJ (5900 Cals). The riders did very well in balancing their energy needs over this period, and data suggested that they managed to balance intake and expenditure remarkably well on a daily basis. This was important, since with the large amounts required to be eaten it would be hard to catch up from one day to the next if intake fell behind. There is only so much that you can put into your stomach each day!

A summary of total dietary intake over the race is presented in the following table. Carbohydrate intake was well looked after, making up over 60 per cent of total food intake. The cyclists churned through 12–13g of carbohydrate per kilogram of body mass per day—further evidence of the remarkable work output during the race. Protein intake was more than adequate, supplying about 15 per cent of total energy during the period, or an intake of over 3g/kg body mass/day. Fat intake, supplying about 23 per cent of energy intake, was well below the typical Western dietary ratio.

Average daily intake of Tour de France cyclists

Energy	24 300kJ/day (5800 Cals)
Carbohydrate	849g/day = 61% of energy = 12.3g/kg/day
Protein	217g/day = 15% of energy = 3.1g/kg/day
Fat	147g/day = 23% of energy
Water	6.7 litres/day

Vitamin and mineral intakes were above requirements, both on the basis of recommended dietary intake levels and from blood measurements of micronutrient status. Not only did these nutrients come from food intake, but from fortified liquid formulas (such as high carbohydrate and liquid meal supplements) and from additional vitamin supplements as well. As would be expected from sweat loss needs, fluid intake was high—an average of 6.7 litres per day per cyclist.

So what did the cyclists eat? The range of foodstuffs listed included sweet cakes (perhaps contributing more fat than the cyclists realised), pasta, bread and breakfast cereals, with high-protein foods including meats, dairy products and eggs. An important contribution to both carbohydrate and energy intake was made by carbohydrate-rich drinks—soft drinks, and more particularly sports drinks, liquid meal supplements and high-carbohydrate 'carbo-loader' formulas. About a third of total carbohydrate intake was provided by these drinks— obviously an advantage in terms of compact and digestible energy.

It is also of interest to note that a substantial part of the day's intake was consumed while actually on the bike. Nearly half the day's energy and nearly 60 per cent of total carbohydrate intake was consumed during the race, presumably thanks to the carbohydrate liquids. An average of four litres of fluid was also consumed while riding.

Thus our cyclists seem to have made good use of sports nutrition information, using special sports products to boost energy, carbohydrate, and total nutrient intake in a compact form. Intake during the race seemed aggressive and designed to avoid dehydration and fuel depletion, and hopefully post-exercise eating was timed to begin rapid recovery at the end of each day.

The human body is a remarkable engine to be able to tackle such a sustained high-intensity workload, and deserves the very best in fuel and maintenance nutrients.

Distance running

Distance runners compete over a variety of race lengths most commonly 10km, 15km, half marathon (21.1km) and the marathon (42.2km). While there is a 10 000m track event, most distance running is done as road races or cross-country runs. 'Fun runs' of various lengths attract community participation, recreational runners joining with elite and club-level runners.

Ultradistance races such as 50 mile, 100km and 100 mile events are not included in the Olympic Games or World Championships, and generally do not attract a large following, particularly at the recreational level. Exceptions to this are races such as the South African 'Comrades' run—a race of 90km which attracts a field of 12 000 competitors each year.

Distance runners mature with age, requiring years of base training to build up to the program of an elite runner. Consequently, most elite competitors are aged from their mid-twenties to late thirties. At a recreational level, running is a great social leveller, and you would expect to find both teenagers and seventy-year-olds competing in the same fun run.

Training

At the recreational level, many runners train primarily for fitness or health, and compete in a number of fun runs, and perhaps a marathon, each year. Daily training sessions might add up to a weekly distance of 50km, perhaps peaking at 80–100km before a marathon.

Elite distance runners typically run up to 200km per week, with two training sessions per day. Some runners include water running and weight training in their programs, but this is the exception rather than the rule, and has traditionally been associated with rehabilitation of injuries. A typical training week includes different types of sessions, each with a specific physiological emphasis. Sessions include longer slow runs for aerobic endurance, with intense continuous runs, fartlek or 'speed play' sessions and track (interval) work all undertaken to improve anaerobic capacity and speed.

Competition

The elite runner may compete in a number of races of varying distance each year, with a few key events being chosen for full preparation and peaking. Many will compete weekly over a season of road races (usually summer) or cross-country runs (usually winter), treating each race as a hard training session. Marathon runners are unlikely to compete more than once or twice a year over this distance.

Events in hot weather are usually held in the early morning to avoid the heat, while cross-country events may be held on winter afternoons. The longer races are normally held as a once-off competition, i.e. without heats or qualifiers. Relay or stage races are sometimes held, requiring competitors to run a series of 6–10km legs, often with only a short recovery time in between. In international events such as the Olympic Games, only rare runners will contest both the 10 000m track event and the marathon, since the races are separated only by a number of days.

Distance running is predominantly an aerobic activity, with elite athletes running from under 30 minutes (10km) to just over two hours (the marathon). Recreational runners can take up to twice as long to complete the same distance, and sometimes even longer. Races above 30km will probably challenge the usual carbohydrate storage capacity of most runners, and steps will need to be taken to increase or supplement muscle glycogen stores.

Physical characteristics

Distance runners typically carry low body-fat levels—an advantage when you have to carry your body weight over many kilometres. In fact, most elite runners have low total body weights, being small in stature and lightly muscled, particularly in the upper body.

Typical physique (elite distance runner)

	Male	Female
Height	172–182cm	not available
Weight	59–71kg	49–55kg
Skinfolds	29–39mm	42–60mm

Other comments

Distance running has for many years attracted the attention of sports scientists. It is a good sport to study, being both popular and predictable—a marathon is always 42.2km, whereas every football match is literally a new ball game. Not only have nutritional and physiological issues been well researched, but the results enjoy good coverage in the popular running magazines.

Thus runners are generally well-educated about their sport. Many recreational runners have read about carbo-loading or what to drink during a marathon, and exercise physiologists, such as Dave Costill and Tim Noakes, are often as well-known as the top runners themselves. Of course, not all the scientific information is understood or turned into good practices, but at least runners have the expectation that scientific approaches to nutrition can aid their performance.

Common nutrition issues

Recovery and carbohydrate—the amount and the timing

Daily and twice daily training sessions call for recovery strategies, especially when two hard sessions are held back-to-back. Even a recreational runner may find that the typical Western diet does not provide sufficient fuel for marathon training. In fact the first time many runners hit the wall is during their first weeks of big training mileage, due to a gradual process of failing to restore muscle glycogen levels.

Recovery will be aided both by the amount and timing of the carbohydrate. Read Chapter 5. Chapters 1.3 and 2.2 will guide you to estimate your daily carbohydrate requirements and build in the dietary habits to achieve your carbohydrate intake goals.

The timing of carbohydrate is crucial for recovery after long, hard training sessions or races. Not only are your muscles depleted of carbohydrate, but running also causes some damage to muscle fibres, which will delay glycogen recovery. Carbohydrate intake immediately after the session or the race will let the muscle take advantage of their most rapid recovery time. Don't leave it too long.

Low body-fat levels

The low body-fat levels of elite distance runners are typically a result of well-chosen parents and high-volume training. However some runners, both elite and recreational, need additional help to reduce body-fat levels.

The first step is to set a realistic target—a body-fat level that is part of good health as well as good performance, and a body-fat level that can be achieved and maintained with a healthy diet and a sensible workload. Read about this in Chapter 3.

Females, fat and food disorders

For some runners, particularly females, setting and achieving a desirable body-fat level poses a problem. Many female runners set unrealistic targets—perhaps below their natural body-fat levels. This can result in a cycle of frustration and problems. Remember that the female body is designed to carry a higher level of fat than a male.

In studies, many female runners report eating a surprisingly low intake of kilojoules—less than you would expect for the training they do. It's not that they don't enjoy eating, in fact, many spend hours each day thinking about food. Rather, to keep body-fat levels down to what they consider to be suitable levels, these runners have to restrict energy intake. Often the situation becomes progressively worse—the more energy they restrict, the less they need to eat. It's almost as if the body is fighting to defend a higher body-fat level.

Some runners complicate the situation further by adding weird and wonderful diets, excessive training, and eating behaviour problems to their weight-loss techniques. Not all runners who practise anorexic (food restriction) or bulimic (bingeing) behaviours have a true eating disorder—many are driven to these actions in a desperate attempt to get on top of their body-fat goals.

If you are stressed or feel out of control with eating and your body fat, then your body-fat goals may not be right for you. The penalties associated with chasing unrealistic goals are twofold—the problems associated with how you get there, and then the problems faced by your body from literally being starved or overloaded. In the latter case, this might include disrupted periods and recurrent bouts of injury, illness or fatigue.

Read Chapters 1 and 2 to convince yourself that the key elements to a healthy diet are variety and an adequate kilojoule budget. If loss of body fat is a healthy option, then Chapter 3 will help you with a sensible plan of attack. If you seem caught up in a cycle of frustration, a sports dietitian, together with a sports psychologist, can help you to break free. You may have to settle for a slightly larger skinfold sum, but with your health and happiness improved, you will perform better in the long run.

Amenorrhea, low bone density and stress fractures

It appears that female runners are more likely to suffer interruptions to their menstrual cycles—called secondary amenorrhea—than other athletes such as cyclists or swimmers. This is no longer regarded as a curiosity or a side-effect of training. Read Chapter 2.6, and the case history of Sharon below. Studies show that low estrogen levels in amenorrheic athletes can lead to loss of bone density—and bone strength—and may increase the risk of stress fractures.

The picture is quite complicated, with many factors to consider. However the bottom line is that you should see a sports doctor if your menstrual patterns become disrupted.

Iron deficiency

Distance runners, particularly females, are at a high risk of low-iron status—perhaps even developing into iron deficiency anemia. As discussed in Chapter 2.5, many iron deficient athletes report feeling tired in training, but it is not until anemia has developed that performance is clearly impaired. Experts still argue about the severity of iron losses from gastrointestinal bleeding, sweat and red blood cell damage, but it is probable that the iron requirements of a runner will be increased. On paper, many runners look like they eat adequate dietary iron but on closer examination, this may be mostly non-heme iron, from plant food sources and it may not be well-absorbed.

Don, below, provides a typical story of a runner who overlooks his iron needs by focusing on carbohydrate intake only. For women runners the risk of iron deficiency is even greater, since their iron needs are increased (to cover menstrual blood loss), but their kilojoule budget is smaller. The iron story is covered below and in Chapter 2.5.

Gastrointestinal problems

Many runners report gastrointestinal problems during hard runs, particularly races. It's hard to do a PB when you are suffering stomach cramps, diarrhea or wind. Some runners experience problems at the top end, with burping and heartburn, and a few even find that they pass blood during races.

The cause of these problems is unknown, but it seems to be related to the intensity of the running, the stress of competition and perhaps, dehydration. Some runners are able to pinpoint certain foods that cause problems, but this is an individual matter. Probably the best general advice is to experiment with the type and timing of food that you consume before running. Often, it is best to run on an 'empty stomach', with pre-race or pre-training meals eaten well in advance. Liquid meal supplements such as Exceed Sports Meal, Gator-Pro or Sustagen Sport make a good low-bulk, pre-exercise meal.

If problems persist, for important races you might need to literally achieve an empty gut, by switching to low-fibre foods and/or replacing meals with liquid meal supplements over the last 24 hours. See Steve's story in the middle distance running chapter.

Alternative dietary lifestyles

When many people take up running, they decide to make some dietary changes as well. Often it is all part of a healthy lifestyle change, but for some there is a belief in better performance with a better diet. It is great to see runners inspired to improve their eating patterns.

Some runners want to sweep through with a new broom, and embark on special dietary programs. Vegetarian diets and Pritikin diets are the most popular, and often claim to have the blessing of well-known runners. Both these dietary patterns have plenty to offer in terms of health and performance since both are based on the idea of increasing carbohydrate and fibre intake, and decreasing fat intake. However, they also have the potential to become very restricted and lacking in variety, particularly in the hands of highly motivated runners. Many runners make the mistake of concentrating on what should be given up rather than on preserving nutritional variety, moderation and flexibility.

Read the comments in Chapter 1 about how dietary changes can be made without sacrificing variety. By all means experiment with these diets, but from many points of view a better approach is to settle for a modified Pritikin or vegetarian diet, picking out the best bits and incorporating them into your own dietary patterns. See a discussion of Pritikin eating in the next chapter, and the vegetarian diet in the gymnastics chapter.

Race preparation

An important dietary preparation is to store sufficient muscle fuel to see out the event. A trained runner should not experience too much difficulty in preparing for events up to the 1/2 marathon. In Chapter 4.2 you will read that adequate muscle glycogen levels can be stored with a high-carbohydrate diet (daily intake of 8–10g per kg of body weight) and 24–36 hours of taper or rest. For weekly events, you may like to reschedule training sessions to achieve an adequate taper at the end of the week.

Carbohydrate loading is almost synonymous with the marathon—and rightly so. Races of this length and further will utilise as much muscle glycogen as you can store. But despite the hype—or perhaps because of it—many runners do not know how to carbohydrate load properly. In the study reported below, some runners did a better job of 'garbo-loading' than 'carbo-loading'. Read Chapter 4.3 for the low-down on loading.

Runners who like to race with a light stomach can modify the fibre and bulk in their diets over the 12–24 hours before the event to reduce their gastrointestinal contents.

The pre-event meal

With early morning races, it is tempting to sleep in for as long as possible—thus skipping breakfast. Other runners worry about gastrointestinal upsets if they eat a big breakfast before a race. However, the pre-event meal should not be sacrificed. It is the last opportunity to top up glycogen stores—particularly liver stores—and to top up fluid levels.

In many cases, a light snack, even a couple of pieces of toast and a drink, might be the best menu. If your race starts later in the day there might be time for a larger meal three to four hours pre-race. Don't forget fluids, especially if the day is hot. Liquid meal supplements provide a compact and quickly-digested alternative to solid food in situations where time is scarce or pre-race nerves are a problem.

Race fluids and fuel

For events up to the half-marathon, you should have all your fuel needs on board. Race nutrition should only need to be concerned with the prevention of severe dehydration. In races of this distance, the major threat of overheating comes from the pace at which you are running—the faster you run, the more metabolic heat you produce. But severe dehydration will add to the problem. So know your sweat losses and replace fluids to keep in touch with this.

In races of less than 10–15km in cool conditions, there may not be any need to drink during the event, and the top runners will not want to sacrifice any time. As the distance increases and/or the temperature rises, however, you will start to find aid stations along the route. Make use of these according to your sweat losses. If you are running for more than an hour, you should aim for a comfortable fluid intake —perhaps, 500–600ml spread over the race. Water is the most likely drink to be supplied, but sports drinks are also suitable.

For the marathon and longer events, performance will be enhanced by taking in carbohydrate during the run. This will be crucial for events of 50 miles or more. An intake of about 50g of carbohydrate per hour is a rough guide for events that go beyond the capacity of your muscle glycogen stores, although you may need to experiment to find what works for you, and to vary the rate of carbohydrate intake at different points of the event. See Chapter 4.7.

For most runners, replacing about 80 per cent of sweat losses will mean a fluid intake of 500–700ml/hr. With a sports drink of 7–8 per cent carbohydrate concentration, and an intake of about 200–250ml at each five kilometre aid station, fluid and carbohydrate needs are generally taken care of (you may need more on a very hot day). The front runners may have difficulty swallowing this amount, but in the middle of the pack you should be able to spare a little more time at the aid station.

In ultradistance races, 50 miles and more, runners even manage some solid food—but then they are often running at a relatively slower pace. Even so, most runners are best served by fluid forms of carbohydrate.

Travelling to races

Many athletes undertake their most important races away from the safety of home. At the elite level, interstate and international travel may be necessary to find suitable competition, or to race in major world events. Even at the recreational level, runners may organise their holidays to provide an opportunity to participate in a well-known marathon or distance event. It can be challenging to achieve your special race nutrition strategies before and during races when you're travelling. You may need to decide whether you trust your special high-carbohydrate needs and pre-race timetable to restaurants, or whether you can choose accommodation that allows self-catering. Be prepared and organise ahead. You may need to bring some of your favourite foods with you if they are not available in your new location. Be wary of carbohydrate-loading banquets and parties that are offered. They may offer a menu that is higher in fat than in fuel. Think about fluid supplies—especially if you are travelling to locations where the local water supply is not safe to drink. It is good to carry a water bottle around with you over the last days of the race, particularly if you are in unfamiliar surroundings. This way you can be sure that you hydrate well, even when taps and fridges are less accessible than at home.

PROFILE: SHARON
The bare bones of running

Sharon couldn't believe her bad luck as she viewed the results of the CAT scan. The sports doctor pointed out the 'hot spot' in her lower leg—her second stress fracture that year. All that hard work and dedication down the drain.

The doctor agreed that it was unfortunate, but suggested that factors other than luck could be involved. He questioned Sharon about her training program and her diet, and listened as she described the lifestyle of a committed long distance runner.

Her training mileage fluctuated between 120 and 150km per week, mixed between track sessions and road running. Eighteen months ago she had had her first taste of international competition, and had come back from Europe with the view that the top women runners were all incredibly lean. Her project since then had been to minimise her body fat, and she worked diligently at this. While it was a constant struggle and required her to eat a sparrow-like and rigid diet, there was now little 'dead weight' on her body. The rewards had been impressive. The more weight she lost, the faster she ran—at least for the first year. Now she was lucky to run at all.

When the doctor asked Sharon if she had regular menstrual periods, she laughed.

'Of course not!' she said. 'Hardly any of the girls do. It's one of the rewards of all the hard work. In fact, often when we line up for a race, we ask around to see who's still having periods, and then you can feel happy that you've trained harder than them.'

The doctor explained to Sharon that amenorrhea in athletes was no longer considered harmless or a reward. As with menopause in older women, the loss of periods is associated with a drop in blood estrogen levels—and he reminded her that an important function of this hormone was to maintain bone mass. Studies have shown that amenorrheic athletes have lower bone density at some bone sites than normally menstruating athletes—and a higher incidence of stress fractures.

While it is tempting to conclude that amenorrhea leads to low bone density leads to stress fractures, the situation is more complicated. Stress fractures result from the failure of a bone to adapt to excessive trauma, and can occur whether bone density is low or normal, though a weakened bone is theoretically more likely to give way.

The doctor organised to sit down with Sharon and her coach and discuss the potential causes of an excessive training load—too much too quickly, hard surfaces, inadequate shoes and poor running style. Next on the agenda was to check her menstrual function and hormone levels, in case some non-sporting factor had caused her periods to stop just over a year ago. Being female, Caucasian and lightly framed was a risk factor for low bone density in itself, so a special bone scan was scheduled to measure her bone density against standards for a female of her age.

The main thrust of therapy to halt bone loss, and perhaps even restore levels, would be to restore low estrogen levels. The ideal situation, of course, would be for Sharon to resume a regular menstrual cycle—but this presumes we know why it happens in the first place. A number of factors have been blamed—low body fat, sudden loss of weight, eating disorders, intense training, stress of all types, and even the type of sport.

However, studies have failed to pinpoint a single or consistent culprit right across the board. Take the low body-fat theory, for example. Studies comparing groups of amenorrheic and normally-menstruating athletes have found no significant differences in the body-fat levels of each group. There are menstruating athletes with low body-fat levels and amenorrheic athletes with relatively high body-fat levels. However, struggling to push your body fat and weight below the level your body seems to prefer seems a critical issue, especially if drastic mea-sures are taken to achieve this.

Some athletes can identify from experience the stress factors that seemed to push their bodies over the edge. For Sharon, trying to achieve a body-fat level that seemed unnaturally low was a possible factor. Before resorting to estrogen replacement treatment, the doc-tor decided it was worth trying to sort out Sharon's menstrual prob-lems from within. He also suspected that her diet was inadequate in a number of respects other than a low kilojoule level, and explained that a low calcium level, in itself, may prevent optimum bone density. However in the presence of low estrogen levels the problem may be significantly worse.

Sharon agreed to see a sports dietitian, who assessed the rigid dietary plan that she had followed over the past months (see table below). A nutrient analysis revealed that this diet was low in kilojoules compared to her estimated energy needs, and low in protein, carbo-hydrate, iron and calcium. Her typical daily calcium intake of about 300mg was below the Australian RDI of 800mg/day, and well below the 1000–1500mg recommended for post-menopausal (and presumably other low-estrogen) women.

Sharon asked if she could remedy the situation with a calcium supplement. She had heard of other runners doing this to prevent stress fractures. The dietitian reminded her that the underlying prob-lems were inadequate nutrition and amenorrhea, and advised that her diet needed total remodelling rather than a 'band-aid' approach.

To cut a long story short, Sharon's bone density was on the low side of the normal range. Nine months later it has improved a little. While reluctant at first to give up her low body-fat goals, she gradually conceded that the situation wasn't working and allowed herself to expand her dietary intake. The dietitian negotiated a daily plan of about 8400–9400kJ per day (2000–2200 Cals), which allowed her greater enjoyment and freedom with food, as well as greater nutrient intake.

Sharon found she could also enjoy a nutritious 'treat' on Sunday afternoons after her long run, without feeling she had binged. A 'skinny' hot chocolate and muffin, or a soft-serve icecream sundae topped off her week—and her calcium intake as well! Even though her body weight increased by 2kg, and her skinfold sum increased by nearly 10mm to 45mm, she agreed that she felt more energetic and less uptight at this level. Her periods resumed after four months—prob-ably due to changes in diet, training and stress.

With careful dietary choices she was able to achieve a calcium intake of over 1000mg/day, eating low-fat, high-calcium foods such as skim milk, low-fat yoghurt and fish with bones. (See table above and Chapter 2.6 for more ideas.) Many of the calcium foods could be turned into high-carbohydrate meals, thus meeting other training nutrition goals.

Sharon's diet before and after counselling

	Before	After
Breakfast	Bowl of fruit salad (2 cups)	Bowl of wholemeal cereal 200ml low-fat calcium-enriched milk
	1 toast + Vegemite Black tea	1 thick or 2 thin slices toast + Vegemite 200ml orange juice
Lunch	Plain salad roll	Large salad roll with reduced fat cheese, or slice of salmon (+ bones)
	Apple	Piece of fruit or small carton of fruit salad
Afternoon tea	Orange packet of sultanas	Carton of non-fat fruit yoghurt Muesli or breakfast bar
Tea	120g lean meat/chicken Medium potato	120g lean meat/chicken 2 cups mashed potato $1\frac{1}{2}$–2 cups rice or pasta
	Small salad Low-joule jelly + Tbsp low-joule icecream	3–5 vegetables or salad Fruit salad + 100g low-fat fromage frais or icecream
Supper	Slice of toast + vegemite	In winter, Milo or coffee made with low-fat milk plus English muffin with jam In summer, banana smoothie made with low-fat milk (300–400ml)
Analysis:		
Energy	5200kJ (1240 Cals)	9300kJ (2200 Cals)
CHO	200g	350g
Protein	60g	135g
Calcium	310mg	1700mg

Sharon's running career has had no further hiccups to date. Her revised training program now includes less total mileage and some on-going water running sessions—she became expert at this while the stress fractures healed. And she frequently lectures her running friends about seeing a sports doctor at the first sign of disruption to their periods.

PROFILE: DON
Feeling ironed out?

Don hadn't been training well for the last month. He felt tired all the time, despite plenty of sleep, and didn't feel as if he was recovering between training sessions. A 'run for fitness' man, he had decided six months ago to try a marathon, and had been doing things by the book in gradually stepping up his program. Strangely, he had coped better with the greater mileage at the beginning, and by now he had expected to be right on top of it. His knees niggled a bit, but one of his training partners kept him well-supplied with anti-inflammatory drugs and these seemed to keep it under control. He decided that perhaps he wasn't getting enough carbos, and decided to see a sports dietitian.

The dietitian questioned him about his symptoms, his training and his diet. Don described his daily meal routine, pointing out that he had put it together himself from a running magazine article. Not being a terrific cook, he had kept things simple—this included eating either rice or pasta each night.

The dietitian questioned him further about specific foods, and found that he didn't often eat meat (he believed it was too fatty for a runner). The same went for fish and chicken, though he sometimes ordered fish when eating at a restaurant. He didn't eat packaged breakfast cereals, but made his own muesli from rolled oats and added bran. As for legumes, silverbeet and spinach, he rarely ventured outside the conventional vegetables his mother had cooked for him at home. Dried fruit? A little in his muesli. Eggs? Too high in cholesterol. Vitamin or mineral supplements were not taken.

The dietitian suggested that iron deficiency, rather than carbohydrate deficiency, might be at the root of his fatigue problem. He was eating plenty of wholegrain bread, rice, pasta and oats for carbohydrate—and this was also his major source of dietary iron. Although his estimated iron intake appeared to be well above the Australian RDI for a male (7mg/day), almost all of his dietary iron was in the form least likely to be absorbed, i.e. non-heme iron. Nor did his meal mixtures make best use of factors to enhance iron absorption.

Additionally, it was likely that Don's iron requirements were increased above the general male RDI level. The increased training mileage, all run on hard surfaces wearing his favourite well-worn shoes, could be causing additional damage to red blood cells. And it was probable that the chronic use of anti-inflammatory drugs was causing a small but consistent loss of blood through gastrointestinal bleeding.

The dietitian organised for Don to see a sports doctor to discuss training and the appropriate use of anti-inflammatory drugs, and to order a blood test to determine his iron status. The results came back a few days later, the hemoglobin level normal, but at the low end of the range, and the ferritin level (a storage form of iron) quite low at 12ng/ml. While these tests are often hard to interpret (what is the best level for an athlete to have?), it seemed likely that Don was in the first stages of iron deficiency.

Experts disagree about the level at which iron deficiency actually affects performance, and it is probable that an athlete would have to become anemic (low hemoglobin level) before a measurable drop in performance could be detected. Nevertheless, many athletes report tiredness in training in the early stages—and the situation deserves treatment, if only to prevent it from continuing into severe iron deficiency.

The doctor and dietitian agreed on a program of high-dose iron supplements for six weeks, to boost iron stores while Don re-organised his dietary intake. Once his iron stores were topped up, Don would support his iron needs with iron from his food. The dietitian outlined the following nutrition plan for Don to follow:

- Continue with high-carbohydrate foods at each meal, but add a small portion of lean red meat, chicken, liver pate or shellfish to the menu. The principle of a low fat intake could still be preserved.

- Add some iron-fortified breakfast cereal, such as Sustain, Bran Flakes or Weetbix to his home-made muesli mix.

- Expand food choices by trying legumes, green leafy vegetables, and low-fat egg dishes.

- Add some vitamin C foods, such as orange juice, to any meal in which non-heme iron was the prominent source of iron.

She provided Don with some recipes and he began to experiment with cooking. While adding oysters and prawns to his stir-fried rice may sound exotic, there were some simple changes he could make also, such as ordering a roast beef and salad sandwich at the lunch shop (saves him cooking a whole roast for one person).

At the end of six weeks, Don reported feeling more energetic and more adept in the kitchen. His ferritin levels had increased to greater than 50ng/ml, so it was agreed to stop the supplement and retest in another six months. Pleased with this success, Don asked if it was all right for his training partners to take iron supplements if they also felt tired.

The dietitian agreed that many runners considered iron supplements a quick 'pick-me-up' for fatigue or else supplemented 'just in case of a deficiency'.

It was true that iron supplements could be bought 'over the counter' at pharmacies. However, the dietitian pointed out that self-prescription and casual use of these supplements often led to an unnecessarily high intake of iron, with the potential for harm including interference with the absorption of other body minerals such as zinc.

However, the real problem lay in seeking a simple solution for a complex problem. For a start, fatigue could be caused by a number of factors—including lack of sleep, overtraining and inadequate carbohydrate intake. These factors would not be rectified with an iron supplement.

Don was reminded that his own iron problem had been carefully assessed and comprehensively treated. His friends who self-diagnosed and self-treated would miss out on such expert advice. They might never discover or treat the underlying causes of the iron deficiency, nor benefit from counselling on all aspects of training nutrition. For example, there could easily be a medical condition causing the iron loss, such as an ulcer. Self-diagnosis and treatment could mean missing the chance for an early diagnosis.

Don went back to his squad with renewed vigour and steadily continued his marathon training program. At the last report, he was confidently counting the days until the big event.

Carbohydrate loading—a load of?

Picture the scene. You have been training hard for six months for the marathon, and there are only three days until the gun sounds. Now for the real fun. Good-bye Pritikin for the next couple of days while you create new records in pizza and chocolate eating. On the final evening, you organise a carbo-loading function with your training buddies, and fill your stomach to within an inch of bursting. Looking at the chocolate mousse, you wish you hadn't eaten so much lasagne. However, you find room on the way home for a couple of donuts convincing yourself that this will come in handy over the last ten kilometres. This carbohydrate loading is great stuff, right?

Wrong. Runners who practise this version of carbo-loading risk a double disservice—an uncomfortably full stomach and a questionable intake of carbohydrate for muscle glycogen storage.

In a study of the carbohydrate-loading techniques used by 76 runners competing in the 1983 Nike marathon in Canberra, the runners were questioned about their training and dietary program over the final week before the race. The results showed a variety of practices, with some depleting in the early part of the week, some tapering their training over the last three days and others continuing to do their normal training right up to race day. Chapter 4.3 explains the modified loading technique that is now recommended.

Of most interest were the high-carbohydrate diets eaten over the last three days before the event. A summary of the results shows the average intake per day:

Dietary intake of runners carbo-loading for a marathon

	Mean	Range
Carbohydrate intake	470g/day	188g–960g
Energy intake	14 600kJ/day	5800–28 400kJ
Proportion of energy as carbohydrate	53%	31–83%

For maximum muscle glycogen synthesis, a daily intake of 8–10g of carbohydrate per kilogram of your bodyweight has been recommended (see Chapter 4.3). For these runners, this would translate into approximately 500–700g of carbohydrate per day, taking up at least 60 per cent of total energy intake. Some of the runners in the group achieved these levels, but at the other end of the scale some managed only 200g or so of carbohydrate per day.

From the proportion of energy that came from carbohydrate in these loading diets, it is obvious that some runners did not understand carbohydrate foods and high-carbohydrate meals. With only 30 per cent of their total energy intake coming from carbohydrates, a few runners managed to eat *less* carbohydrate than would be found in the typical Australian diet—and in Chapter 1 we found that the typical food patterns in this country were already inadequate in carbohydrate intake.

So where did these runners go wrong? Read the hints for carbohydrate-loading in Chapter 4.3. The meal patterns described by the runners in the study showed the following classic mistakes:

- The runners continued to eat large amounts of non-carbohydrate foods at the meal, such as protein foods, and low-carbohydrate salads. Although these are part of a nutritious diet, the main goal of carbohydrate-loading days is to meet carbohydrate intake goals. You can afford to sacrifice some of these other foods (and their nutrients) to make more room on your plate and in your stomach for the carbos.

- The runners fell for the idea that 'junk foods' are good carbohydrate foods. Many ate large amounts of foods they considered to be low in nutritional value—take-aways, chocolate, creamcakes and rich desserts. Most of these foods contributed more fat than carbohydrate to the diet.

- While many foods were correctly identified as high in carbohydrate, when made into a meal, the dish often had only a small amount of this important ingredient. A good example is lasagne: there would be few runners who haven't heard that pasta is a good carbo food, but many forget that lasagne recipes may contain only a few small sheets of pasta, and a lot of meat, oil and cheese. See table below for ways to replace high-fat carbo meals with the real thing.

- The runners continued their healthy habits of eating 'no added sugar' and artificially sweetened foods. While these food items might assist with keeping to a moderate sugar intake in the everyday diet, during the three days of carbo-loading before an event, it is okay to stray outside the usual dietary concerns. Canned fruit with added sugar, sweetened soft drinks and sugary confectionery are easy and compact ways to boost carbohydrate intake.

- Few runners made use of high-carbohydrate fluids—including fruit smoothies, soft drinks and fruit juices, as well as special Sports supplements like sports drinks, high-carbohydrate ('carbo-loader') products, and liquid meal supplements. Don't overlook these as a compact source of carbohydrate.

IDEAS FOR REPLACING HIGH-FAT CARBOHYDRATE FOODS WITH A LOWER-FAT AND HIGHER-CARBOHYDRATE ALTERNATIVE

High-fat carbo food	Alternative
Lasagne	Home-made lasagne—lots of pasta sheets with thin layers of lean bolognaise sauce and a sprinkle of reduced-fat cheese *OR* Pasta—large serve with a small amount of low-fat meat or tomato sauce
Pasta with rich, creamy sauce (very filling)	Pasta as above
Crumpet soaking with margarine	Crumpet with honey or jam
Pancake soaking with whipped butter and/or cream	Pancake with honey or syrup— perhaps a little low-fat icecream
Croissant	Bagel or bread roll
Pizza with the lot	Thick crust pizza—vegetarian, chicken or seafood, with less cheese *OR* Make your own pizza—use commercial bases, muffins or pita bread, with low-fat toppings and a sprinkle of reduced-fat cheese
French fries	Baked potato with low-fat filling
Donut	Coffee scroll (scrape of marg.)

187

High-fat carbo food	Alternative
Cream cake or pastry	Muffin or fruit loaf—low-fat recipes
Ice-cream (particularly speciality or 'premium' brands)	Reduced-fat and low-fat brands of icecream (<4 per cent fat)
Chocolate mousse	Light fromage frais
Toasted muesli	Untoasted muesli and other breakfast cereals
Toasted ham/cheese sandwich	Toasted banana or baked bean sandwich—thick sliced bread and scrape of marg.
Thickshake	Fruit smoothie—skim milk, fruit low fat icecream/yoghurt
Chocolate bar	Plain muesli and breakfast bars—especially low-fat brands, or low-fat sports bar
Chocolates/toffees	Jelly beans and jubes

In this study, the group of runners who finished the marathon in less than three hours reported significantly greater training mileage and achieved a higher percentage of carbohydrate in their loading diets, than the runners who took more than 3.5 hours. This is of course only an observation and cannot prove directly that the extra carbos improved performance. It is just as likely that the good runners knew more about what they were doing, than that a good loading diet improved race times.

The moral of the story is that carbohydrate loading might be on the tip of every runner's tongue, but to get it right you need to carefully consider which foods go into your mouth.

Middle distance running

In this chapter running events ranging from 800 to 5000 metres are covered, with the common link being that each is run as a track race, and each requires the development of both aerobic and anaerobic energy supply systems.

Competition begins with school athletics, and continues through from club level to the international scene. In addition to World Championships and the Olympic Games, an international Grand Prix circuit of track and field meets is held each year, with a selected program of events rotating each season.

Training

Middle distance runners often train similarly to their long-distance counterparts in the off-season (traditionally winter) although total weekly mileage and the distance of their 'long runs' may be slightly less. Training is undertaken twice a day, with a mixture of continuous runs and track interval work. Some runners include weight training when time and facilities permit.

As the competition season approaches, greater emphasis is placed on track work and improvements in speed. There may be a drop in mileage as the quality of the sessions increases. Training is normally reduced over the days leading up to the race, depending on the importance of the event.

Competition

Middle distance athletes normally specialise in one or two distances, such as the combination of 800m and 1500m races. At national and international level, an athlete will rarely compete in more than two races on the program, although at the interclub level some athletes will try themselves over a variety of distances. At specialised meets, such as the Grand Prix circuit, the restricted program will usually offer only one event suited to each runner. For example, in one year's program a 1500m race may be offered, while the previous year, the 800m race was featured.

The competitive season is traditionally summer. Athletes wishing to compete overseas, particularly in the opposite hemisphere, may have to organise their training to extend their competition peak, or to peak out of time to their own domestic scene. Interclub meets are held over a day, usually in the afternoon, with some athletes competing in a couple of different races. Some national and international track meets are held over a number of days, often with heats and semi-finals (if needed) on the same day, and the final on the following day. Events at such meets are generally held in the afternoon or evenings, although heats may be scheduled for mornings. Other European and Grand Prix meets involve a single evening's program of selected events, with a straight final between invited runners.

Middle distance events are not long enough to challenge the normal glycogen stores of a well-trained athlete. However, with athletes competing up to 15 to 20 times over a season, especially on the European and Grand Prix circuits where mid-week competitions can entice runners to compete three times in a fortnight, recovery of glycogen stores between races becomes an important issue. In general, the limiting factors during middle distance events result from the build-up of the products of anaerobic metabolism—including hydrogen ions.

Physical characteristics

The physical characteristics of a middle distance runner are quite similar to the long distance runner. Perhaps because middle distance runners are not required to transport their body weight so far, there is less penalty from being slightly heavier—particularly in terms of height or muscularity. However, body-fat levels continue to be low.

Typical physique (elite middle-distance runners)

	Male	Female
Height	176–186cm	168–172cm
Weight	66–74kg	52–64kg
Skinfolds	34–42mm	43–81mm

Common nutrition issues

Many of the nutritional issues of middle distance running are similar to those of long distance running, and only the differences will be discussed in this chapter. From the Distance Running chapter read the first seven points which cover shared features of the training diet. Case histories are provided below to explore Pritikin eating, and gastrointestinal upsets during running—common concerns in both sports.

The following competition nutrition issues are important to the middle distance runner.

Race preparation

Middle distance runners do not need to carbohydrate-load for competition, since their normal glycogen stores will be more than adequate to see them through the event. With 24–36 hours of a high carbohydrate diet combined with rest or tapered training, a runner should be well-prepared for a race. Since races can be run at various times of the day, pre-race plans will vary. A breakfast or brunch-type meal will be suitable for events early in the day. If you are running in an evening race you might like to continue your normal meal plans until lunch and then finish with a light pre-race meal. Read Chapter 4 for more details.

Post-race recovery

Hard running causes muscle fibre damage, and impairs the refilling of glycogen stores. Muscle glycogen storage is aided by providing a rapid supply of carbohydrate to the muscle. The first few hours are an important recovery period for a depleted muscle, and a damaged muscle will also make better use of carbohydrate during the first 6–24 hours than over the next 24–48 hours.

Make use of this window of opportunity to maximise your recovery, especially if you have a busy race calendar. Don't presume that race organisers will look after your needs. Bring your own supplies of fluid and carbohydrate—see Chapter 5 for ideas.

Travelling on the circuit

For those lucky enough to compete on an international circuit, particularly the Grand Prix or European circuit, there are many challenges. Some of these relate to being a travelling athlete, such as living out of suitcases and eating at restaurants. Another challenge comes from the compact competition schedule, which can mean ten big races in as many weeks. This timetable requires a quick recovery and preparation between events, over and over again. Juggling training and racing, not to mention transport schedules, accommodation details and money, can be exhausting. It is often hard to hold your peak—both physically and mentally.

The travelling athlete needs to plan well in advance, and to be aggressive about meeting nutritional goals on the road. An efficient preparation and recovery plan requires careful attention to finding the local carbohydrate foods, and clever scheduling of training between events. Look after immediate post-race recovery by consuming fluid and carbohydrate straight away. Again it may be wise to have your own recovery food supply—don't rely on the post-race party or a late-night meal in a foreign town. Get recovery on the road, and then take part in post-race celebrations—sensibly of course!

PROFILE: STEVE
Runner's trots

At the finish of his last 5000m race, Steve doubled over with stomach cramps. It happened quite often in big events—pain, wind and the threat of diarrhea. Frequent pit-stops used to interrupt evening training, but he had gradually learned to control this by cutting out any afternoon snacks. However, the competition situation was still out of hand, and he feared that he might become another statistic in his running club—those who had to respond to an urgent 'call of nature' during a race.

His sports doctor organised a series of tests of his gastrointestinal function and reported that there were no obvious abnormalities. He suggested that an anti-diarrheal drug might help out in important events, but also that a session with the clinic's sports dietitian might result in a more comprehensive solution.

The dietitian placed the following checklist in front of Steve and invited him to look back over his experiences, searching for any common threads.

Steve considered this list carefully. There was no doubt that nerves played a role—he was often agitated before important races and could almost feel his stomach tie itself up in knots. He also remembered how anxious he had been before hard track sessions in his early days at the running club. There were plenty of problems in those days—

FACTORS POSSIBLY ASSOCIATED WITH RUNNER'S DIARRHEA

- Stress and nerves: do your symptoms get worse when you are nervous or stressed?
- Intensity of running: are symptoms worse during intense running— e.g. racing and training at or above race pace?
- Dehydration: a recent study has reported that dehydration increases the incidence of gastrointestinal complaints. Could this be adding to your problem—especially if you are withholding fluids in the belief that it could be the cause of your distress?
- Intake during exercise: do you consume concentrated drinks or solid foods during exercise? Perhaps you should experiment with a different program of fluid and carbohydrate intake. Does your sports drink contain a significant amount of fructose?
- Timing of pre-exercise meal: have you experimented with changing the time of your last food intake before training or racing?
- Size of pre-exercise meal: have you experimented with changing the amount of food eaten in the pre-exercise meal?
- Type of food in pre-exercise meal: have you experimented with changing the foods in your pre-exercise meal?
- Foods in your everyday diet: have you identified whether certain foods, or large quantities of certain foods, cause gut problems that become worse when you run?

  Examples: too much fibre

  too much lactose (milk, icecream and milk-based products)

  too much fructose (fruits, some sports drinks)

---

just like last year around tax time when work had been incredibly busy and stressful. It didn't seem to matter how fast he ran, but how much he worried about how fast he ran.

Looking further down the list, Steve discounted the contribution of dehydration to his problems, explaining that he was careful to keep his fluid levels topped up. Intake during exercise was also not relevant to Steve as a middle distance runner. Changing the timing and amount of food eaten before exercise to minimise gastrointestinal contents helped to reduce the diarrhea to a certain extent, although this tactic seemed to be self-limiting. He couldn't give up eating altogether and he worried about fuelling up before important races. As for specific foods that caused problems, Steve could remember a couple of bad experiences before races—one with a bowl of untoasted muesli and another with a generous intake of stone fruit straight from the orchard. He'd learnt that too much fruit and too many raw oats didn't agree with him, at least not on the day of a race.

Steve described his usual meal patterns—seemingly a varied and moderate food schedule. The dietitian enquired further about Steve's intake of milk and milk products, and decided that there did not seem to be any evidence of intolerance to lactose (the sugar in milk).

Thus it seemed no single food or dietary factor was at fault. Rather, Steve's nervous state made his gut more active or susceptible to upsets. From the dietary view the dietitian suggested that he trial a program of reducing gastric contents before less important races. It would be hard to simulate race stress in training, so Steve prepared to experiment with some of the early races in the competition calendar.

For the 24–36 hours pre-race he would eat only low-fibre foods, and on the day of the race he would consume a liquid meal supplement as his pre-race meal. A low-lactose product was recommended, such as Exceed Sports Meal, to avoid any complications from a sudden increase in lactose intake. By race time—late afternoon—he should be feeling light and untroubled.

Steve tried this on a couple of occasions and reported an improvement, not just in his gut symptoms, but in his pre-race anxiety levels. Worry about his gut problem was indirectly adding to the problem. The thought that medication provided still another avenue was comforting, but for the moment Steve decided to leave this as something to fall back on. In fact, a stress management course offered at work has since taken his fancy, and he has decided to work on relaxation techniques for pre-race as well as everyday stress relief.

PROFILES: TOM, DICK AND HARRY
Pritikin eating

The late Dr Nathan Pritikin wrote a series of best-selling books in the early 1980s promoting his diet and exercise program, which claimed to reverse coronary heart disease, achieve weight loss, and improve vigour and mental acuity. For endurance athletes he promised improved performance, specifically covered in the 1985 book *Diet for Runners*. At a wider level, he caused a great number of people to rethink their eating habits, and to take greater responsibility for their health and performance. His work has produced off-shoots such as special Pritikin foods, Pritikin-style restaurants, recipe books and health resorts—all devoted to helping achieve a low-fat, low-salt, high 'complex' carbohydrate diet.

While these principles agree with the dietary guidelines for good health, not to mention the optimum training diet for an athlete, Pritikin preached a more extreme message than nutrition experts would have liked. He recommended that fat intake be kept below 10 per cent of total energy, with 10–15 per cent of energy coming from protein and 80 per cent from 'complex' carbohydrates. In addition he advocated that people abstain from any alcohol, caffeine, sugar and added salt, and that vitamin supplements were unnecessary and even dangerous.

Pritikin's message and his writing are emotive—full of dramatic warnings about the health consequences of eating the American or Western diet, and full of inspiring testimonials from people whose lives were enhanced by following his program. And although his program requires quite dramatic and rigid changes to eating and lifestyle habits, self-discipline is a familiar and often-prized characteristic of many athletes.

While the principles of the Pritikin diet can be appraised, it is probably more relevant to appraise an individual's *interpretation* of the diet. There are as many versions of 'Pritikin eating' as there are Pritikin followers, and in many cases, what makes the diet helpful or harmful to an athlete, is how the individual has put theory into practice.

For example, let's say that a year ago, Tom, Dick and Harry joined an athletics club with the goal of racing middle distance in interclub competition. They had all been successful at school athletics, and looked forward not only to the health and fitness benefits from training, but to carving their niche in Master's level competition. They threw themselves into their sport, enthusiastically adopting the training, the equipment, the language and lifestyle of runners. Pritikin's *Diet for Runners* was purchased by each and taken home. Twelve months later, we check their progress.

Tom, a perfectionist, has followed the Pritikin book almost to the letter. The very day the book was purchased he cleaned out his fridge and pantry of all 'illegal' foods. Out went cheese, egg, toasted muesli, icecream, the salt shaker and his after-work beers. He liked the simplicity of the 'seven survival staples' and basically formed his diet around these foods—wholemeal rice, kidney beans, steamed chicken, tomato-vegie sauce, frozen bananas, stewed apples and berries, and cottage cheese 'mock cream'.

Tom's wife was sceptical at first but has now resigned herself to his regimented diet, even if she does call it a 'desert island menu' or 'army rations' behind his back. On the nights that he is late home from training, she lets him cook his own meals. However, on weekends when the family eats together, she pores through recipe books to come up with low-fat, low-sugar meals that they can all eat. Entertaining guests is quite difficult. She misses her gourmet cooking, and complains that Tom's coffee substitutes don't finish off the meal with the same flourish as a brew of freshly ground coffee. They no longer dine out as regularly. Their friends seem a bit reluctant to fiddle around

195

with menus and restaurants to suit Tom or perhaps they have tired of his lectures on how they are poisoning themselves with their eating habits.

Strangely enough, Tom doesn't actually look the picture of health that he promotes. He is pale, gaunt and drawn, having lost seven kilos in the first two months of the diet. To prevent further weight loss he has had to ignore some of the food quotas on the Pritikin maintenance scheme, and increase his intake of fruit and low-fat dairy products. His running is progressing adequately, but he doesn't always feel as 'supercharged' as the book promised.

Dick began his diet as enthusiastically as Tom, and for the first six months matched him rice cake for rice cake. He lost weight, his running progressed and then with an air of complacency he began to lose interest in the dietary regimentation. Some aspects were easy to keep up. He had successfully banished red meat, eggs, dairy products other than skim milk, and most packaged foods from his menu.

But gradually he began to reintroduce some of the foods that he missed. Treats included margarine on his toast, a weekly meal of fish and chips or a well-known burger chain meal, and Homer Hudson Icecream (after all, it comes in a pretty small tub). Everything in moderation, he told himself, so an occasional chocolate nibble wouldn't upset the good work achieved by the rest of his diet. And at the bakery after Sunday's long run, he often slipped a few choc-iced donuts in with the Pritikin buns.

Dick hasn't noticed the creeping weight gain, nor has he connected the occasional fatigue in training with his diet. He still considers himself a Pritikin devotee, and ordered a Pritikin meal at the Club Christmas Dinner.

Harry also believes in moderation, but his interpretation is different to Dick's. He read the Pritikin book, followed by a couple of other books on sports nutrition and nutrition for health, and he noticed that many of Pritikin's ideas overlapped with the views of the dietitians and nutritional scientists. Instead of overturning his diet completely, he decided to work on gradual improvements using some of the Pritikin strategies as a guide.

He began by concentrating on lower-fat meals, replacing fatty meats and dairy products with trimmed and low-fat versions and experimenting with low-fat cooking methods. He reduced the size of his protein serve, leaving room to explore the world of carbohydrate foods. His wife cooked some new dishes from Pritikin recipe books, and used the principles to successfully modify some of the family's favourite recipes as well. Rather than moving along a pathway of increased food restriction, Harry found that his diet was actually expanding.

Harry and his wife eat out regularly, finding that with careful selection from the menu, and occasionally special requests, they can enjoy a healthy meal. However, they often try Pritikin-style restaurants, looking for new ideas for family meals. The transition has been gradual and painless, though Harry can mark his success by his trim figure and his training vigour.

Harry's modified Pritikin diet has an energy spread of 65 per cent carbohydrate, 12 per cent protein and 23 per cent fat, with all nutrients exceeding the recommended dietary intakes. Harry achieves the best of all possible worlds—nutritional goals for training and health, food enjoyment, support from family and friends and a flexible outlook.

Tom's diet, on the other hand, is modelled strictly on the Pritikin principles—with an energy intake ratio of 80 per cent carbohydrate, 8 per cent fat and 12 per cent protein. However, he has trouble meeting total energy needs from his unchanging and bulky food choices, and sometimes even fails to eat enough carbohydrate. With such a limited food range, his diet may also be limited in minerals and other nutrients. He has had to sacrifice the social and enjoyment aspects of food, although he is still too enthusiastic (or obsessed) to notice it.

Interestingly, Dick's diet has the same energy distribution as Harry's diet—about 65 per cent carbohydrate and 25 per cent fat. However, his vitamin and mineral intake is much lower, and has the same potential inadequacies as Tom's. And unlike Harry, who used his extra fat intake to allow him to eat nutritious foods such as reduced-fat dairy products and red meats, and to increase his social flexibility, Dick's dietary lapses have been splurges on high-fat, lower-nutrient value foods. Since his diet is erratic, switching from high-fat days to rigid Pritikin days, he sometimes fails to meet his carbohydrate needs for training or racing. And his weight will generally follow an upward trend as he grows fonder of his treats.

Hopefully, Tom and Dick will update their reading with the new books from the Pritikin Foundation, written by Nathan's son, Robert. The message has moved towards greater moderation and flexibility— practices which are already part of Harry's world. The Pritikins do not have a monopoly on healthy eating for runners or any other athletes, and it is not necessary to follow their diet completely and faithfully. However, we do owe a debt to the Pritikin influence for helping to commercialise and popularise attention to the way we eat.

Jumps, sprints and hurdles

Track and field competition includes a number of events of short duration that rely primarily on the development of power through anaerobic energy. At Olympic-level competition, sprint events include the 100m, 200m and 400m, as well as 4 × 100m and 4 × 400m relay events. Hurdle events are contested over 100m (women), 110m (men) and 400m. The jumps consist of high jump, long jump, triple jump and pole vault.

Competition begins with school athletics, and an amateur athletics career can continue through club competition to international events—the most important being the Olympic Games, the World Championships and the expanding international Grand Prix circuit. While a full program of events is included at major competitions spanning a couple of days, at specialised meets such as Grand Prix competitions there is a selected program which rotates each year.

Sprint running also has a strong professional competition circuit, but in recent years we have seen a dismantling of the traditional barriers between amateur and professional running. A number of former professional runners have crossed to amateur competition to compete in state, national and even international competitions. Similarly, amateur athletes now compete in professional races.

Training

The competitive season usually spans five to six months over the summer period. At the school and club level, many athletes will not train specifically during the off-season. Many are involved with other sports or study, and turn their attention to athletics only a month before the start of the interclub season. During the competition season they may train three or four evenings a week and compete on the weekend.

At the elite level, athletes train all year round with the base or off-season training involving around eleven sessions per week. Since an important component of success in these events is the ability to generate power relative to body weight, off-season training usually involves a considerable commitment to weight training, with about one-third of the total training load being carried in the gym.

The other emphasis of off-season training is the refinement of technique. In addition to running sessions on the track, drill sessions are conducted, for example, to improve leg speed or knee lift. As the competitive season approaches, track work increases to include more intervals and sprints, although technical work and weight training are still maintained.

The pre-competition taper does not need to be as severe as that practised by middle and long distance runners, since sprinters are already training for quality rather than quantity.

Competition

Sprinters and jumpers can compete regularly at weekend or mid-week interclub meets during the season, but usually target three to six events in their calendar as being of greater importance. Athletes wishing to compete overseas must be ready for an additional season, requiring them to work towards double or even triple peaks in their competition preparation.

At the interclub level, athletes often compete in a number of events conducted on the same day of a meet—for example a couple of sprints of different lengths, a jumping event and a relay race. At national and international level, athletes will only be qualified to compete in their major event and perhaps one relay, and events may be spread out over days of a meet. Depending on the size of the field there may be heats, semis and finals in the sprints and hurdles, and a qualifying round leading to the jump finals. The finals may be held on the same or next day to the qualifiers, depending on the length of the meet.

Even though the event itself involves a brief explosion of energy, a competition such as a jump may drag out for many hours while all competitors take their turn. The athlete's fuel stores are not a limiting

199

factor in competition. Muscle ATP and creatine-phosphate systems are the most important energy source for events lasting seconds and are quickly regenerated between bouts. Anaerobic metabolism of carbohydrate plays a greater role during events lasting up to a minute, but muscle glycogen stores are not limiting in events of this duration.

Physical characteristics

Sprinters and jumpers typically share the low body-fat levels of distance runners, since power-to-weight ratio is an important determinant of performance. Muscle mass is typically higher, accounting for some of the higher total body weight. However, these athletes, particularly the jumpers, also tend to be taller than distance runners.

Typical physique (elite sprinters)

	Male	Female
Height	172–185cm	166–181cm
Weight	67–81kg	60–69kg
Skinfold sum	32–52mm	45–88mm

Typical physique (elite jumpers)

	Male	Female
Height	178–190cm	172–183cm
Weight	67–83kg	55–71kg
Skinfold sum	41–73mm	41–73mm

Common nutrition issues

Low body-fat levels

Low body-fat levels usually occur naturally for male athletes, thanks to the cumulative effect of training on the right genetic stock. Some female sprinters and jumpers may have to manipulate their food intake and training to achieve their desired body-fat levels, but there is generally not the same desperation as seen amongst female distance runners. Club-level athletes of both sexes who reduce or cease training over the off-season may need to lose body fat at the beginning of the next competition season. Where help is needed in this regard, read Chapter 3 for sensible and successful methods.

Training nutrition

The goals of training nutrition are discussed in Chapters 1 and 2. Matching carbohydrate intake to training needs is still a priority for sprint-type athletes, although understandably, carbohydrate requirements do not reach the levels of endurance-type athletes.

If you are unsure whether your eating plans meet your nutritional goals, a sports dietitian is the best person to assess your diet and guide you. Even if you think you are eating well, you may learn new ways to expand and enjoy your nutritional horizons—and getting a stamp of approval can be a great confidence boost. See Andrew's story below.

Preparation for competition

Since jumps and sprints will not deplete muscle glycogen stores, increasing these stores by strict carbohydrate loading before a competition, provides no advantages. In fact the gain in body weight from additional glycogen and water is simply extra weight to carry, and is therefore a possible disadvantage to performance—especially in jumps and hurdles where you must lift yourself off the ground as well as propel yourself forward.

The day of competition is best tackled with glycogen stores topped up to their usual resting level. With a high-carbohydrate diet already in place for training needs, glycogen levels can be restored before competition with 24–36 hours of rest or very light training.

Competition day food and fluid

The role of the pre-competition meal is discussed in Chapter 4.4. Choose a high-carbohydrate meal that suits the time of your event and your personal preferences. If you are competing early in the morning, for example in a heat, you may only have time for a light breakfast. Late afternoon and evening events may allow you to eat your everyday breakfast, and even lunch, finishing off with a small snack two to three hours before the event. Experiment in training if an important competition is coming up and you are programmed to compete at an unaccustomed time. Take care to drink plenty of fluids when you are competing in hot weather.

Although your sport technically lasts only seconds or minutes, competition may be a drawn-out affair. Your day can become a number of all-out efforts interspersed with variable amounts of waiting around in between. What should you eat and drink between events, or during events that sprawl out over hours?

Your nutritional goals are to keep hydrated, to maintain blood sugar levels and to feel comfortable—avoiding hunger but not risking the discomfort of a full stomach. How you will do this largely depends on the time interval between events or efforts. See Bernadette's account below for ideas, and like her, be organised to look after your own needs.

Travelling to competition

Track and field athletes, like other athletes, frequently find their competition opportunities interstate or overseas. It requires forward thinking to ensure that competition eating goals can be achieved while away from home—particularly if you are eating at restaurants or hotels. The challenge is considerably greater if you are travelling on a Grand Prix circuit and away from a home base for a long time. It may be appropriate to bring some of your own supplies, particularly if you know that important foods will be missing in a new country, or that catering arrangements at the competition venue are not ideal. The tennis chapter provides some ideas for frequent travellers. Otherwise, think ahead to arrange appropriate food and be assertive in restaurants and hotels when ordering meals (see golf chapter).

PROFILE: BERNADETTE
A long day on the track

Despite being the most promising sprinter in the region, at last year's interschool athletics carnival, Bernadette could only manage one bronze medal. Her program had been busy—heats of the 100m at 9.15, long jump at 12.30pm, final of the 100m at 3.00pm and the 4 × 100m relay at 4.15pm. The morning of the meet was rushed, hurrying to get across town to the sports ground of the host school. Bernadette had forced herself to swallow a mouthful of toast as she raced out the door. She consoled herself that she was too nervous to eat anyway.

By mid-morning, with the 100m heats out of the way, Bernadette was ravenous. She eagerly scoured the sports ground kiosk for something light to eat—after all, the long jump was not far off. The offerings were limited to pies, hot dogs, soft drinks and chocolate bars. She chose the chocolate 'for energy' and made her way to the jump pit. With so many competitors, the long jump stretched out for nearly two hours and as she sat out on the oval awaiting her next jump, Bernadette felt herself become hot and sunburnt. It was hard to concentrate and she jumped badly.

There was barely enough time to warm up for the 100m final, let alone get to the amenities block on the other side of the sports ground to find a tap. She ran, feeling tired from a dull headache. She finished the day with a third place in the relay event—small comfort for the hours of training she had completed over the past three months.

This year the story was quite different, although her training was unchanged and the meet program was almost the same as the previous year. The difference was a careful plan for competition day, organised in collaboration with the school's new athletics coach.

Bernadette rose earlier than usual to allow herself to have a light but relaxed breakfast of cereal and fruit juice before leaving for the sports ground. Not willing to rely on the ground catering, she brought with her a picnic basket of provisions for the day—foods that she had tested out in training over the previous month.

Once the 100m heats were over, Bernadette had a small meal of honey sandwiches and fruit juice, knowing that these would be comfortably digested before the jumps started in two hours' time. Once they called for competitors in this event, she set up a 'camp' on the oval near the jumps pit, bringing with her a drink bottle full of cold sports drink, and a small beach umbrella for shade. Some of the other competitors laughed at the sight but were soon feeling the heat of the midday sun and wishing they had done the same.

With a victory and a personal best in the long jump, Bernadette commenced her warm-up for the 100m final and followed up soon after with her second gold medal for the day. With just over an hour before the relay event there was little time to eat solid food. Feeling a little empty, Bernadette was glad she had a 'ready-to-go' liquid meal supplement on ice in her picnic basket. Refreshed and revitalised, she prepared for the last event and helped her team win a silver medal.

While Bernadette knows that her medals were not just the result of particular food or drinks, her careful organisation did allow her to do justice to her talent and training, rather than see it wasted with careless race-day mistakes.

PROFILE: ANDREW
How does a dietitian assess a diet?

Andrew, a 400m hurdler, is aiming for selection in next year's World Cup athletics team. He has been interested in sports nutrition for the last two years, gleaning information from his coach, from articles in *Runner's World* and from the occasional sports medicine seminar. He has tried to incorporate these ideas into his own diet, although he is not always sure which foods are involved.

Wanting to leave nothing to chance in his running career, Andrew decided to seek professional opinion on whether his diet was as good as he thought it was. He made an appointment to see the sports dietitian at the nearby sports medicine clinic, and his first question was: 'How will you tell if I'm eating well? Will you do a hair analysis or something?'

The dietitian explained that hair analysis, along with practices such as live-cell microscopy and iridology (eye examination), fall into 'alternative' medicine therapy and are not generally regarded as valid measures of nutritional status. The results are open to misinterpretation and do not fit in with the conventional scientific view of nutrition.

A dietitian's major assessment tools are body composition measurements (usually skinfolds), information on lifestyle and exercise patterns, and a careful assessment of food intake patterns. Medical information may be needed, including an examination for signs and symptoms of various nutritional conditions. Sometimes the dietitian will also require biochemical tests in order to confirm a suspicion of a nutritional problem.

Since biochemical tests are expensive and occasionally a nuisance to the subject, they are best undertaken only when the other information points to a possible problem. For example, it is not necessary for athletes to have hundreds of tests to see if they are deficient in one or more of the vitamins or minerals. However, if symptoms of iron deficiency are apparent, and the athlete's usual eating patterns were assessed to fall short of their estimated iron requirements, then it would be useful to take the appropriate blood tests to confirm iron status.

Andrew's nutritional assessment began with a discussion about his sporting commitment—his goals, training and immediate competition plans. The dietitian then asked about his interest in nutrition and any special dietary ideas he was already following. Did he live at home with his family, in an institution, alone, or in a shared house? Who did the shopping and cooking? What else did he have to fit into his day apart from training—university, full-time work or part-time job?

The discussion turned to body weight and body fat, with Andrew explaining that his body weight never fluctuated more than one or two kilograms at any time of the season. He showed her the results of a recent body-fat check, taken by an exercise physiologist accredited in skinfold measurements procedure. His score for the sum of eight skinfold sites was 38mm—very lean.

Next, the dietitian took a dietary history from Andrew, asking him to recount a typical day's eating plan. She led him through the day, noting his activities—particularly training—and typical food habits. It was a gentle but thorough interrogation, drawing a detailed account of the types, timing and quantities of foods and drinks consumed, noting how it was cooked or prepared, and why it was chosen. Special attention was focused on intake before, during and after training.

Weekends were described separately, looking for any changes to usual weekday patterns. Separate questions looked at eating out, takeaways, and other changes to the routines just described, such as differences in summer and winter eating. Competition nutrition was then explored, looking at any special dietary preparation, pre-race meals and tactics for race-day food and fluids.

'What can you learn from this?' Andrew asked. The dietitian explained that, providing Andrew had been able to accurately describe his usual eating patterns, this profile could provide a good general assessment of his success in meeting his nutritional goals. Not only did it look at what was consumed, but it helped to explain some of the reasons why it was chosen. This was important to know, especially when improvements were advised. For example, knowing that food availability or finances stood in the way of a better food choice would call for different tactics than if lack of nutrition knowledge was the only problem.

To complete the picture, Andrew was asked to keep a food diary. The dietitian explained that this was like having a video made of a person's golf swing or swimming stroke. By recording food intake over a period of time, Andrew could step back and look at it objectively, comparing actual intake with what he thought he was eating, and with what he should be eating for optimal performance. Once an accurate description of usual food intake was collected, a computerised dietary analysis could be undertaken, estimating daily intake of kilojoules and nutrients.

Of course, to do justice to the exercise, special skills must be applied both by the athlete and the dietitian. Andrew was instructed in the special tactics of keeping a good food record. Firstly, he needed to make sure that the period of recording reflected his usual eating patterns, and secondly he needed to learn techniques to accurately describe the type and amount of food and drink consumed. He then completed a diary for seven days using these skills, describing a full week of training and an interclub meet.

For her part, the dietitian utilised her special nutrition knowledge and training in using the computer dietary analysis program to estimate Andrew's daily nutrient intake. Although she scrutinised day-to-day variation in intake, most interest was focused on the average daily nutrient intake—a reflection of his typical diet. The results of this are presented in the table below along with a description of typical meal plans and the recommended dietary intakes set for Australians (RDIs).

To evaluate Andrew's diet, the dietitian worked through the checklist of goals of training and competition nutrition.

- Suitability of body weight and body fat: Andrew's daily kilojoule intake is appropriate, maintaining his body fat at a low level to suit his sport.

- Adequacy of nutrient intake: The intake of all nutrients included in the analysis is well in excess of the RDIs even where requirements may be increased by heavy exercise. This is partly due to Andrew's generous energy intake, but is also due to his careful choice of nutritious foods. His enjoyment of a wide food variety is an important asset.

- Recovery: Andrew has done well to make carbohydrate his principal energy source, thus supplying plenty of fuel to restock his muscles after each training session. Although his carbohydrate requirements do not reach the extreme levels of an endurance athlete, training twice a day still places a load on muscle glycogen

205

stores. As well as looking after his total intake of carbohydrate, Andrew cleverly promotes recovery by timing a carbohydrate meal or snack to immediately follow each training session. Fluid replacement is also well looked after.

- Long-term nutrition issues: Andrew's diet meets the dietary guidelines for good health being moderate in fat and salt intake, and focused on a variety of nutritious carbohydrate and fibre foods. As well as looking after his immediate sporting goals, this diet should lessen his risk of nutrition-related diseases in later life.

- Competition nutrition: Andrew uses interclub meets to practise strategies that he will use in more important competition. He has fine-tuned his preparation and pre-race meal and takes his own food when he travels to an interstate meet. It is better to be safe than sorry!

- Social and enjoyment eating: Although Andrew chooses wholesome foods and meals most of the time, he enjoys eating out with friends and occasionally scans the dessert menu for his all-time favourite—sticky date pudding with icecream. Careful but not fanatical, he feels happy with his menu.

A nutrient analysis of a typical day's eating for Andrew (hurdler, 78kg)

Typical food patterns

Training: water or sports drink

Breakfast: straight after training at home
Wholegrain cereal—e.g. Weetbix, Sustain, Just Right
large bowl (75–120g) + 300ml low-fat milk + sliced or canned fruit
2 sl. of wholemeal toast + scrape of marg + jam
250ml fruit juice
Plenty of water

During morning: water, particularly if warm day

Lunch: at work
(Summer) 2 wholemeal rolls with scrape of marg OR mayonnaise (never both)
low-fat filling of chicken, salmon, egg or roast beef
Salad
(Winter) Soup plus 2 rounds jaffles/toasted sandwiches with banana, baked beans,
ham + tomato or 'left-overs' for fillings
Scone or muffin, unbuttered
250ml fruit juice
Piece of fruit

Training after work: water or sports drink

On way home from training: 500ml fruit juice
Plain bagel

Dinner: home, later in evening
Medium serve (120–150g) of lean meat, fish or chicken
Large serve of potatoes, rice, pasta or noodles (2–3 cups)
3–4 other vegetables
(all cooking low-fat)

Dessert: fruit or fruit salad with low-fat yoghurt or
low-fat icecream
1–2/week pudding or cooked dessert
(low-fat cooking)
Water or juice

Average daily energy and nutrient intake

	Andrew's diet	RDI
Energy	13 930kJ	
	3330 Cals	
Protein	145g	
	= 1.8g/kg body weight	1g/kg[a]
Carbohydrate	540g	
	= 6.9g/kg	6–8g/kg[a]
Fat	65g	
Alcohol	—	
Vitamin A (retinol)	2675µg	750µg
Vitamin B1	3.5mg	
(thiamin)	= 0.26mg/1000kJ	0.10mg/1000kJ
Vitamin B2	4.3mg	
(riboflavin)	= 0.32mg/1000kJ	0.15mg/1000kJ
Vitamin B3	69mg	
(niacin equivalents)	= 5.2mg/1000kJ	1.6mg/1000kJ
Vitamin C	525mg	40mg
Iron	33mg	7mg[a]
Calcium	1120mg	800rng
Zinc	20mg	12mg

Energy contribution—general training

Carbohydrate	60%	50–60%[a]
Fat	22%	20–30%
Protein	18%	12–15%

Notes: [a] taken from Chapter 2—estimated requirements for a moderate training load
Sources: Nutrient analysis: NUTTAB 1991–92; Australian Department of Community Services and Health
RDIs: *Recommended Nutrient Intakes, Australia*, NHMRC, 1990.

The dietitian congratulated Andrew, assuring him that his diet met his nutritional goals as a hurdler. All that was left to make his diet ideal was confidence that he was eating well, and enjoyment of his food. Not only would such a diet meet his physiological needs but it would give him a psychological edge. In top competition, Andrew would be well served by these advantages.

Strength sports: Olympic weightlifting, powerlifting and throwing events

In lifting and throwing events, performance is based on the generation of explosive power for a couple of seconds, relying almost completely on anaerobic energy. Muscle ATP and creatine-phosphate are broken down to supply the energy for a single effort, and are quickly re-generated between bursts.

The throwing events include the javelin, shot put, discus and hammer. Athletes compete openly against each other in these field events. Weightlifting is also an Olympic event, with competitors being grouped into categories according to their bodyweight. There are ten body-weight divisions ranging from flyweights (below 52kg) to the super heavyweights (over 110kg). Olympic weightlifters perform two lifts—

the snatch and the clean and jerk. The competition recognises both individual lifts as well the combined total.

Powerlifting is not an Olympic event. It uses the same body weight categories as the weightlifters, and judges the overall weight lifted during three lifts—the bench press, the squat and the dead lift. Although women compete in all lifting and throwing events, powerlifting and weightlifting are dominated by men.

Training

At school or club level, athletes may not train all year round. However, as the level of competition increases, so does the training commitment, both in terms of a year-round program, and in terms of an increased number of training sessions per week. As with endurance sports, it is not possible to maintain a peak for prolonged periods of time, so training is organised into a series of cycles leading to a peak during the competition season, usually summer. Athletes competing internationally may have to peak for two or three competition seasons each year.

The training focus of power athletes varies with the skill demands of their event and the time of the season. Lifters concentrate on weight training, and in the case of Olympic weightlifting (which involves greater technique), flexibility. Throwers divide their training time between weight training, running and speed work, flexibility work and technique training.

In the off-season or in base training, the main focus is on increasing muscle bulk and strength through more general weight training. The number of sets and repetitions undertaken in a weight training session is larger at this time of the season, providing stimulus for muscle hypertrophy and strength gains.

As the competition season approaches, the repetitions are reduced and the weights increased to increase power output. More time is spent fine-tuning the technique of events.

Competition

The throwing events allow three throws per competitor, with the leading eight being given a further three throws to decide the placings. The competition is conducted without a break and may take one or two hours to complete. In large international competitions a qualifying round may be held on the day before the final, with a qualifying distance being set for entry into the final.

The lifting events allow each competitor three attempts at each lift category, with the competitor nominating the weight they wish to lift.

There is a break between each section of lifts. Weigh-in occurs about an hour before the commencement of the competition.

Physical characteristics

Since strength is related to muscle mass, the typical thrower or lifter has a large body weight and muscle mass. In the throwing events, where there are no body weight limits, body-fat levels can also be high—even by community standards. Unless body-fat levels become so high that body shape interferes with technique or general health is at risk, there seems less penalty for throwers to carry extra body fat than for other athletes. The exception is javelin throwers who have a longer run-up prior to throwing, and who need to generate as much speed as possible over this distance. Javelin throwers would be expected to have the lowest body-fat levels amongst throwers.

Lifters, being classified into weight divisions, will show a great variety of body weights and body-fat levels. In the lower weight divisions, maximum strength will be achieved by maximising muscle mass and minimising body-fat levels. Thus a weightlifter in the fly and bantam weight divisions should strive for low body-fat levels. As the weight divisions increase, body-fat levels increase along with muscle mass, although it is not until heavy weight and super heavy weight divisions that lifters can be less concerned about their power to weight ratio. Typical physical characteristics will not be presented as they vary widely between sports and weight divisions.

Common nutrition issues

Bulking-up—how much protein do you need?

In Chapter 3.6 the necessary ingredients for a successful bulking-up program were listed as:

- the right parents
- the right training load
- the right diet.

Hopefully the first two ingredients have been taken care of, and all that stands in the way of you and success is your diet. What constitutes the right diet is a point of difference between strength-training athletes and most sports scientists. The folklore in strength sports is that a high protein intake is required—up to 3g/kg of body weight, or up to 20 per cent of total energy intake, figures that are supported by Eastern bloc scientists.

However, as discussed in Chapter 2.3, the consensus of most sports scientists is that while the protein needs of strength-training athletes are increased, such high levels are not necessary. A figure of around 1.2–1.6g of protein per kilogram of body mass is recommended during times of muscle growth, although adolescents may require 2g/kg during total body growth spurts. Dietary surveys of strength-training athletes generally report that these protein intake levels are easily reached. For example, the weightlifters studied below were estimated to consume an average of nearly 160g of protein per day, supplying 1.8g/kg body weight.

Unfortunately, many strength athletes who chase protein foods end up eating high-fat diets. The diets of the weightlifters below, and diets of other strength athletes reported in studies, contain just on 40 per cent of energy from fat—which contributes neither to protein nor carbohydrate needs. Read Chapters 1 and 2 to reorganise your ideas about the optimum training diet. In particular, Chapter 2.3 lists protein foods that are low-fat or high-carbohydrate, suggesting ways to achieve all nutritional goals simultaneously.

The key issue for bulking up is really energy intake. A high energy intake from nutritious food will also be high in protein, carbohydrate, vitamins and minerals. The account of Paul below illustrates that some athletes still find difficulty in consuming sufficiently high energy intakes. Read how to overcome this by being organised, and planning frequent compact meals and high-energy drinks.

Dietary supplements

Another area of folklore in strength sports is the need for dietary supplements, both to meet physiological nutrient needs and to provide direct ergogenic benefits. Many studies of strength athletes have reported heavy use of various dietary supplements. Read Chapter 6 and the account of the weightlifters below so that you can make up your own mind.

Body fat—optimising power to weight ratios

Although in some lifting and throwing events, a high body-fat level is not a great disadvantage, there are some instances in which athletes could benefit by reducing their body-fat levels. The best example of this is in the low and middle weight divisions of weightlifting and powerlifting, where you will derive an advantage over your opponents by being at the greatest muscle mass (and therefore lowest body-fat level) that is possible for your weight limit—a higher power to weight ratio.

Many lifters do not seem to appreciate this. It is almost a universal practice to compete in a lower weight division than usual training weight, theoretically to compete against smaller and weaker opponents. Like wrestlers and boxers, most lifters lose weight just prior to competition through dehydration and fasting. However, unlike wrestlers, studies of lifters report that many are at higher body-fat levels than necessary for an athlete, and could shed weight through loss of body fat. This could provide a long-term and safer way of making weight than previously practised, as well as ensure that lifters are in their most competitive weight division.

Read Chapters 3.1–3.4 to learn about setting and achieving an ideal body-fat and body-weight level.

Making weight

Read Chapter 3.5 about making weight before competition and the case history in the boxing/wrestling chapter. These warn of the disadvantages and dangers of dehydration and severe food restriction practices. Unlike wrestlers, most lifters may only need to use such drastic measures at three or four major competitions per year. Many compete in higher divisions or not at all outside these occasions. And unlike wrestlers and boxers, lifting events, being brief and power-related, are less likely to be impaired by dehydration and carbohydrate depletion than sparring events.

Nevertheless, there is a healthier and safer way to attack making weight. As explained in Chapter 3.5, you should keep within reach of your competition weight while in training by using sensible weight control techniques. The final kilo(s) can be shed easily in the later stages of preparation. No more saunas, spitting and diuretics!

Lifestyle

Some strength athletes take advantage of their bulk when looking for employment, by taking jobs as 'bouncers' or security guards. On one level this can look like a handy part-time or full-time job, particularly if it is a night-time job that leaves you with your days free for training.

However, there are some traps involved with nocturnal work, particularly in places such as night clubs and discos. It can be difficult to maintain your nutrition goals and a proper sleep pattern. It is also tempting to get caught up in heavy alcohol intake, irregular meals based on convenience foods, and inadequate rest. Beware of throwing away your sporting goals because of this lifestyle.

It will take dedication and good planning to organise training and eating needs around a shift-work schedule. Be focused on your goals—read Chapters 1 and 2 to remind you of the principles of the optimum training diet.

Blood lipids

Several studies of blood lipid measurements of throwers and lifters have reported high levels of cholesterol and triglycerides, and low levels of HDL-cholesterol (the protective form of cholesterol). This indicates an increased risk of coronary heart disease, and is in contrast to studies of endurance athletes that generally show quite low-risk profiles.

There are a number of reasons to explain the poor lipid profiles in these strength athletes. Firstly, some athletes are overweight, with body-fat levels that are obese even by community standards. Many athletes follow high-fat bulking up diets in search of high protein intakes. And finally, the use of anabolic steroids is known to disrupt lipid levels.

If you share any of these characteristics, particularly if you have a family history of heart disease, then a blood lipid screening should be undertaken. Even if the results are okay, you may be persuaded to change to a healthier lifestyle. There are other benefits to performance from following the principles of the optimum training diet in Chapters 1, 2 and 3. Be at your ideal body weight and body-fat level, and eat a high-energy diet that is high in carbohydrate and moderate in fat intake. High protein levels can easily be achieved with such a plan.

PROFILE: PAUL
Get massive? Get organised!

Paul weighed six kilograms less than the shotputter he wanted to be. At the end of last season he set a goal to be 95kg by his next competition, and his efforts over the following four months produced a gain of 1kg. For someone with his dedication this seemed slow progress. He trained hard in the gym, ate constantly and until he was uncomfortably full, and supplemented his diet with amino acids, herbal steroids and weight gain powder. Finally, in desperation, he consulted a sports dietitian.

The dietitian began by reviewing his goals. Had he set himself a realistic target? Had he allowed himself sufficient time to achieve this? Although a shotputter pays less penalty for having a high body-fat level than other athletes, Paul's target was to gain muscle (and strength) rather than pure body weight itself. His coach assured him that he had the body characteristics and a training program to bulk up well. It was theoretically possible to gain 1–2kg of lean body mass per month under circumstances such as this. Could the weak link be his diet?

Paul described a typical day of eating to the dietitian. A late but hearty breakfast of cereal, toast and eggs, followed by a session in the gym. Then it was home for a cooked lunch and off to afternoon lectures at the technical school. A quick dash to training, the evening workout, and home again to an evening of eating. His mother would have dinner number one ready when he walked in the door, and before

213

he went to bed he would sit down to another sitting of left-overs and a weight-gain milkshake. His family marvelled that each of his evening meals totalled more than that of his mother, father and young sister combined.

On weekends, Paul explained that the routine changed due to his job as a 'bouncer' at a night club. Working 9pm–4am on Friday and Saturday nights meant having naps on Friday afternoon and between training sessions on Saturday. Sunday, a non-training day was spent catching up on lost sleep.

The dietitian suggested that Paul should keep a food diary during a typical week. The results came as a surprise to him, but it was quite easy to see his problem when it was written in black and white. Although he spent some parts of his day eating a lot, there were many hours that were quite devoid of food intake. Paul had many activities in his day—school, training, work and sleep. All these turned his attention away from food.

Weekends were a complete upheaval of his lifestyle, breaking up any routine that he might have developed during the week. Not only did he waste good 'eating time' during the day catching up on rest, but during the night at work he took only a couple of sandwiches to eat on his short rest-break, representing almost eight hours of wasted opportunity for energy intake.

The dietitian concluded that Paul's problem was simply an inadequate energy supply to support the maximum gain of muscle mass. She explained that an increased energy intake would bring with it increases in protein and all the other nutrients that were part of building new muscle. The solution was to find more efficient (and nutritious) ways to get kilojoules into his mouth, and the keys were planning and frequency.

Planning meant having foods on hand—for example, taking a supply of foods to eat on the way from school to the gym, and to eat while at work. Instead of taking a couple of rounds of sandwiches to the night club, Paul was advised to take a couple of frenchsticks made up into giant meat, cheese and salad rolls. He could work his way through these, inch by inch, over the night.

High-energy drinks would also be part of the plan. The dietitian explained that there was nothing magical about the weight gain powder that he had bought from the health food shop. The trick was to use it more frequently, even three times a day between meals. She showed him several cheaper options in the form of homemade thickshakes and smoothies, using a less expensive commercial product or skim milk powder to boost the nutritional value. These drinks would be a mainstay on week-ends when Paul was trying to catch up with sleep. A snack and a drink could add up to plenty of kilojoules, and yet be quick and non-bulky so as to conserve his nap time. There is nothing worse than trying to sleep with a huge meal sitting uncomfortably in your stomach.

A meal plan was negotiated for Paul that consistently achieved six meals a day: breakfast as soon as he woke up, to be followed by a mid-morning milkshake before he left for training. Home for lunch, as before, but a couple of rolls and a thermos of his milk drink would accompany him to school for a snack between classes. In the evening he was to have two meals, one being the family dinner and the other a lighter snack and a high-energy fruit smoothie. This way he went to bed feeling less bloated, and ready for breakfast as soon as he woke up. A different, but nevertheless planned, routine was organised for weekends.

With his energy intake spread more evenly throughout the day, Paul was able to increase his total intake by almost 30 per cent. This kick-started his muscle gain program within a fortnight, and Paul achieved his target weight within six months. Since the herbal steroid and amino acid supplements did not seem to be part of the achievement, he was quite happy to abandon them along the way.

Paul found that his new body weight could only be maintained with dedication to his meal routine. For example, in celebrating the end of exams at school, he led a rather nomadic life for a fortnight—going out with friends at night and sleeping in later in the mornings. The scales showed a 2kg loss and reinforced the lesson that gains are made through a carefully planned diet rather than haphazard eating. Paul now appreciates that while he wants to continue his shotput career, he needs to treat his food intake with the same rigour and organisation that he shows in his training sessions.

PROFILE
Food or pills?

In 1984 an extensive dietary study was carried out on a group of national and international-level Australian Olympic weightlifters. The nineteen lifters were interviewed about their typical eating patterns and kept careful food diaries of a week's food and fluid intake. One of the most interesting features was the use of dietary supplements, with all lifters reporting daily use of supplements—often five or six different products at a time.

In order of popularity, supplements included multivitamin and B-vitamin formulas (used by 16 lifters), vitamin C (13 lifters), protein powders, liquids or tablets (12 lifters), calcium (12 lifters), 'vitamin' B15 (7 lifters), and herbal preparations including comfrey, ginseng and chlorophyll (7 lifters). Vitamin E supplements were taken by 6 lifters, electrolyte drinks or potassium tablets by 4 lifters, vitamin B12 (3 lifters), minerals such as iron or magnesium (2 lifters), amino acids (2 lifters), ATP powder (1 lifter) and ATP injections (1 lifter).

The reasons given for the use of these supplements were:

- that training increases nutritional requirements beyond the scope of dietary sources
- that certain supplements can directly improve training or competition performance.

The lifters quoted other lifters and health food shops as their major source of nutrition information, and those who had travelled to international competition were eager to swap secrets and supplements with Eastern Bloc athletes. This even extended to taking supplements with labels written in Russian and Bulgarian. Not knowing exactly what the contents were was no deterrent!

What can be said about these supplement practices? The first charge to be explored is that food cannot supply adequate nutrient levels for a weightlifter. The table below summarises the group average daily intake of selected vitamins and minerals, comparing intake from food with the intake supplied by supplements. To put this in perspective the recommended dietary intakes (RDIs) are presented.

Nutrient intake from food and supplements compared in a group of 19 weightlifters

Nutrient	Number using supplements	Mean daily intake Supplements	Food	RDI
Vitamin A	10	2060µg	2002µg	750µg
Vitamin B1 (thiamin)	15	93mg	2.1mg	1.5mg
Vitamin B2 (riboflavin)	15	53mg	3.5mg	2.3mg
Vitamin B3 (niacin equiv.)	15	122mg	52.5mg	24mg
Vitamin C	16	1945mg	199mg	40mg
Iron	10	8.0mg	22.9mg	7mg
Calcium	15	473mg	1567mg	800mg

Average daily intakes of protein and energy
Total intake of energy: 15 200kJ/day (3640 Cal)
Contribution from supplements: 200kJ/day (48 Cal)

Total intake of protein: 156g/day (= 1.8g/kg body weight)
Contribution from supplements: 6g/day

The lack of confidence in food seems unfounded according to these results. Although most weightlifters chose a high-fat diet, the vitamin and mineral intakes from food sources exceeded the RDIs. Imagine what the results would look like if more nutritious lower-fat, higher carbohydrate diets were in place! The use of vitamin and mineral supplements provides a very haphazard nutrient intake profile. In some cases (e.g. thiamin and vitamin C) supplement intake provided nutrient levels far in excess of the RDIs. On the other hand, the intake of calcium and iron from supplements was small compared to that from food sources. And supplements were an insignificant source of energy and protein intake in this group. Hopefully a better appreciation of nutrient levels in food would help the weightlifters to re-think the need for protein, vitamin and mineral supplements. If nothing else, money could be saved on the supplements that provide an irrelevant nutrient supply.

Many of the other supplements used by these lifters fall into the nutritional ergogenic aid category (see Chapter 6), and into limbo with regard to proof that they work. In most cases there is no support for the assertion that such supplements can assist training and competition performance, despite the 'scientific' theories put forward for some supplements. For example, it sounds clever to take ATP—getting right to the business end of the muscle's energy production. However, it is by no means certain that ATP, eaten or injected will make its way inside the muscle cell to where it is needed—in fact it seems highly unlikely. Therefore such supplements are unlikely to have a physiological effect.

Perhaps the major point of interest in the ergogenic aid supplements is to see how fashion changes. In 1984, the big sellers were B15 and herbal preparations. In the 1990s these have been replaced by amino acids, chromium picolinate and Frac. Even without the verdict of scientific trials, what does the swing in (sports) public opinion tell us?

While these lifters may have enjoyed a psychological boost from their use of supplements, it is not possible to tell whether this translated into better performances. It would be interesting to see whether the weightlifters would change these practices, if their information sources were sports scientists and nutritionists, rather than health food shops, 'muscle magazines' and each other.

Bodybuilding

Bodybuilders are primarily concerned not with strength or other parameters of athletic prowess, but with their physique. Muscular definition, balanced development of different body parts and symmetry of development are the criteria upon which bodybuilding competitions are judged. Not all bodybuilders compete, however. Many simply enjoy the challenge of improving their physique and appearance through training and diet.

Training

The year of a competitive bodybuilder is broken into three phases. In the off-season, training is targeted at bulking up, or increasing overall muscle size. The result is that most bodybuilders are well over competition weight, and body-fat levels can be relatively high. As the competition season approaches, bodybuilders begin to 'cut up'—aiming to lose body fat in order to increase muscle definition without losing muscle mass or size. Finally, in the days or week prior to competition, bodybuilders undertake special methods to achieve cosmetic changes that will make their bodies appear 'pumped', with clearly defined muscularity and vascularity. Bodybuilders who do not take part in competitions may simply train to bulk up.

The exact training methods used by bodybuilders are diverse and dramatic, and there are as many enthusiastically recommended programs as there are articles in bodybuilding magazines. In general, both elite and recreational bodybuilders can spend many hours in the gym each day, usually following 'split routines' where different parts of the body are trained at different sessions. Training typically involves three to five exercises for each of the six major muscle groups (chest, back, arms, legs, shoulders and abdomen). Each exercise normally comprises three to six sets of lifts or repetitions. Bodybuilders usually perform a greater number of repetitions per set (6–15) than do power and weight lifters (1–5) since this provides for greater muscular hypertrophy.

In the cutting-up phase many bodybuilders incorporate more aerobic exercise into their programs to help reduce body-fat levels.

Competition

There are three stages of judging involved in bodybuilding competitions: the structural round in which all competitors are judged on stage together while in relaxed pose, the individual posing routine in which competitors display their own routine of poses lasting about two minutes, and the compulsory poses which are judged comparatively.

Depending on the number of age or weight divisions, judging can take six hours or more.

Physical characteristics

The physical characteristics of bodybuilders are striking and well-known—almost needing no explanation. Bodybuilders have a large total body weight due to pronounced muscle development. Depending on the time of the year, body fat levels can vary from normal–high during the bulking-up phase, to minimum skinfold sums during the competition phase.

Other comments

The world of bodybuilding is flamboyant. Bodybuilders have a unique lifestyle and beliefs that are often viewed as bizarre and even unattractive by those outside the sport. They are a close-knit group, with information being spread pervasively and persuasively through their circles, by word of mouth and through bodybuilding magazines. Perhaps the most well-known of these is Joe Weider's *Muscle and Fitness* magazine, which claims a readership of over eight million people, worldwide. Understandably, those at the top of the empire have great power to shape the beliefs, as well as the muscles, of those below.

Most of the 'science' of bodybuilding comes from other body-builders —champions maybe, but non-scientists nevertheless. While there are a few bodybuilders or followers of the sport with legitimate scientific qualifications, there are others who quote qualifications that are at best unorthodox and unrecognised. Thus, many bizarre and occasionally dangerous practices have been used and promoted in bodybuilding, including the use of drugs.

Probably more than any other sport, bodybuilding has placed emphasis on the role of nutrition in performance and bodybuilders are unique in their fastidious attention to food. However, not all the nutrition philosophies—and there are as many as there are training philosophies—agree with established scientific views.

It is hard to compete against the typical bodybuilder's nutritional beliefs and practices. For a start, it is hard to compete against the powerful communication and merchandising networks, and the testimonials of the champions. And, sadly, it is sometimes hard to measure up against the undeniable results that can be gained through the use of anabolic steroids and other drugs, or other unsafe practices. Healthy or safe dietary practices which are offered as an alternative are at a clear disadvantage if they cannot match these results. Nevertheless, it is hoped that with time and with access to scientific and health-minded nutrition information, at least some bodybuilders will make the transition.

Common nutrition issues

Who is a nutrition expert?

Almost every bodybuilding magazine carries a number of articles in which top competitors share their dietary and training secrets. Other articles are written by people with 'scientific' qualifications which do not fit within the mainstream academic program. Who should you listen to? How do you know who the real experts are?

Most people, athletes or otherwise, give each other advice or comments about their diets, and it has been suggested that some nutrition 'experts' have as their only qualification the fact that they have eaten food almost every day of their lives. The ideal nutrition advice is something that has been rigorously studied and tested, and the results scrutinised by a variety of objective scientists. And it will probably be found to complement the general nutrition guidelines for health and athletic performance, rather than oppose them.

In Chapter 5 the basis of scientific proof was discussed in relation to dietary supplements. This theme can be extended to all nutrition issues. Testimonials from successful athletes and scientific theories can provide the material for ideas to be tested. However, until the idea is adequately tested, no judgement can or should be made. Many of the dietary philosophies of bodybuilders remain on the drawing board, awaiting attention. Interestingly, they can't all work, since some ideas flatly contradict others.

What are the problems with using practices that are not yet tested and approved? In some cases, there may be no major disadvantages and even some benefits—the practice may actually work, you may get a psychological edge from your belief in it, or you may simply enjoy the feeling of being part of the scene. On the other hand, some dietary practices are expensive, and some are unhealthy—even dangerous.

When trying to evaluate dietary advice or the credentials of the nutrition expert promoting it, the checklist below may be useful. Read all the articles in your bodybuilding magazine with interest, but learn to distinguish the columns that carry more weighty material. You'll probably notice that some magazines are now regularly including information from more legitimate sources.

CHECKLIST TO EVALUATE DIETARY ADVICE

- What recognised qualifications does the nutrition 'expert' have? Check with a sports dietitian if you are unsure.
- Does it promise results that are too good to be true? They probably are!
- Is the advice based only on an idea or case histories—regardless of which famous athlete swears by the advice or how 'scientific' the theory sounds?
- Have the ideas been scientifically tested and reported in a reputable journal? (See the profile at the end of the chapter.) These journals accept only those studies that have been adequately conducted and the results handled by proper statistical methods. Check with a sports dietitian if you're not sure.
- Is the advice generally compatible with healthy nutrition guidelines, or is the advice supported by recognised nutrition authorities? Again, check with a sports dietitian.
- Is anyone going to make money from this advice?

Nutritional ergogenic aids

Studies of bodybuilders have reported that, despite nutrient intake from food being up to 400 per cent of the recommended dietary intake levels, there is widespread use of dietary supplements. Numerous supplements are taken in large doses, sometimes with nutrient intakes reaching levels that are regarded as toxic. Other supplements do not provide nutrients, but large doses of strange and rare substances found in food.

Apart from the advice or observation of everyone else in the gym, the best support for supplements comes from bodybuilding magazines.

Magazines can carry up to 30 pages of advertisements in each edition, not to mention unpaid testimonials and articles which all proclaim the virtues of various products—from traditional favourites such as weight gain powders and vitamins to the latest trends in amino acids, carnitine and Frac. The supplements promise a variety of wonderful achievements—some claiming to help you 'get massive', others to promote fat mobilisation and loss to help you 'get ripped', and still others to give you more energy in training. Some supplements are directly promoted as an alternative to steroids, dramatically claiming that they will pass all drug tests.

It should come as no surprise that the supplement industry makes millions of dollars from bodybuilders—and makes millions of dollars *for* some bodybuilders. Interestingly, a huge supplement range is marketed by the same person who owns and publishes the largest-selling bodybuilding magazines. Cynics might see the magazine almost as a manufacturer's catalogue, although the advertisements are more powerful and emotive than the junkmail that you normally get in your letterbox.

Chapter 6 gives the low-down on supplements, with most bodybuilding supplements falling into the nutritional ergogenic aid group. The bottom line is that we don't know whether such supplements work, since they have not been adequately tested. By the same token, we can't be sure that they do not work. Whether you experiment for yourself is an individual decision, but realise that you may be paying to be a guinea pig in an uncontrolled experiment.

Meanwhile, there are *some* dietary supplements that can be of proven help to bodybuilders. Bulking up often requires a bodybuilder to consume more food energy than is practical or comfortable. High-energy, nutritious fluids can be a useful way to boost energy intake—see Chapter 3.6. Although you can make your own low-fat milk shakes and smoothies, supplements such as weight-gain powders can help to fortify a drink with extra kilojoules and nutrients. Note that you do not need a high-protein formula, but rather a high-carbohydrate complete nutrition formula.

If you check the price of bodybuilding supplements, you will find that the cheapest commercial supplements are pharmaceutical products such as Sustagen Sport, Gator-Pro or Exceed Sports Meal. They are also formulated with a balanced nutrient profile that mimics recommended dietary intakes, rather than 'special' ingredients such as gamma-oryzanol, free-form amino acids and carnitine.

Bulking-up

While there are many variations on a theme, the typical bodybuilder undertakes a rigid and quite unusual dietary pattern during the bulking-up phase of training. Typically, bodybuilders believe in high-energy, high-protein diets. The traditional high-protein diet is also high in fat, since these nutrients are often found simultaneously in foods. However, in recent years the role of carbohydrate as a muscle fuel has been recognised. Thus the contemporary bodybuilding diet is now high in protein, moderate-to-high in carbohydrate and low in fat. Some competitors make these ratios more extreme.

It is not just the principles of the diet that can be rigid. Many bodybuilders set themselves a narrow range of foods, and an unchanging meal plan to meet their dietary targets. Many make meals from large quantities of a few chosen foods—particularly low-fat, high-protein types and repeat the same meal plan day after day. In fact, you can often pick a bodybuilder not just from their muscle-bound appearance, but from the contents of their shopping trolleys. Look for lots of chicken breasts, cans of tuna (water-packed), cartons of eggs (they eat only the whites) and skim milk powder. For carbohydrates, rice cakes, rice and pasta are popular.

The high-energy diet is eaten in a series of meals, often six to eight over the day. This is a practical way to ensure that large energy intakes are managed, and may also maximise the metabolic gains from food. See Chapter 2.7 for more details. However this philosophy can also be taken to extremes. There are reports of bodybuilders who set the alarm clock to go off every three hours during the night, allowing them to get up for another 'food fix'. Don't forget the importance of adequate and restful sleep!

Chapter 3.6 summarises the principles of gaining muscle mass: the right parents, the right training, and a diet that supplies adequate energy and all other nutrients. Protein requirements for maximum muscle gain have long been debated, with the current consensus being that they are likely to be elevated above normal (sedentary) requirements, but still within the range of a high-energy diet of normal protein-to-energy ratio.

Nutrition experts argue that even the highest protein intake that can be justified scientifically, that is 1.5–2.0g/kg of body weight per day, can be achieved in a high-energy diet. However, studies of bodybuilders report that actual intakes are often twice as high, with protein being elevated to more than 20 per cent of total energy intake. Because many bodybuilders are unable to translate food into nutrients, they may be unaware of their total protein loads. Some will even add a high-protein supplement to a diet that already exceeds the level of possible protein utilisation.

While bodybuilders are to be congratulated on their dietary concern and motivation, there are perhaps three areas for improvement of present typical meal plans:

- Protein intakes need not be as high as often achieved.
- By virtue of high-energy intakes and the nutritious choice of foods, the vitamin and mineral intakes of most bodybuilders are also expected to exceed the recommended dietary intake levels. With

223

this confidence, some bodybuilders may re-think their use of vitamin supplements.

- There are many ways of choosing and enjoying foods to achieve a healthy dietary intake. Most bodybuilders could enjoy a greater range and flexibility with foods, including greater variety and versatility at meals.

Cutting-up

The length and severity of the cutting-up phase will vary between bodybuilders. Some competitors remain in shape during the bulking-up phase and leave adequate time before competition for a consistent and moderate rate of body-fat loss (0.5–1.0kg/week). Other body-builders set out to lose large amounts of body fat in a short time (2kg/week)—perhaps because they have budgeted only a short contest preparation period, or because they believe that dramatic weight loss will achieve a more dramatic 'ripped' or 'shredded' appearance. Unfortunately, rapid weight loss has the disadvantage of sacrificing muscle mass.

Typically, body-fat loss is achieved by increased aerobic exercise and restriction of dietary energy. Some bodybuilders cut back on the total quantity of all foods, while others severely restrict carbohydrate intake. In any case, the typical cutting-up diet is even more regimented and inflexible than the bulking-up phase. Certain supplements are promoted as 'fat burners'—particularly carnitine—and may be added to the weight loss diet.

For a guide to safe and healthy body-fat loss, which aims to preserve total nutritional goals and minimise loss of muscle mass, read Chapter 3.3. It is both unnecessary and a disadvantage to become too rigid and restrictive in dietary energy intake and variety.

The pre-competition diet

A bodybuilder aims to enter the contest with his or her muscles looking 'pumped' and fully defined, with clear detail of the striations and vascularity in each muscle. A number of techniques are used to achieve the last fine-tuning. Many bodybuilders carbo-load over the last week, depleting their muscles of carbohydrate over the first part of the week, and switching to a high-carbohydrate diet over the last couple of days. The aim is to store extra glycogen (and water) in the muscles, making them look 'pumped' and massive. There are many stories of when and how to achieve loading, without overshooting the mark, and making the muscles look too smooth.

Fluid and electrolyte balance is also manipulated in the last couple of days, with the aim of dehydrating the skin and making it appear tightly stretched over the muscles. Techniques include fluid and sodium restriction, and the use of diuretics and potassium supplements. Many of these practices are harmful and there have been stories of bodybuilders collapsing on stage due to dehydration and electrolyte imbalances—for example, Albert Beckles in 1988.

The best advice is to experiment with your pre-contest strategies to find a loading practice that puts you at your best—not just in appearance but in overall health. Avoid techniques that are severe and drug-based.

Post-competition blow-out

After months of a strict and restricted diet, many bodybuilders see the post-competition phase as a time for 'letting their hair down'. Many spend the next days or weeks bingeing on food and sometimes alcohol. For example, one case study noted the following menu for a female bodybuilder on the day after a competition: 2 brownies, 2 cups milk, 2 donuts, 375ml beer, 1 icecream, 2 cups of potato chips, 30g dip, 1 bacon/egg/cheese burger, 1 Big Mac, 1 cup hashbrowns, 4 biscuits, 1 litre of soft drink, 60g barbecue ribs, 9 scallops, 1 cup steamed shrimp, 4 crab legs, 1/2 cup seafood casserole, 1/2 cup corn, 1 piece pineapple cake, 1 piece strawberry shortcake, 1 piece of cheesecake. This is a big change from a diet based on fruit, cottage cheese and rice cakes!

Post-competition bingeing obviously leads to a big jump in fat and kilojoule intake. Depending on the duration of the binge, the nutritional implications could include large gains in body fat, stomach and gut upsets, and nutrient inadequacies. Bodybuilders often jump from one limited bunch of foods (high nutrient, low fat) to another limited bunch of foods (low nutrient, high fat). Going from one extreme to another is not good for body or soul—by the time the bodybuilder gets back to the straight and narrow, they may have a legacy of guilt and a number of unwanted kilograms to get over. In the long run, the extremist never learns the pleasures of eating well and feeling good about eating. Take a more balanced approach to all phases of the season—enjoy a more liberal but well-chosen training diet, follow a food plan that will look after your real competition needs (rather than following the fads that take the fancy of other bodybuilders) and, enjoy some time-out after it's over. Time-out may mean indulging yourself with some different foods and some different activities—but at a level that you can enjoy rather than regret later.

Blood cholesterol levels

Studies of bodybuilders have reported blood cholesterol and triglyceride levels that are unfavourable in terms of heart disease risk. Low levels of HDL-cholesterol—the 'good' cholesterol that helps to protect against coronary heart disease—are a particular concern.

In the case of old-fashioned bodybuilders, an unfavourable blood-lipid profile may be partly explained by a high-fat intake. However, the major cause of such disturbed cholesterol levels is steroid abuse, perhaps sentencing long-term users to a greater risk of heart disease. Fortunately, the abnormal cholesterol levels appear to be quickly reversed when steroids are discontinued.

PROFILES
Exploring the myths

Although well-meaning advice is given by one bodybuilder to another, there are many myths and misconceptions spread through bodybuilding circles.

Dear Muscle-Magazine,
    I am the original 10 stone weakling—65kg to be exact. I'm tired of everyone laughing at my puny body and kicking sand in my face at the beach, so I've decided to do something about it once and for all. I joined Silver's Gym last month and got a weight training program written for me. Can you advise me what sort of diet I need to help me to bulk up.
    Ronald

Dear Ronald,
    Congratulations on joining the sport of bodybuilding. I used to be just like you, so take heart. Of course it has taken me many years to build up to this level, but you are right about the importance of diet. Superior nutrition was my secret weapon in winning the Mr World title last year—it's the only way to push yourself over the edge.
    I have refined this plan over a number of years and stick closely to it when I am bulking up. A typical day's menu is:

Breakfast: 10 egg whites + 1 egg yolk, made into an omelette
              100g oats + 50g raisins + cup skim milk
Meal 2: (after training) 200g tin of tuna (water packed)
              200g boiled rice
              cup of broccoli
Lunch: 250g lean steak
        1 cup cooked pasta
Meal 4: 250g lean steak
        100g boiled rice
Dinner: 200g tin of tuna (water packed)
        100g boiled rice
Meal 6: 10 egg whites cooked into omelette
        2 rice cakes

I change this round by having different green vegies or salad each day, and by interchanging chicken breasts and the lean steak. This diet is extremely low in fat and high in protein and carbs. Good luck with your training,
    Mr World

Comment   Photos of Mr World attest that he is indeed massive, with the identifiable factors in his success being years of hard training and

226

the right genetic potential. Mr World's diet will not achieve a similar success for Ronald in the absence of these ingredients. It is difficult to predict how much diet has contributed to Mr World's physique. Certainly, a diet that is inadequate in energy, carbohydrate, protein or any of the vitamins and minerals involved in growth and exercise metabolism, will hold back the progress and results of training. But can extra protein and vitamins increase muscle mass? Current scientific knowledge says no.

An analysis of Mr World's typical daily intake reveals the following estimations: 14 060kJ (3355 Cals), 350g of protein, 330g of carbohydrate, and 77g of fat. Protein intake provides over 40 per cent of his total energy intake—slightly more than his carbohydrate intake. Mr World weighs in at 100kg, giving him a protein intake of about 3.5g/kg body weight. If Ron were to eat the same diet, he would achieve a protein intake exceeding 5g/kg/day. Conventional science says that it is not possible to utilise such high protein intakes. At best, this protein becomes an expensive energy source. At worst, there may be health penalties to pay for chronic intakes of such high protein loads.

Read Chapters 1 and 2 to find the principles and food aspects of healthy training nutrition. Mr World's diet is not really as high in carbohydrates as he imagines—less than 3.5g/kg/day to fuel his workouts. He might be surprised to find that swapping some of his protein budget for carbohydrate energy will increase his training performance. Above all, it is unnecessary to maintain such a rigidness with meal choices, and to eat the same thing day in, day out. Variety adds nutritional depth as well as food enjoyment.

Dear Muscle-Magazine,
Can you give me some tips on good nutrition for the intermediate bodybuilder? I want to be a champion like Arnold someday,
Larry

Dear Larry,
The best advice I can give you about diet is to keep it simple and natural. This way you won't overload your body's digestive system, and will get full value from the food you eat. Have many small meals rather than large meals. Eat food raw and whole as much as possible—for example, raw vegetables and salad rather than cooked vegetables, whole meat rather than minced meat, whole fruit rather than juices.
Don't eat too many foods at the one time. It is better to have two or three different foods at a meal and another three at your next meal than to bombard your intestines with too many foods all at once. The worst combinations are protein foods mixed with acidic foods such as oranges, and protein mixed with carbohydrate foods. Digestive enzyme supplements are an excellent aid if you have already overstrained your system. Regards,
Mr Galaxy

Comment The human body has remarkable powers of adaptation, otherwise there would be no rewards from training. Your digestive system is quite sophisticated and well-equipped to handle the challenges of a varied diet. Think back to your school biology lessons—you may remember that your small intestines work like a long conveyor belt. Food is passed down its length, firstly being broken down to its smallest molecules, and then passing to the special site programmed to absorb particular nutrients. Everything is well organised—various sections are specialised for each duty, so there is no worry about overloading or overstressing the system. Additional 'digestive enzymes' are not needed, and anyway the popular supplements marketed for this purpose are unlikely to pass through the acidic stomach environment without being inactivated.

In Chapter 1 the benefits of food variety were discussed, including the advantages of mixing and matching foods at the same meal. In general, nutrients and food factors interact to improve the nutritional quality of the meal. Rather than follow Mr Galaxy's advice, Larry should aim to include many different foods in each meal. This makes for more interesting and enjoyable eating as well. Despite the publicity, there is *no* danger in combining protein and carbohydrate—it already happens inside foods such as bread, pasta and rice. Concern over acidic foods is also unfounded since the acid content of the stomach far outstrips any dietary source.

In general, foods that are minimally processed or cooked will maintain their maximum nutrient value. Thus it is good to include foods that can be eaten raw or in as natural a state as possible. However, it is not necessary or even helpful to insist that all foods are left raw and whole. There are many ways to prepare and cook foods that minimise the loss of nutritional value or the addition of less desirable compounds such as fat, sugar or salt. Practise moderation and flexibility in all aspects of nutrition.

Dear Muscle-Magazine,
    Help! I'm confused. First I read that bodybuilders should eat high protein diets, then I read that they should eat plenty of carbs. What's the correct advice?
    Laura

Dear Laura,
    Yes, there is a lot of conflicting information about this area of nutrition. My own experiments have allowed me to work out a solution—at least one that works for me. I favour the high protein look since that helps me to look hard and chiselled. However, when I say high protein I don't mean fish and chicken. I mean beef—two to three pounds a day.
    Beef is meat muscle. It's already full of glycogen, so you don't have to eat much other carbohydrate. Besides, the glycogen is already processed, so it doesn't need to go through digestion and absorption. It can go straight to your muscles.
    I have used this approach in my training this year and the results of the Ms Globe contest speak for themselves.
    Ms Globe

Comment   As interesting as Ms Globe's theories sound, they contradict both food composition information and the laws of human physiology. There is negligible carbohydrate in meat, whether beef, chicken or fish. Meat is technically animal muscle, accounting for its high protein content. However, muscle glycogen stores do not account for a great mass of carbohydrate—at least not in the quantity of meat that you are likely to eat at the one time. Additionally, most of the glycogen is broken down in the slaughtering process.

Even if glycogen could be consumed in appreciable amounts, it would have to go through the same digestion processes as any carbohydrate in food. You body will not discriminate and send it to reform in the muscle either. It will simply add to the body carbohydrate pool, and its fate will be decided according to the body's immediate requirements.

If you are still confused about the body's requirements for protein and carbohydrate, go back to Chapter 2 (sections 2.2 and 2.3). A high-energy diet will be high in all nutrients, but for athletes in heavy training the most important fuel source is dietary carbohydrate.

Dear Muscle-Magazine,

I have been training for three years and plan to enter competition soon. I have very little spare money and want to know if it is possible to get to the top without taking supplements. Also, what supplements are the best value?

David

Dear David

I sympathise with you. The more advanced you become, the more important and significant is the role of nutrition. The blasting training sessions typical of champion bodybuilders place a great stress on normal nutrition stores. Without adequate nutrients you will not get maximal gains. Supplements are your best health insurance, since they will provide all the nutrients needed in quantities not possible through ordinary foods. My own program includes Smash Weight Gain powder, amino acids, megaformula multivitamins, gamma-oryzanol and inosine. When cutting up I use extra doses of carnitine.

If you are on a tight budget, go for the Smash Weight Gain formula and a multivitamin product. When taken as directed and in conjunction with your workouts, it can help you to gain up to a pound a day. I use it in my training to bulk up quickly. You can do the same.

Mr International

Comment   Read about supplements in Chapter 6! It is not possible to gain a pound of muscle—or even fat—each day. Set your sights on a more realistic goal. The Smash Weight Gain formula, being a high-energy nutritious drink, can help you to boost energy intake while on a bulking up program (see Chapter 3.6), but there are less expensive ways to achieve the same result. The least expensive commercial supplements of this type are the pharmaceutical brands such as Sustagen Sport, Gator-Pro and Exceed Sports Meal. However, you can make a cheaper version yourself by blending together skim milk plus extra skim milk powder, banana or other fruit, and some ice cubes.

Optional extras are low-fat yoghurt or low-fat icecream.

PROFILE
Amazing results in muscle growth? Reading a 'scientific study' critically

An article in a recent edition of a popular magazine claimed to provide scientific proof that a combined supplement and training program promoted accelerated muscle gains—approximating those normally only associated with drug programs. The article was written in the style of a scientific report and carried the credentials of a well-known bodybuilding expert who has extensive qualifications in education. Unfortunately, the scientific jargon used in this article merely disguised a 'study' with many flaws.

Details of the 'study' described in the article are summarised below:

- 5 bodybuilders, chosen at random, followed a 12-week trial in which they undertook exercise program X and supplement program Y. Both programs were said to be standardised; however no details were supplied in the report.

- Body weights and body girths were measured at regular intervals during the 12-week trial, and photographs were taken.

- At the end of 12 weeks, 'all subjects exhibited significant gains in body part measurements' and 4 out of 5 had increased body weight. Selected results from individual subjects were given, representing the maximum gain in weight or girth at a particular site. Results included a weight gain of 10.5kg, a chest gain of 14cm, and a 14cm loss at the waist.

- The report concluded that it is 'clear that Supplement Y can be used in conjunction with specialised exercise programs to achieve maximum muscle gain'.

How could a bodybuilder fail to be impressed—both by the individual results quoted and by the 'scientific' flavour of the article? But what about a bodybuilder with some knowledge of science and of the tools of rigorous scientific investigation? Hopefully they would make the following critical comments:

- A muscle-building magazine is not a peer-reviewed journal with a respected scientific reputation. Of course, many lay magazines do carry reports of scientific studies. In many situations studies which have been published through a suitable critical review process will then be rewritten for a lay publication. This is to be encouraged since it helps to spread the news to athletes who might make best use of the results, in a language they understand and with practical guidelines to boot! It may be necessary to simplify the description of the study methods and the statistical analysis of results. However, the original publication should be cited so that these details can be followed up for explanation or verification. Our present article does not appear to have been published in the scientific literature, so it appears to have escaped the opportunity for proper scrutiny by experts.

• Since the article contains only a brief description of the 'study' design, some important information is lacking. It is possible that some of the issues discussed below were addressed in the study but were omitted from the report. However (and unfortunately), it is probable that these issues were not properly handled in the first place. Current weaknesses of the study design and the report include:

1 There are no details of the characteristics of the subjects (age, sex, bodybuilding background and prior level of training). Were these controlled for, since they will have an effect on the way that a subject responds to a treatment?

2 There appears to be no control of other factors that may influence muscle or weight gain (e.g. other training, diet, use of drugs, level of training).

3 There are insufficient details of the Supplement program or the Training program. Why were these programs chosen?

4 Were the techniques used to measure the results up to the task? There were insufficient details provided on the methods of body measurement or body photos. These methods, unless carried out with expensive equipment by expert technicians, would not generally be accepted as a valid way to measure body composition and its changes. Generally they would be regarded as imprecise and subject to large errors. There are more scientific ways to measure body changes, such as underwater weighing, labelled water techniques and DEXA scans. And what about measurements of strength changes in these subjects. Could they also be measured with some precision and used to judge the success of the treatments?

5 Why test out two treatments at once when you don't know what each of the treatments (the training program and the supplement program) does by itself? How can you interpret the results properly and give credit where it is due? For example, even if the overall results are positive it is possible that one of the programs had no effects, or even negative effects, but these are disguised by the results from the other program.

6 Why weren't the results scrutinised by an appropriate statistical method? Good research projects are designed so that statistics can be used to draw the Big Picture—to determine the overall effect of a treatment and whether this is the result of a real change or pure chance. One subject's results may be unusual and may not tell the overall story. Anecdotal reporting is particularly open to abuse—after all you can pick out the subject whose results most suit the story you want to tell.

7 Finally—leaving the biggest problem to last—there were no 'control' or 'placebo' groups in the study. Back in Chapter 6 we discussed the limitations of 'testimonials'—the 'I did X and it worked for me' stories. We noted that changes often simply happen over time (for example as the result of ageing or going through adolescence, or from maturing in a training or sports program). We also noted that the power of positive thinking can allow up to half of a group of subjects to really feel or see a change simply because they think it might occur. How do we know that the subjects in the present study didn't go through a normal growth spurt? Perhaps they simply trained harder than usual because they were excited about the attention they were getting or because they really thought the supplements were giving them power. In other words, perhaps the gains were the result of harder work, rather than any special training techniques or exotic supplements.

To answer these questions and gain some credibility, this study would have to be done again with a larger number of subjects, including groups who would reflect changes that occur independently of the program or supplements—changes that occur because of the power of positive thinking (the placebo effect). In other words, in addition to the group of subjects who would receive the test programs, there would be another group of subjects with identical characteristics to the first who took a 'dummy set' of supplements (but believed these to be real) and/or perhaps another group who did a 'dummy' training program (believing it to be the special Program X). Measuring changes in each of the groups accurately, with each of the groups following their programs under identical conditions, would help you to tease out the real effects of the Supplements or the Special Training Program. Obviously the proper design for this study becomes a little more complicated if you want to look at the effects of the two treatments separately. And if the researcher wants to make a valid claim that his program is better than another one (even a drug-related program), then he really needs to include a group that follows the comparison program. Otherwise the claims are still speculative.

This is a brief critique of the present study. Of course it would be difficult and expensive to conduct the 'perfect' study—even to examine the claims made in this article. But the bodybuilding industry is encouraged to carry out such studies. It is a shame that the present study has added to the puzzle about supplements and not the solution.

Wrestling and boxing

Wrestling and boxing are male-dominated combative sports which share a similar competition structure in terms of having both weight divisions, and a marked division between amateur and professional codes.

There are ten divisions in wrestling, from light flyweight (below 48kg) to heavyweight plus (100–130kg). Boxing is run by a number of governing bodies, with at least eleven or twelve weight divisions depending on the federation. In general, divisions range from light flyweight (below 48kg) to heavyweight (above 80kg).

The duration of an amateur wrestling bout has undergone many changes, and is currently contested over one five-minute round. An amateur boxing match is fought over three 3-minute rounds. Professional bouts in both sports can be up to twelve 3-minute rounds. Both sports feature relatively short bursts of high-intensity anaerobic effort against a background of continuous low-intensity activity. Although aerobic fitness is important to both wrestlers and boxers in helping recovery between bursts, it is the ability to generate muscular force quickly that is the primary requirement for successful competition.

Training

The training of wrestlers and boxers will depend on their mode of competition, whether in weekly bouts, in multi-day tournaments, or as a single fight. In the latter situation, for example in the case of a professional boxer, there may be long periods between fights during which time specific training and even general fitness work may be suspended or reduced.

However in the lead-up to a competition, wrestlers and boxers train daily, supplementing skill and technique sessions with various forms of aerobic training such as running and skipping. Weight training may be undertaken to increase muscular strength and power, but becomes less important just before or during the competition phase.

In the competition phase, attention turns to making weight, and the athlete may increase the aerobic training load to help reduce body-fat levels. Often, food and fluid restriction and other rapid weight-loss techniques are employed to assist in achieving weigh-in targets.

Where weekly competition is undertaken, then a mini-cycle will operate, with heavier training during the first part of the week, and weight-loss activities dominating the end of the week prior to the weekend match.

Competition

Competition may be organised as a single bout, a weekly competition, or a multi-day tournament. Weigh-in is normally completed on the morning of a competition, which in the case of a major fight, may leave eight hours to rehydrate and prepare for the evening bout.

Recovery from bouts—and from repeated efforts to 'make weight'— is especially important in multi-day tournaments and weekly competitions, and athletes who fight at their natural weight have an advantage over athletes who must continually cut weight. In single fights, the effects of cutting weight may increase with the length of the bout, and a fighter may try to force an early conclusion before his stamina is tested.

Physical characteristics

There are a wide range of body sizes seen in these combative sports, with the weight divisions attempting to level out the physical inequalities between competitors. Top wrestlers and boxers tend to low body-fat levels, trying to maximise power and strength for their weight limit. In the heavyweight divisions of boxing, higher body-fat levels are seen. Typical physical characteristics will not be presented as they vary markedly between weight divisions.

235

Common nutrition issues

Training nutrition

Many wrestlers and boxers do not set themselves a routine training diet. Rather they move between extremes of eating everything and eating nothing depending on the phase of their competition. This may happen over a weekly cycle for those in a competition season, or on a more extended level for those who compete sporadically in major fights. Clearly this is not ideal for either nutritional status or weight control.

Why not take a completely different and more long-term view of your sport and your diet? Read Chapters 1 and 2 for an overview of the healthy training diet. A balanced and stable program will be better for body and soul, avoiding the physical and mental stress that goes with the current practice of jumping from one extreme to another.

Choosing a fighting weight

Combative athletes choose their fighting weight for many reasons, few of which are based on healthiness and optimum performance level. In the case of professional athletes it may be to chase an opponent or a title, and these athletes often fight at a number of weight divisions depending on what is on offer. Wrestlers may select their weight division because it is the only available spot on the school or club wrestling team. Adolescents may be chosen or certified at one weight division at the beginning of a season, and then fail to take into account growth and weight gain in the subsequent months.

There are two philosophies, integral to combative sports, that continue to support these decisions. The first is the belief that it is necessary to gain an advantage of strength, speed and leverage by fighting against a smaller opponent. By coming down from a weight that is above the limits of their weight division, wrestlers and boxers feel that they have achieved this goal. Of course, the advantage is wiped if their opponent has done exactly the same thing, and if the methods used to cut weight actually impair performance.

The second factor is the acceptance of rapid weight-loss techniques. Not only have they become a means to an end, but they have become ingrained in the language and the culture of these sports. The restricted eating, the excessive training and the saunas are almost part of the romance of being a wrestler. They have become a shared experience or common interest that bonds people within the sport—despite the disadvantages to health and performance. Read the account below to see just how institutionalised these practices have become, and the price that must be paid in return.

Numerous calls have been made to clean up this aspect of wrestling and boxing, particularly where adolescents are involved and particularly where competition (and therefore weight-loss practices) are frequent. The first step is to set realistic competition weights, based on a weight and body-fat level that is healthy and achievable for the athlete. For growing adolescents this may need to be continually reassessed. If you have body fat to spare there may be leeway for weight loss. However, if you are already at a low body-fat level you should think carefully about the weight division you choose. See Chapter 3 for a more detailed discussion.

Making weight

The study of the wrestlers below highlights the wrong way to approach weight-limits and weight loss. The physical and psychological disadvantages, both short-term and long-term, are clearly outlined. From a distance, it seems obvious that better selection of weight divisions and healthier weight-loss or weight-control programs would benefit combative sports, both in presenting athletes at their peak for competition, and in reducing the negative side-effects in general. Of course, it is hard when you are close to a sport to see the total perspective, or to see how major changes in attitude can come about. Nevertheless, it is up to all those involved—coaches, athletes and administrators— to slowly push for change.

Read Chapter 3 for a clearer account of healthy weight-loss, including both long-term weight control and last-minute fine-tuning before a competition. If you can maintain a general training weight within a kilogram of so of your competition target, it is possible to 'tickle' off the last grams without fuss or detriment (Chapter 3.5). This can be practised both in a weekly competition, and as in the case of Ross below, for a special one-off fight. While these healthier techniques might strip combative sports of some of their tradition and some of the locker-room talk—who really needs it? The wrestler's world can sound brave and wonderful in books and films, but the reality of diuretics, induced vomiting and sweat-boxes is hardly glamorous.

PROFILE
The life of a college wrestler

Amateur wrestling has a large following in high schools and colleges in the USA. Typically, the wrestling season involves weekly competition, with athletes certifying in a weight class that is below their off-season weight in order to gain a theoretical advantage over smaller opponents. Weigh-ins are conducted before each competition bout, requiring a weekly struggle to cut weight to the competition target. Following a match, wrestlers typically consume large amounts of food and drink, relaxing their end-of-week restrictions and gaining excess kilos that must be shed by the next weigh-in. This pattern of weight loss and regain is repeated throughout the competition season.

The rapid loss of body weight is achieved through one or more of the following: very restricted nutrition, artificial means of dehydration, and excessive exercise. A survey of large number of high school and college wrestlers was recently conducted to paint a picture of the typical lifestyle involved.

The mean age of the wrestlers was sixteen years (high school) and twenty years (college). The average age at which cutting weight began was fourteen years. On average, the high school wrestlers reported cutting weight nine times a season, with the college wrestlers needing to do this fifteen times in their competitive year. Weekly weight fluctuations ranged from 3–9kg/week for the college athletes, with smaller amounts being reported by their high school counterparts. Looking over their careers, a third of the college wrestlers estimated that they had to cut 5kg at least 100 times, and 20 per cent reported that they had lost 5–10kg between 20 and 50 times.

Details of the weight-loss methods used by wrestlers were provided. About a third of the group dehydrated using a sauna or rubber/plastic suit while exercising, at least once a week. Eighty per cent restricted fluids at least once a week, with half this number restricting fluids three to four times each week. Food was restricted by half the group, three or four times a week, and daily by a fifth of the wrestlers. More than half the group completely fasted once a week. Vomiting, laxatives and diuretics were used by smaller numbers on a less frequent basis.

Most of the wrestlers reported that it was difficult to make weight, and reported severe fatigue (75 per cent), anger (66 per cent), anxiety (33 per cent), feelings of isolation (23 per cent), depression (24 per cent) and low self-esteem (12 per cent). They reported that they were often or always preoccupied with foods, and many felt out of control with eating.

Apart from the psychological problems and the unhappiness associated with cutting weight, there are physical effects on both health and performance that need to be considered. Rapid weight loss is achieved through loss of body water, glycogen and perhaps protein (muscle). There is insufficient time between weigh-in and the event in most sports for adequate recovery of fluid and fuel stores to take place, leaving the athlete at a competitive disadvantage. During the training week, chronic weight-loss efforts may also take their toll.

While dehydration may not impair strength for short-duration exercise of seconds, it has been shown to impair exercise of two to three minutes or more and to decrease recovery, thus reducing performance in most competition situations. In the training situation, lack of concentration and loss of muscular endurance will interfere with training for improved fitness and skill acquisition. Loss of strength may eventually result if muscle is sacrificed.

Some of the weight-loss techniques also cause other side-effects, such as the loss of electrolytes with vomiting and laxative use. Restrictive diets will eventually impair nutritional status, perhaps with vitamin and mineral deficiencies, and with an effect on energy metabolism. Weight cycling is believed to depress energy requirements, making it even more difficult to shed real body fat.

Just because these weight-loss techniques are an accepted part of wrestling, does not mean they are acceptable practices. It is hoped that with time and education, a fairer approach will be taken in such sports—fairer to the basic idea of matching equal opponents in competition, and fairer to the athlete in allowing him to reach optimum health and performance.

PROFILE: ROSS
Fighting fit and light

Ross consulted a sports dietitian when things looked bleak twelve weeks before his next title fight. Life had been a little up and down in the past year. Twice he had had title fights cancelled, although the last time—a last-minute cancellation—it was probably a blessing in disguise. With four weeks to go, he had still been 6 kg overweight, and had been making poor progress with either his training or his weight.

It was hard, when the competition schedule was so infrequent and so uncertain, to keep himself motivated. After his last fight nine months ago, he had been so glad that the battle was over (both in the ring and with the bathroom scales each morning) that he had slipped gladly into a life of sloth and gluttony for a couple of months. This had left a legacy of an additional 9kg above his weight division, a figure that had gone up and down between the training come-backs and false starts. Losing weight was becoming increasingly harder with each fight, and Ross was becoming tired of the pressure it put on his career. Could a dietitian get him down to 59kg in twelve weeks, without costing him his sanity and his sweet tooth?

The dietitian firstly assessed Ross's body-fat levels to determine what excess baggage he had to shed. With skinfold levels of 92mm, she agreed that body fat could be safely lost. A loss of 50mm of body fat could well equate with the 9kg that he needed to lose, meaning that Ross need not jeopardise muscle mass to get down near his fighting weight. She listened to his training program, and advised him that a slow but steady rate of loss would be needed—not only to ensure that fat was lost preferentially, but to ensure that adequate carbohydrate and nutrient intake would be supplied to support his exercise needs. Eight kilograms in twelve weeks would be hard work, but could be achieved without the usual problems of fatigue, irritability, and mental stress. His wife and his coach were also pleased with this news.

Typical day's eating for Ross (boxer)—weight loss diet

Breakfast (after training)	Medium bowl of wholegrain cereal Low-fat milk 2 slices wholegrain toast + jam Unsweetened fruit juice or piece of fruit Tea with skim milk
Lunch	Thick sandwich or large roll—wholemeal bread, no margarine Small amount of chicken, cottage cheese, salmon or lean roast meat Plenty of salad Fruit scone or muffin—unbuttered Low-joule drink
Afternoon tea (prior to training)	Low-joule drink Piece of fruit Carton of low-fat fruit yoghurt or light fromage frais
Tea	Lean meat, fish or chicken—100–120g serve Cup of wholemeal rice, pasta or large potato Plenty of other vegetables or salad Medium serve of fruit salad or low-fat fruit yoghurt

Once a week treat of chocolate bar or icecream in cone

Energy: 7500–8000 kilojoules (1800–2000 Cals)
Carbohydrate: 320g (60–65% of energy)
Protein: 90g (20% of energy)
Fat: 25–30g (15–20% of energy)
Vitamins and minerals: all above RDI level

The dietitian devised a menu plan of 7500kJ (1800 Cals), including a high carbohydrate intake, plenty of nutrient-rich foods and a sprinkling of 'treat' foods that helped to put a sparkle in his day. The outline of this plan is presented in the table below. Ross's wife worked with the dietitian to prepare different recipes and variations on the theme. Ross was astounded—he'd never lost weight before without having to face endless nights of steamed fish and boiled chicken. He felt more energetic in training than ever before, and enjoyed his sweet treats without feeling guilty.

After four weeks he had lost 4kg (skinfolds down by 18mm), and at eight weeks was within 3kg of his weigh-in limit (skinfolds down by a total of 35mm). At the beginning of the title fight week, he was within 1.0kg of his target (weight 60kg, skinfolds 43mm), and under the dietitian's instructions he began to move into competition mode to shake off the last grams.

For the four days until the weigh-in, Ross restricted his salt intake, making sure that body fluid accumulation would be avoided. All salt was cut from his meals (pepper helped to flavour the cooking), and he was careful to avoid salty foods such as cheese, nuts, chips, processed meats and salted crackers (not that these foods had been part of his diet for a while). On the Thursday, he ate his normal breakfast, and then switched to drinking a Sustagen Sport low-fat milkshake for lunch, afternoon tea and dinner. He woke up on the Friday morning feeling nervous, but light and trim—and his flat stomach showed-off the ripplemarks of all his recent training.

Weigh-in was conducted before Ross had eaten or drunk anything, and the scales rewarded him with a reading of 58.7kg. For the remainder of the day, he rested and ate light snacks of carbohydrate-rich foods, topping up his fluid levels at frequent intervals. A final light meal of pasta with a tomato sauce was eaten at 4.00pm, about $3^{1}/_{2}$ hours before he had to step into the ring.

And the fight was great. He felt confident and strong both physically and mentally. Hearing that his opponent had spent two hours in the sauna that morning before weighing-in had given him a great psychological boost. He remembered all the times that he had resorted to that himself, and how dreadful he had felt on the occasion that he had taken a diuretic. It was no surprise that the title became his—as the rounds progressed he became stronger and more confident, while his opponent was gradually worn down.

While basking in the glory the next day, Ross made himself a few promises. First, he decided to continue with some training even when no fights were in the wind. After all, he felt and looked good and it would be a shame to throw that all away. And there was no trouble in keeping to his new dietary principles as a year-round plan. There was room and the excuse for a few celebratory meals for the next couple of days, and he could afford to increase his total kilojoule intake now that he was down to his target weight. But gone forever was the on-again, off-again feasting and fasting approach that had been part of his earlier career. He felt on top of the world, and he had the title to prove it!

Gymnastics and diving

Artistic gymnastics and diving are highly skilled sports in which performance is evaluated subjectively by a panel of judges. There are six events in an Olympic men's gymnastic program—floor, pommel horse, rings, vault, parallel bars and the high bar—while the women's program features four events—floor, vault, asymmetric bars and the beam. In each of these disciplines there are compulsory routines, set every four years on an Olympic cycle, as well as optional routines selected by the athlete. There are separate titles for team competition and for individual performers, with the individual prizes being awarded for each event as well as the overall score.

All events in artistic gymnastics are anaerobic in nature, the longest being the floor (about a minute) and the shortest the vault (a few seconds including the approach run). Skill, muscular strength and power relative to body weight are important components of success.

Diving is separated into springboard (1 and 3 metre) and highboard (3, 5, 7.5 and 10 metre) events for men and women. There are a set number of compulsory and voluntary dives which each competitor must perform. Each dive is marked separately. Numerous combinations of starting position, flight movements and twists differentiate the degree of difficulty of each dive. As in gymnastics, depletion of fuel stores is not a contributing factor to diving performance, with skill and power being the important determinants of success.

Male athletes peak at a much later age than females in these sports. While most top male divers and gymnasts fit within the 18–28 year age range, elite female competitors are much younger. In fact, rules are now in place to restrict females under certain ages (e.g. 14 or 16 years) from competing in international level gymnastics or platform diving.

Training

The development of gymnastic skills takes years of intense practice and requires gymnasts to totally commit their lifestyle to the sport. Training begins at an early age, and even by nine or ten years gymnasts in elite development programs may be committed to a training load in excess of twenty hours per week. These programs now begin to prepare athletes four to eight years in advance of specific competitions, gradually building up to a full training load of 30–40 hours per week. Typically, eleven or twelve training sessions are undertaken each week, with daily training sessions before and after school or work lasting two or more hours each.

The training load of an elite diver can be equally demanding, with three to four hours per day spent on water work, and another hour of dry-land training. Training generally starts at an early age, reflecting the years of skill and strength development that are required. Occasionally, elite divers emerge from a gymnastics background, changing to diving at a later age after injury or lack of success halt their gymnastics career.

In the non-competitive season, or in the early development of the gymnast or diver, much of the training time is spent on acquiring skills through technique work and body conditioning. Supplementary weight training is often undertaken, particularly by male athletes, and may make up to 25 per cent of total training time.

As the athlete matures or as the competitive season draws closer, progressively more time is spent on the development of the compulsory and optional gymnastic routines or dives.

Competition

There are four separate components in a gymnastics program:

1 Set/compulsory routines on each of the apparatus.
2 Optional routines on each of the apparatus.
3 Individual combined finals, where only the optional routines are performed again.
4 Individual apparatus finals, where the top performers on each apparatus compete again.

This program is spread over four days, with the duration of competition being about two hours per day for each competitor as they rotate between apparatus. A warm-up of a similar length is usually completed before the start of competition, and between performances (from five to 30 minutes apart) competitors may perform stretching exercises.

In diving contests, preliminary rounds are held when there are more than sixteen competitors, and the top twelve competitors proceed to a final. Preliminary rounds may be held on the morning and finals in the evening of the same day. Men perform eleven dives and women, ten dives in springboard events, and in highboard events ten and eight dives are performed respectively. Four or five dives in each event are compulsory, with the remainder being dives selected by the athlete. A diving meet can last four to six days with the competition for each board being held on separate days.

Physical characteristics

Gymnasts are a physically homogeneous group, the characteristics for elite performance being very marked. The skill and agility of gymnastics requires that an athlete should be small and well-muscled, with a low body-fat level. The physical profile of the female gymnast has changed since the 1970s, with champions such as Olga Corbut and Nadia Comanechi turning attention away from mature female physiques to a youthful almost pre-pubescent look.

In addition to the physical advantages of increased mechanical efficiency and power-to-weight ratio, being small and light conveys a more favourable visual image to gymnastic judges.

Divers share similar physical characteristics to gymnasts, with a compact frame and low body-fat level being important both for physical and aesthetic advantages.

Typical physique (elite gymnasts)

	Male	Female
Height	160–174cm	154–162cm
Weight	56–70kg	43–51kg
Skinfold sum	31–47mm	37–51mm

Common nutrition issues

Body fat and size—are goals realistic?

Athletes in aesthetically-judged skill sports—gymnastics, diving, figure skating, ballet dancing etc.—are set strict guidelines about weight and skinfold levels. Females, especially, face an uphill battle to achieve or maintain the sparrow-like dimensions that are expected of them. They may have to combat the fat deposition that accompanies puberty, as well as to achieve body-fat goals that are more applicable to endurance training athletes. Although these athletes spend many hours in training each week (or each day), the training load is focused on skill and technique rather than kilojoule-burning aerobic exercise.

The secret of body-fat loss is explained in Chapter 3 and involves increasing the amount of aerobic exercise and/or decreasing food energy intake. When athletes are already training many hours each day, there may be no time for extra aerobic exercise, or the coach may be reluctant to allow an extra training load with a high risk of injury. This leaves the athlete with only one choice—to resort to a low-kilojoule intake. Even with a well-chosen meal plan there may be difficulties to be faced—from inadequate intake of some nutrients to depression of metabolic rate and increased energy efficiency. In some cases the athlete may actually be in a state of chronic low-grade starvation. And this is the best-case scenario. Many athletes enter the cycle of fad diets, disordered eating and eating disorders as they aim to meet their body-fat goals. The disadvantages are then those of undernutrition as well as the side effects of the weight-loss methods used.

For males the problem is not so critical. Males are more likely to naturally arrive at low body-fat levels associated with these sports. However, some will face similar challenges to their female training partners.

Regardless of the sex, it is important that realistic weight and body-fat targets be set for these athletes. While low body-fat levels confer a physical advantage to skill, there is nevertheless also a component of aesthetic value and peer-pressure involved. Why should extremely thin or pre-pubescent athletes be judged as better performers, simply because of their appearance? Above all the health and happiness of the athlete should be taken into account when setting body-fat goals. See Chapter 3 for more details.

Body weight worries

Because of the worry about remaining lean and trim, many gymnasts and divers weigh themselves many times a day. Sometimes weighing-in is a routine part of the training session. Coaches have valid reasons for fearing sudden and major increases in body weight. It is dangerous for an athlete to attempt an intricate dive or gymnastics routine with the sudden addition of an extra three kilograms—obviously this upsets their balance and centre of gravity and other aspects of their finely tuned skills. Coaches want to know if their athletes are at such a risk at any single training session, and to be prewarned of creeping weight gain that might need to be checked.

However, scale watching can lead to an overconcern about weight. Add a few misconceptions about body weight and its fluctuations and you can end up with worried athletes who take unhealthy measures to achieve impossible goals. For example, some athletes (and their coaches) do not realise that it is normal and healthy (and necessary) for weight to fluctuate each day—as much as a kilogram in small-bodied athletes. This is because of weight losses through sweating, temporary weight of food and fluids consumed (weight gain equal to the weight of the food/drink) and weight lost after going to the toilet. And this is without counting the weight of clothes and shoes that you may be wearing when you hop on the scales. Of course, none of these issues has anything to do with your body-fat levels.

Set yourself body-fat goals and an eating strategy that keeps you trim, performing well, and happy. A good plan will not allow great weight increases or decreases (2kg or more) to occur, and you won't need to resort to eating and drinking extremes (starving and not drinking, then overindulging later). Read the case history of Samantha below. Coaches: work on promoting these happy and healthy eating strategies in your gymnasts, rather than using the scales as a threat or a big stick. Even in an elite program, periodic weight checks (one or two per week) may give you all the information you need and will reduce the panic and misery of being tied to the scales.

The nutritional needs of adolescence

Gymnastics and diving begin at an early age, following athletes through late childhood, adolescence, and—if they survive in the sport—into adulthood. Growth and puberty exert special nutritional demands, including increased needs for energy and protein for growth, and iron and calcium for the building of bones and blood supply. Where a chronic low-energy intake exists, there is the possibility of nutritional deficiencies and delayed growth and maturity.

A recent study of the physical characteristics of junior elite female gymnasts reported that those in the 7–10 year age group were of average height and weight for their age (around the 50th percentile), but that the 11–14 year olds had slipped back to the 20th percentile in these measures. Muscle mass was high but body-fat levels were below average in these groups. The drop in height and weight could indicate:

- that nutritional deficits exist, causing a delay in puberty and growth failure;
- that sports-specific factors are selecting the gymnasts—that is, that the smaller and lighter gymnasts are progressing while heavier and bigger gymnasts drop out of the program; or
- that both factors are operating.

Obviously, there is a need to follow the same group of gymnasts right though to determine which factor is most important. However, a warning is sounded that young gymnasts are nutritionally vulnerable, and that health and growth may be compromised if dietary intake is restricted. It is hoped that gymnastics programs are not so dogmatic that they consciously 'bonsai' their young athletes—that is, consciously restrict their growth by keeping them undernourished. Poor growth patterns are associated with greater disease morbidity, including impaired bone development.

Amenorrhea, calcium and bone impairment

Athletic groups with low body-fat levels, particularly those that seem artificially contrived, may be at an increased risk of amenorrhea. Amenorrhea may be in the form of a failure to start periods altogether, or the cessation of an already established menstrual cycle. The former condition appears to be a common pattern with elite gymnasts. A complication of amenorrhea is reduced bone density, and perhaps an increased risk of stress fractures now, and osteoporosis later.

It is important that delayed onset of periods be reported to your sports medicine doctor so that issues such as bone health can be monitored. In many cases a healthy-eating gymnast will have good bone density which appears to benefit from the bone-stimulating effects of exercise, rather than poor bone density due to hormone deprivation. A healthy high calcium diet (1000–1500mg/day) should be part of the program for all gymnasts. There is some evidence that high calcium intakes, usually achieved by use of a calcium supplement on top of a good diet, can increase bone density in pre-pubertal children.

Training nutrition—an overview

It has already been established that many gymnasts and divers are at risk of inadequate nutrition, because of their restricted energy intake. Indeed dietary surveys of female gymnasts have reported inadequate intakes of many vitamins and minerals. Read Chapters 1 and 2 for an overview of the nutritional goals of an athlete in heavy training.

Another factor that greatly influences the eating habits of these athletes, is the great time commitment involved in their sport. With the day divided between school, training, homework and, later on a job, there is often little time for cooking and preparing meals—for the athlete or their family. The only people busier than young gymnasts are their mothers—driving them to and from their training, and struggling to meet the needs of all the family members. Meals are often eaten in the car on the way to school, or on the way home from training, and Mum must be creative to organise food that is nutritious, transportable and easily eaten.

Competition nutrition

Athletes need a meal plan that will fit in with their competition schedule, often spread over a number of days. Competition is not likely to threaten fluid and fuel stores, since it is quite brief and low in intensity. However, each athlete needs to find a plan that sits comfortably —both in the stomach and with their confidence. Challenges include the risk of weight gain if energy intake is not kept relative to the reduced energy expenditure of a very reduced training load. When gymnasts travel away from their parents and personal coaches, lack of supervision at meals can also increase the risk of poor eating and weight gain. There is no need to carbo-load or undertake severe dietary preparation for an event. Read Chapter 4.2 about general preparation for competition, and Chapter 4.4 for ideas about pre-event meals. The timing of meals will need to be organised to fit the daily schedule of training and competition sessions. This may vary from day to day.

Eating disorders

With so much pressure to be light and low in body fat, it is not surprising that much of the life, the conversation and the hobbies of female gymnasts and divers revolve around food and weight loss. There is constant attention to what the athlete looks like, how much she weighs or how large her skinfold sum is, all of which are reinforced by other athletes, and often unfortunately, by coaches and parents.

In this environment it is not surprising that eating disorders and disordered eating become apparent amongst female athletes. How else can unrealistic goals be met? And how do you resist when everyone else is doing it? Read the account below to see how the problem covers a spectrum from shared weight-loss activities to desperate and pathological disturbances in eating behaviour. The hazards and the treatment will vary accordingly, but budget for great patience and support and the input of various professionals. The problem also occurs with male athletes but there is a much lower incidence.

PROFILE: CAROL
Starving for success?

When Carol took up her new position as head gymnastics coach at the college, she immediately consulted a sports dietitian. She explained that her last job had caused her some unhappiness because of suspected eating disorders amongst some of the female gymnasts. In a new setting and with new students she wanted to tackle the issue with a fresh mind. What could be done to prevent the problem? Was there anything that she did to cause or provoke the situation? How could she detect which girls were having problems and what did she do if difficulties were found?

The dietitian summarised the symptoms of the two major eating disorders, anorexia nervosa and bulimia. While anorexics deny themselves food and generally lose large amounts of body weight, the major feature of bulimia is uncontrolled eating followed by purging, through vomiting or laxative use. In the case of the bulimic, great swings in body weight can be seen. While the syndromes can exist separately, many sufferers show both symptoms, either simultaneously or in tandem. In all cases, there are very clear psychological problems —including disorders in body image and in feelings about food.

The dietitian then explained that eating disorders are not always clearcut. Not every athlete who skips a meal is anorexic, and not everyone who induces vomiting on one occasion is a true bulimic. Instead, there is a spectrum of eating behaviour problems amongst athletes.

At one end of the spectrum are people who suffer with anorexia or bulimia as a primary disorder—that is, a classical psychological disturbance with nutritional consequences. What causes these disorders is unknown, but the symptoms are well recognised and the health implications can be serious. Death is the most extreme outcome—from starvation in the case of the anorexic, from severe electrolyte disturbances in the case of the bulimic, and from suicide in the case of related depression. These disorders also occur in the community, and their numbers include some athletes who then bring the nutritional implications into the sports arena. Extensive treatment is required for both these eating disorders, involving specialised counselling from both psychologists and dietitians, and exploration of interpersonal relationships.

At the other end of the spectrum are athletes with 'occupational' eating disorders—those who have problems with their eating behaviour because they are under pressure to achieve unrealistic nutritional or sporting goals. Achieving or maintaining a low body-fat level is the most common issue, and disordered eating may be expected more commonly amongst athletes or sports that emphasise low body-fat levels. Having been set an unrealistic target of too much or too soon, many athletes turn to bizarre diets, vomiting, laxative use or other problem practices. The other factor that supports the behaviour is peer acceptance. In some sports, body-fat phobia is almost institutionalised, with athletes swapping ideas about weight-loss techniques and making problem eating behaviours seem normal by the virtue of 'everybody' doing it.

The difference between this disordered eating and eating *disorders* is the focus. For the true anorexic, starvation is the end, while for an athlete with an eating behaviour problem, it is the means to the end.

SIGNS OF EATING DISORDERS

Weight changes	sudden loss of weight
	wide fluctuations in weight over a short time
Food behaviour	consumption of large amounts of food that are inconsistent with the athlete's weight
	evidence of eating in private (food wrappers or food disappearing etc.)
	avoidance of eating or refusal to join in social occasions involving eating
	excessive interest in handling food and in preparing food for others
Self-image	worry about being too fat
	constant self-examination and comparison with others
Personality	withdrawn, anxious
	mood swings
Evidence of problem behaviours	admission or evidence that athlete uses diuretics, laxatives or diet pills
	admission or evidence that the athlete vomits after meals
	excessive exercise often in addition to set training program
Physical signs	amenorrhea (cessation of periods, or failure to start menstruating at all)
	tooth decay/acid erosion of teeth from vomiting
	stress fractures
	cold intolerance
	jaundiced skin (carotenemia)
	lanugo (fine hair on body)

In many cases, the athlete when removed from the pressure or the environment that condones the behaviour will revert to better eating practices and the problem will disappear. Others, however, may get caught up in a powerfully-sustained cycle and become enmeshed in a true eating disorder. When the athlete loses the ability to stop the behaviour, even when there is no longer a need and the behaviour is causing harm and injury, then a real problem is evident. Athletes seem to be at greater risk of developing eating disorders than non-active people, partly because of the pressure and the environment that supports control of eating and body weight/fat levels, but also because of their personalities. An obsessive, perfectionist person who likes to tackle tasks with focus and determination has the psychological characteristics which help athletes to make it to the top. At the same time, however, this is considered a 'high-risk' personality for the development of eating disorders.

After listening to this explanation, Carol thought back to her gymnastics career and the memories of her own weight obsession returned. She agreed with the dietitian that the environment had certainly supported disordered eating practices. Having been set unreasonable body-fat targets—by herself, her coach or the sport—she had become driven with the desire to be lean.

'We all thought about food all the time,' she said, 'We weighed ourselves a thousand times a day, and looked at our tummies every time a mirror or shiny surface was passed. The only time I stopped thinking about my next meal, how many Calories, and how much exercise I'd have to do to burn it up, was when I started thinking about my friend and whether she was thinner than I was.

'We were certainly very miserable, although at the time I didn't know any different. We were always trying the latest diet, and one day we bought some diet pills, though they were short-lived and didn't seem to make any difference. Some of my friends could make themselves sick, but I was too frightened to try, in case my mother found out. One girl in the class eventually ended up in hospital after taking too many laxatives, and that gave us all a scare.

'Funnily, I never considered I had a problem, and in fact when I stopped competing in gymnastics I stopped worrying so much. I still like to keep myself in trim, but it's not like the consuming passion that it used to be.'

The dietitian agreed that this was part of the range of eating behaviour problems, and that at any level the athlete experienced disadvantages to physical and emotional health, and to athletic performance. Even if it does not become a life-threatening condition, many athletes worry too much about their food and their body-fat scores. While definite causes of disordered eating and eating disorders can often not be pinpointed or eradicated, it is important to recognise the contribution of both a perfectionist personality on the part of the athlete, and a pressurised environment created by coaches, parents and other athletes.

PROFILE: SAMANTHA
The scales—a friend or an enemy?

Samantha joined a new elite gymnastics program when her family moved interstate. As a young gymnast, she had shown a lot of promise, however since her sixteenth birthday Samantha's performances had become less and less consistent—both in training and in competition.

251

HINTS FOR DEALING WITH EATING DISORDERS—for coaches, training partners and parents

- Recognise athletes with compulsive and perfectionist personalities. While self-drive and motivation are good characteristics for success, many athletes would benefit from counselling in skills of goal setting and achievement rather than behaving as their own worst enemies.

- Create an environment that supports healthy nutrition and weight control principles. Allow athletes to set realistic body weight and body-fat targets, and make healthy nutrition advice accessible—both at a group and individual level.

- Be aware of early signs of disordered eating behaviour (see table on p. 250). Recognise that you may be over-reacting, and try to be objective in collecting evidence of a suspected problem.

- If appropriate, confront the athlete carefully. Express concern, and talk only about objective data—changes in performance, signs of unhappiness, etc. Do not label the athlete or try to diagnose. The athlete may attempt to deny the problem, so stick to discussing hard evidence.

- If it is not appropriate for you to talk to the athlete, speak to someone who can—perhaps the coach or the team doctor, or someone in the athlete's family.

- Seek professional help. It is not your problem—and you are not trained to deal with it. You may have the consent of the athlete to organise this step. Alternatively you may have to wait for the right moment before the help is accepted. Sometimes you may need to withdraw your support of the athlete until this step is taken. Make sure that they are clear that you still care for them, but you do not support their behaviour.

- Professional assessment and counselling should probably involve both a psychologist and a dietitian—make sure that you know of services that specialise in this field.

- Support the professional advice and treatment plan. Try not to become embroiled in the problem, but remain caring, supportive and objective. Be prepared to be patient and flexible—the athlete may need constant reassessment of their goals.

What's more, she no longer seemed to enjoy her sport. The long hours of training restricted her social life and her school activities. Of course, that was nothing new. It was just that everything had become a pressure, rather than a pleasure—especially the whole business of eating. She remembered the days when she could 'eat anything' without worrying about her weight. Then almost overnight it had changed and the scales had taken over her life. The last year had been misery; trying hard in the gym and at the table, but getting nowhere. Perhaps a new club would give her a fresh start.

Samantha found the routine of the new club to be quite different. For a start, there were scales at the gym, but only the older gymnasts were required to 'weigh in'—and that was once or twice a month instead of once or twice a day. Of course, you were free to weigh yourself more frequently if you wanted, but no-one seemed to be in a panic about it. Body fat ('skinfolds') and body weight were monitored and reviewed every month by the sports dietitian who worked with the club. Samantha was surprised to hear that she would negotiate her personal 'ideal skinfold' with the dietitian after 6 months of monitoring, and that this would include a small range for movement up and down that was still considered OK. At Samantha's old club, everybody had to keep their skinfold sum below 40mm, and the number loomed large in the lives of all the gymnasts. In Sam's case, it seemed the more she worried about her skinfolds, the more there was to worry about—literally. Her skinfold sum had hovered around 32–34mm for 7 sites back in the good old days, but had gradually inched higher until it had reached 45mm.

Determined to do better with her fresh start, Samantha threw herself headlong into the 'skinfold action plan' she had followed on and off at her old club. These strategies had been the way of life for all of her friends there. It was a tough life, made bearable only by sharing the struggle with the other gymnasts. The day started with breakfast—the menu varying according to whether Sam had been to the toilet on rising and thus felt 'light'. If so, she enjoyed a decent-sized bowl of cereal with low-fat milk and a small glass of orange juice. However, if the trip to the toilet had been unproductive and left her weighing 'heavy', Samantha would eat a small bowl of cereal, 'dry', and skip the drink. The total weight of this breakfast: about 50g. This was worth a few brownie points at the weigh-in before training. By comparison, her full breakfast with milk and juice weighed about 450g—which could put her bodyweight above 35kg on a 'heavy' morning.

During the day you had to work hard to minimise the weight of all food and drink consumed. If successful, you could weigh-in at afternoon training at around the same weight as at the morning session. Although her mother sent her off to school with a packed lunch, Samantha usually threw this out. After all, a sandwich weighed 200g or even more if full of salad, an apple almost the same, and a carton of orange juice was a luxury at 250g! Who could afford to consume a 650g lunch and face the scales and the coach with most of that still on board at afternoon training? A chocolate bar (60g), or a packet of chips (50g), provided a smaller and lighter alternative. It was hard to

253

keep yourself to only a mouthful of drink though. You got pretty thirsty over the day. You might be able to steal away for a drink during the training session, but the coaches usually watched to make sure that only a few sips were taken. Once, one gymnast had drunk so much that she gained nearly a whole kilo on the spot. Water sure was fattening!

With afternoon training over, there was a brief time to relax about weight—although Mum was pretty careful about the evening meal. You could count on a small serve of meat or chicken and vegetables, followed by some fruit or fruit salad, and icecream twice a week. Of course, Samantha still felt hungry, and raided the secret stash of biscuits and chocolate hidden in her bedroom. She and her friends made raids to the 24-hour supermarket on the weekends to replenish their stores. The stash provided some joy in a day of self-discipline, and you could feel comforted that Tim Tams and lollies were small and unlikely to weigh you down.

Saturday afternoon was the best time of the week. Once you left the gym there was a whole 36 hours of freedom. Saturday night was a night at the movies (family pack of sweets and an icecream instead of dinner), or a sleep over at a friend's house (baking slices or cakes). Sunday morning meant a special breakfast at home—pancakes. By Sunday afternoon the fear of facing the scales next morning usually brought on an attack of the guilts, followed by a run (all rugged up to help you sweat more). One of Samantha's friends had a sauna at home, and sometimes they all met there to spend a couple of hours sweating off their weekend's excesses. Of course, sometimes there was no way to avoid facing a weight jump—a kilogram or even two. And then the week started again.

However, at the new club, Samantha found herself alone in this ritual. In fact, her gym mates were so concerned about her strange eating patterns that they took their concerns to one of the coaches. The coach had a small talk to Samantha and arranged for both of them to talk to the club dietitian. The dietitian listened sympathetically to Samantha's story and agreed that it was a hard way to be a gymnast. What's more, she suggested to Samantha that she was not just making herself miserable, but dooming herself to continued problems with her weight and her performance.

First, the coach explained to Samantha the reason for the concern about body weight in her sport. She explained that gymnastics requires precise skills and balance—factors that could be thrown out by a sudden gain in weight. For example, try doing some of your routines with 2 kilograms of sand in a backpack strapped to you! Gradual changes in height and lean body mass through growth could be accommodated, although at the end of the line there was a mechanical bias towards gymnasts who remained small and lean even after the completion of growth and puberty. These days talent identification programs in gymnastics concentrated on selection of children who were genetically destined to fit these physical characteristics. Monthly checks on weight, height and skinfolds helped to keep an eye on progress. If problems were noted, such as a steady increase in skinfolds and corresponding weight, then steps could be taken to address the situation in its early stages. In Samantha's new club, great pains were taken to make skinfold goals realistic and healthy for each gymnast— and to help rather than to harass each gymnast if skinfolds became much higher or lower than their ideal range.

'But if I'm only weighing myself once a month, won't I get fat?' Samantha questioned, unconvinced. The dietitian assured her that the scales were available whenever she wanted to get some feedback, but that weighing yourself didn't stop you gaining body fat, or help in losing it when necessary. These results came from healthy eating strategies, sound exercise practices and happy thoughts. In fact, in the dietitian's experience, the more people weighed themselves the more they worried about the results, instead of the process needed to achieve the results. The situation often developed into a vicious and unhappy cycle of weighing, worrying, thinking about food, eating food, then weighing, worrying . . .

The twice-daily weighing had actually distracted Samantha from the real issues. What's more, it had confused her into following the very patterns that made it easy to gain body fat. Samantha had been tricked into thinking that quick weight changes over the day reflected her body-fat levels—and nothing could be further from the truth.

The dietitian reminded Sam of what she had learned in biology at school—that gaining body fat is a long-term project. Each kilogram of body fat is equal to about 30 000 kilojoules of surplus energy. To lose that or gain that from your body takes 1–2 weeks of consistent energy imbalance. Daily weight changes are largely due to the normal fluctuations of food and fluid coming in and out of our bodies. Most people eat between 1.5 and 4 kilograms of food each day. Our notional '8 glasses of water each day' weigh about 2 kg and many athletes need to drink two or three times this amount to replace daily sweat losses. If we are exactly eating our energy requirements, this food will be processed over the day, and the waste products eliminated. Fluid is also in dynamic balance in the body, being lost through sweat, breathing and trips to the toilet. In the case of athletes who train in hot weather for long periods, 'weight' can drop 2–4 kilograms by the end of the session if fluid isn't being consumed during the session. So, at the end of the day nett weight gain may be nil, even though there have been constant 'deposits' and 'withdrawals'. In a small gymnast who is eating and drinking healthy foods and spreading this intake over the day, body weight may fluctuate up to a kilogram from lightest to heaviest each day. This will not be a problem for training performance.

But when gymnasts weigh themselves too often and react (especially with panic) to every small fluctuation, they can confuse the short-term with the Big Picture. In Samantha's case, she had been confusing the weight of her meals and drinks with their kilojoule value and their overall contribution to her nutritional requirements. Unfortunately, size doesn't correlate to kilojoules. For example, some foods that are 'small' and 'light' are also full of fat and kilojoules, and not necessarily full of vitamins and minerals (chocolate, chips, biscuits). Fat content is a particularly tricky issue because fat is such a compact kilojoule source and because fat itself may be more 'fattening' than other nutrients per kilojoule. On the other hand, some 'heavy' foods, like fruit and vegetables, are low in fat and kilojoules and full of nutrients. Water is 'heavy' but has no kilojoule value. What's more, plenty of fibre and fluid are part of regular bowel habits.

When it was put this way, Sam could see how her 'small foods diet' had some flaws—but it was hard to comprehend that you could eat a lot of food and actually be eating less kilojoules. The dietitian prepared a computer analysis of a typical day of the old diet, and a typical day of a new eating plan. The new eating plan included cereal, fruit, reduced-fat milk and a piece of toast for breakfast, a yoghurt for morning recess, some fruit and a roll or sandwich chock-a-block with various fillings for lunch, and Mum's dinner with some extra vegies after training. Healthy snacks before bed included some air-popped popcorn or a carton of yoghurt (frozen to make it take ages to eat). There were even some treats for the weekend, and some new dessert ideas including fruit kebabs with low-fat milk custard. Water was to be drunk at every meal and during training—constantly topping up rather than drying out and then drinking like a camel. It sounded too good to be true—she would not get hungry or empty like before, it would help to make her trips to the toilet regular, and it would give her more energy for training and school. It was designed to be just a little lower in kilojoules than her present needs, so that a small and constant loss of skinfolds would result.

Despite the bright outlook, Sam found it hard to change her ways at first. It was such a total change in everything she had believed and she had to constantly remind herself that her future eating plans needed to be different if her gymnastics future was to be successful. Her coach and the dietitian were encouraging and patient—weaning her down to a weekly check-in on the scales, then fortnightly, then monthly. Once she couldn't help herself and tried the scales at the local pharmacist. The results were a bit scary—and prompted her to skip dinner that night. But her weekly appointment with the dietitian gave her an opportunity to talk through her fears and regain her confidence. After six months on the new program, Samantha received some great rewards: a skinfold measurement back below 40mm and the award for best new gymnast at the club. At her end-of-year review she felt happy to discuss a long-term skinfold goal with her coach and dietitian—and felt confident that 35–40mm was a good target.

Samantha is looking forward to her next year at the club, and has set herself a number of personal goals. There are some important competitions to do well in, and perhaps an overseas trip to aim for. But part of her program is to keep working on her food attitude—to reduce her fears about each meal so that she can enjoy it more. At the end of the road she hopes to stop thinking about food at all—knowing that with a healthy eating program in place, she doesn't need to worry.

PROFILE: MAUREEN
A vegetarian adventure

When Maureen's older sister came back from a year overseas as an exchange student, she announced to her parents that she had decided to become a vegetarian. One of her foster families had been Seventh Day Adventists, and she had enjoyed their vegetarian lifestyle. After becoming involved with an ecological interest group at her new school she decided that she was ready to take a personal stand on the killing of animals.

Maureen, a state-level diver, was enthusiastic to join the cause. Over the past six months she had become very picky with her food, and the family mealtime had become a bit of a battleground. She explained that being vegetarian would help her keep her skinfolds down, 'I'll never get to the top being this fat,' she said.

The response from other people was less favourable. Maureen's father was aghast at the thought of eating 'hippy food' and warned her that she would be unable to keep up her strength for twenty hours of training a week, let alone her school work. Her diving coach was also tentative—the only vegetarian athlete he had trained had become anemic and dropped out of competition. Finally her mother mediated in the dispute and took Maureen to see a sports dietitian. She had two questions:

1 Is a vegetarian diet healthy? and
2 Can a successful athlete be a vegetarian?

At the world level, there are millions of people who eat vegetarian diets, and for many cultures and populations this is the normal way of life. By contrast, in Australia, it is more often an individual choice rather than an organised eating pattern.

People choose to be vegetarians for a variety of reasons—because of cultural or religious backgrounds, due to moral or ecological beliefs, because of food availability or financial considerations, because they think it is healthy, and sometimes, simply because it is trendy.

257

Whatever the reasons, the advantages and disadvantages of vegetarian eating are not clear-cut. Vegetarianism is used to cover a wide variety of food patterns which may have quite different outcomes on health and athletic performance. To most people, being a vegetarian simply means not eating meat, but this is a gross simplification of the total dietary plan. In fact there are many levels of vegetarian eating, including:

- lacto-ovo-vegetarians who eliminate meat, fish and poultry, but who eat dairy products and eggs;
- vegans who eliminate all animal products; and
- part-time vegetarians, who rely on vegetarian meals most of the time but freely depart from this pattern, particularly on social occasions.

The best examples of vegetarian eating are seen in communities or established groups which have practised it for generations, such as Seventh Day Adventists, certain religious orders and the Hare Krishna sect. These people have developed alternative eating patterns and food uses to replace the animal foods that we normally eat. Extensive use is made of nuts, seeds and legumes (beans and pulses), and a greater variety of cereals, fruits and vegetables is explored. Many food products, for example, can be derived from soya beans, including soya milk and tofu curd.

Recipes, clever food combinations, and other healthy nutrition secrets are passed between members of the vegetarian community, and the food supply is usually geared to make a variety of vegetarian foods available and cheap. Amongst such well organised groups it is rare to see nutritional deficiencies, since their food patterns have been been carefully thought out and developed over long periods of time. The emphasis is not on what they are giving up but on how they can enjoy a wider variety of other (vegetable) foods to supply their nutritional requirements.

Compare this with a modern vegetarian who thinks that the message is simply to give up meat. In the worst-case scenario, we see people sitting down to a pile of steamed vegetables minus the traditional lamb-chop, or pulling the ham out of their ham sandwich and thinking that this is a healthy way to eat. Many 'nouveau-vegetarians' make no attempt to replace the nutrients that have been eliminated along with the foods they have given up. Maybe they are too busy feeling virtuous from the thought of giving up fat and chemicals (or the other 'nasties' they think are in animal foods). Maybe they do not know how to explore the world of grains and legumes, and their cooking skills are limited. Or, maybe these new food supplies are hard to get and expensive, because they are going against the tide of the general community eating patterns.

How healthy a vegetarian diet is depends on the individual vegetarian. When vegetarian eating is planned and adventurous, it has the promise of being low in fat and salt, and high in carbohydrate and fibre. This should sound familiar, as it is the blue-print for healthy eating and the optimum training diet for an athlete.

Studies of established vegetarian communities generally show lower rates of heart disease, obesity and high blood pressure than seen in meat-eating Western groups. Of course, these problems are not entirely the result of eating animal foods per se, but from the tendency of the modern Western diet to be high in fat and salt, and low in fibre and carbohydrate. The Western diet can be modified to turn around this profile without removing all animal foods. The important point is that a well-planned vegetarian diet can be as healthy as a well-planned meat-containing diet, but that badly-planned diets of both types are unlikely to fulfil the nutritional goals for health and athletic performance.

What are the traps of a hit-and-miss vegetarian diet? Firstly, there are the problems of inadequate nutrient intake, and of eating insufficient kilojoules because of the bulkiness of plant foods. Eliminating animal foods leaves a vacuum in terms of protein (meats, eggs and dairy products), iron, zinc and other trace elements (especially red meats and shellfish) and calcium (dairy products). Finding suitable replacements from vegetable foods is sometimes tricky, since the vegetable food source may be lower in nutrient content, and the availability of the nutrient (how well your body can absorb and use the nutrient) may be lower than in the animal food form. This is true for protein (read Chapter 2.3 about mixing and matching vegetable proteins to improve their amino acid profile) and for iron (read Chapter 2.5 about making vegetable iron sources available to the body). Occasionally other nutrients, such as some of the B-vitamins, fall into short supply in a restricted vegetarian diet.

In general, the risks of nutrient deficiencies are greater for those who have increased dietary requirements and for those who restrict their food range to the greatest extent. Into the former category go females (iron), adolescents (protein, energy, iron and calcium) and heavily training athletes, while the latter group includes vegans and the unimaginative vegetarian eaters mentioned already.

The other problem, especially in the case of new players, is that vegetarian food is not necessarily healthy. While plant foods are generally carbohydrate-based, heavy use of vegetable oils in cooking, high-fat pastries and batters on food, and the addition of cream and cheese to recipes, all produce a high-kilojoule, high-fat meal. Some vegetarians, while refusing meat because they believe that it is high in fat, will continue to use full-cream dairy products and to cook with high-fat methods. For example, a 'vegetarian pie' made with greasy stir-fried vegetables in a pastry case and topped with a thick layer of melted cheese packs in a lot of fat. Clearly, such a diet will not achieve

SPECIAL ISSUES IN VEGETARIAN EATING

Nutritional issue	Sources	Comments
Variety	all foods	Choose to be lacto-ovo-vegetarian (eating eggs and dairy products) rather than vegan, *or* enjoy a range of both vegetarian and meat-based meals—the more variety the better.
Energy (kilojoules)	all foods	To keep up a high kilojoule intake: — spread food into six or seven meals, rather than three large ones — make high-energy drinks such as fruit smoothies or make use of liquid meal supplements — avoid excessive fibre intake, and include some less bulky refined carbohydrate foods such as juices, white bread and white pastas (see Chapter 3.7). To avoid excess kilojoule intake: — watch the total quantity that you eat ('healthy' doesn't necessarily mean low-joule) — limit intake of fats and oils.
Fats and oils	• oils • margarine • cheese • pastry • nuts & seeds • cream	Limit fat and oil in cooking, and vegetarian recipes based on pastry, cream and cheese (see Chapter 1.2 for general ideas).
Carbohydrate	• grains • cereals • fruits • starchy vegies • legumes • flavoured low-fat dairy foods	This is your chance to try new foods and learn different ways of cooking. Make nutritious carbohydrate foods your first choice—they will also be an important source of protein, vitamins and minerals.

Nutritional issue	Sources	Comments
	• liquid meal supplements and fruit smoothies	
Protein	• low-fat dairy foods • eggs • legumes • nuts & seeds • wholegrains & cereals • soy products • liquid meal supplements	The quality of vegetable protein can be improved by mixing with a small amount of animal protein (dairy food or eggs) or by matching with another vegetable food. Good matches are cereals/grains and legumes, or legumes and nuts/seeds (see Chapter 2.3).
Iron	• wholegrain cereals—esp. breakfast cereal • legumes • nuts & seeds • tofu & soy products • eggs • green leafy vegies • dried fruit • liquid meal supplements	Add a vitamin C food to the meal to increase the iron absorption, avoid excessive fibre intake (see Chapter 2.5).
Zinc and trace minerals	• eggs • other iron-rich foods	Generally, if you look after iron intake, other minerals will also be looked after.
Vitamin B12	• dairy products • eggs • fortified soy milks or soy meats	Lacto–ovo–vegetarians will have no problems finding an 'animal' product to provide their small daily B12 requirement. Strict vegetarians will need to find a fortified soy product or a B12 supplement. While vitamin B12 is traditionally considered to be found only in foods from

Nutritional issue	Sources	Comments
		animal sources, B12 deficiency due to poor intake is rarely found even in vegans.
Riboflavin (Vitamin B2)	• dairy foods • Vegemite • breakfast cereals • legumes	Dairy products are the most important source of riboflavin in typical Australian diets. Lacto–ovo–vegetarians should be able to meet their riboflavin needs easily, but vegans should ensure that alternative sources are found.

the health and performance advantages that they seek. In fact, some new 'vegos' actually gain weight with this high-fat intake and end up worse off than before.

So, vegetarianism: to be or not to be? For moral, religious or cultural reasons the choice may be clear cut, and athlete or not, such a decision should be respected. Maureen's sister fits into this category, and in making the choice to be vegetarian she must also accept certain responsibilities. It may be harder for her to meet her nutritional needs, especially living amongst a meat-eating community, and she will need to be organised to make this happen. The preceding table presents a summary of some of the issues of vegetarian eating.

From the health or athletic performance perspective, the choice doesn't need be so black and white. There are both nutritional advantages and disadvantages to vegetarian eating, but the best of both worlds can be easily achieved—as Maureen found out. With the blessing of her parents and the help of her sister, she has started to explore the world of vegetarian food. Twice a week, they experiment with different recipes, from vegetable and tofu stir-fries and lentil burgers, to bean sauces for pasta.

Learning about these foods has helped her understand more about nutrition in general, and on the nights that she eats meat, fish and chicken meals she uses some of the ideas from her vegetarian cook books to add plenty of carbohydrate foods and cut down the fats. Not only has she begun to enjoy food and nutrition, but her skinfold problem has slowly started to look after itself, with much less panic than before.

Rowing

In international competition, both male and female crews race over a distance of 2000 metres. Crews are distinguished by the number of members in the boat (singles, doubles, fours and eights), whether there is a coxswain steering (the pairs and quads may be coxed or coxless), and whether the boat is sculled (two oars per person) or rowed (one oar each).

In some competitions, there is a separate lightweight division in which male rowers or scullers are not permitted to exceed 72.5kg with a crew average of 70kg, and in which the weight limits for women are 59kg (maximum) and 57kg (crew average). Lightweight competition has been recently added to World Rowing Championship, and Olympic Games programs. Weight limits also exist for the coxswains.

At elite levels, the time taken to complete the 2000-metre race ranges from over seven minutes for the singles to around 5.5 minutes for the eights. Since both arms and legs are active, representing a large proportion of total body muscle mass, considerable cardiovascular and metabolic demands are made. Rowing places great demands on both the aerobic and anaerobic energy systems, with the mean oxygen consumption for a race being not far short of the maximum achievable.

Training

Rowing training is long and intense. For eight to ten months of the year, rowing training consists of about twelve sessions per week, with nine on the water and three in the gymnasium. At times some crews make an even greater commitment, with two water sessions and a gym session in the one day. A typical rowing session covers about twenty kilometres at a heart rate high enough to stress both aerobic and anaerobic (lactic) metabolism. Weight training sessions are often undertaken to improve muscular endurance. It may seem a discrepancy that such long hours of training are spent in preparation for a 5–7 minute event, however rowing requires a unique mixture of technique, power and endurance of both aerobic and anaerobic energy systems and this time is required to optimise the level of each individual component.

Competition

Depending on the stature of the regatta, competition may last from three days to a week. Scullers and crews are first drawn in heats, with successful competitors progressing to semi-finals or finals, and the remainder to a repechage. Competitors successful in the repechage may progress to a semi-final. In large competitions, rowers will be required to race only once per day, however they may be required to race as hard on the first day as in the finals, to keep progressing through the competition. Light training is undertaken on rest days.

In lightweight competition, weigh-ins are conducted on the mornings of the events.

Physical characteristics

Heavyweight rowers are tall and heavy, with strong muscles and long limbs being favourable characteristics. Since the load is held constant (weight limits for the boat and coxswain), a larger and heavier crew has an advantage over a physically smaller crew. While muscle mass should account for most of the athlete's increased weight, body-fat levels are often relatively high among heavy-weight rowers, particularly females.

Lightweight crews are obviously smaller and lighter than their heavyweight counterparts, with lower body-fat levels showing the importance of a high power-to-weight ratio. As in most sports with weight divisions, many athletes 'sit on the fence' of the weight limits—being too small and light to compete successfully against bigger and stronger athletes, but nevertheless struggling to fit naturally into the lower weight limit.

Typical physique (elite heavyweight rowers)

	Male	Female
Height	187–195cm	174–181cm
Weight	87–93kg	65–76kg
Skinfold sum	38–56mm	72–114mm

State level lightweight rowers

	Male	Female
Height	—	165–177cm
Weight	70–76kg	59–63kg
Skinfold sum	38–51mm	60–87mm

Common nutrition issues

Training nutrition—high energy and carbohydrate requirements

Rowers can face enormous energy and carbohydrate requirements to support their heavy training loads and body weight/strength goals. Males especially fight to keep their body weight up while all rowers must work hard to recover from one day to the next. The lifestyle of the rower can also interfere with meeting these huge requirements. The time spent at training is time that isn't spent eating, and as in the case of Terry below, many rowers find it difficult to chew and stomach the amounts of food they need in a day.

Read Chapters 1 and 2 for details of the optimum training diet. A high-energy, high-carbohydrate, highly nutritious diet should be on the menu to achieve all the goals of heavy training. A pattern of small frequent meals, including a carbohydrate snack immediately after training, is the best plan of attack—allowing high energy goals to be achieved (Chapter 3.7) and recovery to be maximised (Chapter 5). Of course, this means being organised—see the case of Terry below.

Matters of physique

Higher body-fat levels are not as great a disadvantage to a rower as they are to a distance runner. After all, it is an advantage to be heavy and strong, and body weight is supported in the boat. However, there is a limit to the excess baggage that can be carried. It is better to be 80kg with body fat of 50mm, rather than 80kg with a body fat of 100mm. Lightweight crews have a definite need to optimise their power-to-weight ratio.

At some stage you may need to undertake special programs either to gain lean body mass or lose body fat. See Chapter 3 for advice.

Females and iron status

Female rowers face the risk of poor iron status, reflecting both their sex and their training commitment. Read Chapter 2.5 for advice about a high-iron diet that is also high in carbohydrate. Regular checks of iron status are recommended, especially where a previous history of iron deficiency exists. Male rowers may also need to be aware of possible problems with iron, particularly during adolescence when iron requirements are increased to cover growth costs.

Fluid needs

Long training sessions on the water in hot weather lead to significant sweat losses, particularly when undertaken twice a day. Learn good hydration practices in training—drink before sessions, take a water bottle to training, and rehydrate fully afterwards. Weighing yourself before and after training sessions will give you a clear picture of your body's fluid swings (see p. 29). A sports drink will provide carbohydrate during and after long training sessions—experiment to see if your training performance is improved.

A study of fluid balance during rowing training by the AIS reported average sweat rates of 2 litres/hour for elite male and 1400 ml/hr for female rowers in hot conditions (30°); in cool conditions (10°) average sweat rates were about 1160 ml/hr and 780 ml/hr respectively. Even though the rowers came prepared with their own water bottles they were unable to drink enough fluid to keep pace with their sweat losses—especially in the hot conditions. Even in cold conditions the rowers did not drink enough—perhaps they thought that they would not sweat much. Problems included the need to carry large amounts of water on the boat (despite being surrounded by water, rowers can only drink from their own provisions), and the need to stop training to drink (two hands are needed on the oar to row!). Better hydration might only be achieved in hot conditions by working on a special plan with your coach. The coach could bring extra fluid out in the speed boat so that empty water bottles could be topped up or replaced, and they could allow more drink breaks during the session—a few seconds every 15 minutes or so would not disrupt the session too much, and might produce better performances.

Competition nutrition

Rowers should go into each race with fluid and fuel stores topped up, and feeling comfortable after the last meal. With the regatta or competition lasting a number of days, the challenge is set to recover between each day's sessions and to repeat these goals for the next race.

Read Chapter 4 for advice about competition nutrition, and Chapter 5 for strategies to promote rapid recovery. Special care may be needed with pre-event eating—it can be very uncomfortable to race with a full stomach. Liquid meals may come in handy as a low-bulk pre-event meal or snack. With much of the day tied up in preparation and the race itself, there is usually neither time nor opportunity for rowers to meet their usual high-energy intake. Consequently, some rowers find that they quickly lose weight over the course of the competition.

Whether it be for an energy boost, or for a well-timed post-race recovery snack, it makes good sense for rowers to have nutritious food supplies at their finger-tips at all times. This might mean organising suitable supplies both at the rowing site and at the competition accommodation. Don't rely on the event organisers to have thought of your needs. Liquid meal supplements are again useful, being low in bulk, nutritious and portable. Use your creativity to think up other snacks as well.

Finally, don't neglect fluid needs. You may be dehydrated through your rowing efforts, through your making-weight practices (see below), or just from sitting out in the sun watching the rest of the competition. Carbohydrate-containing fluids such as sports drinks can be useful for both fluid and carbohydrate top-ups.

Lightweight rowing

As in other weight-matched sports, many rowers attempt to row in lightweight competition when their training weight is well above the event limits. For many lightweight rowers, obsession with food and weight, leading to disordered eating and eating disorders, becomes part of the way of life. This is topped off with severe dehydration and food restriction in the days leading up to competition—practices which may be repeated over the duration of the rowing competition. Females seem to be most at risk, although these problems are also experienced in male crews.

There is no doubt that these measures are harmful—physically and mentally—and affect both health and performance. From the performance perspective, a rowing competition is an extremely severe exercise challenge that should not be attempted at less than optimum preparation. The long-term consequences of a rowing career include the potential for disturbed metabolic efficiency. It is not unusual to find rowers complaining of increased difficulty in losing weight as time progresses, eventually reaching the point that, even with heavy training and sparrow-like intakes, they seem to be in energy balance. There are many additional disadvantages to health and nutritional status.

Read Chapter 3, and the account of Maree below for alternative ways to deal with the issue. Commonsense is often overlooked because crazy weight control practices become entrenched in the sport. Unfortunately, they can even be glorified. From the commentary box during the 1990 World Rowing Championships in Australia came the following encouragement 'And let's give a big hand to the crew from

X—these girls have not eaten anything for four days to make it into this final. What a heroic effort.'

The life of the cox

The coxswain's life is not easy. There is usually the pressure of making weight (the crew obviously wants the cox to be as light as possible), as well as the responsibility of keeping the crew together in stroke and spirit. It takes a distinctive sort of personality to rule over the boat. Weight control is made a little more difficult for coxes given that their job is not energy-burning—they are more or less there for the ride.

Since a cox may be involved in many hours of other people's training each day, there is often little time or incentive to take on additional aerobic exercise to aid their own weight control goals. This puts more emphasis on reduced energy intake to reduce body-fat levels. Many get caught up in the vicious cycle of making weight through dehydration and starvation, and in a general obsessiveness about food and weight. As in other sports this will have a detrimental effect on health, and like the lightweight rowers, an energy efficiency may develop, making the weight situation worse.

The issues of making weight have been dealt with for lightweight rowers, and in the wrestling and boxing chapter. The same advice is repeated below, and can be followed up in more detail in Chapter 3:

- make sensible decisions about weight targets;
- try to achieve body-fat loss through healthy nutrition and exercise plans, even if that means additional aerobic training; and
- avoid severe dehydration and food restriction practices before competitions.

If you won't do it for yourself, do it for the team. The last thing a top crew needs to face before important competition is an irritable and fatigued cox!

PROFILE: TERRY
Fitting enough food into the day—and into your stomach

Terry was living in a university college and rowing with the university coxed fours. The training schedule leading into the competition season was intense—ten water sessions and three weight training sessions each week. The energy requirements were obviously enormous, because Terry was fighting a losing battle to maintain his weight. Not only was he becoming tired, but he was starting to give away over five kilograms on the average crew weight. He was careful to eat a high carbohydrate diet. He had learned all about that in the nutrition classes of his physical education degree at university. But where he could find the time, the stomach room and food to increase his intake, he didn't know. He was already suffering from heartburn, especially when he bent over the oars, and on a couple of occasions he had actually vomited. Naturally, he was reluctant to increase his meal size any further.

He sought help from a sports dietitian after the third consecutive drop in his skinfold readings. She took a detailed account of his typical daily training and eating habits, as summarised below.

The dietitian was pleased with Terry's level of nutrition knowledge. He had a good understanding of carbohydrate foods and was able to make these the focus of all his meals. However, he simply wasn't eating enough, and the dietitian picked out two reasons for this.

- He was limited to eating three times a day, firstly because the university dining hall catered for this, and secondly because his time was tied up between meals. Training took up four or five hours a day, but he was also confined to class or study for a similar time.

A day in the life of Terry (rower)

5.30–8.00am	Rowing at river Often has heartburn from too much food the previous evening.
8.30am	Back to university college for as much breakfast as can be scoffed in 25 minutes: Cereal + tinned fruit + milk Fruit juice Toast + baked beans or spaghetti
9.15–12.30pm	University classes Indigestion and heartburn
12.45pm	Lunch at University cafeteria (Packed lunch provided by university college): Sandwiches/rolls with meat and salad fillings Fruit bun Fruit juice Sometimes has to cut back the amount if heartburn is bad—can't risk too much discomfort for evening session
1.45–4.30pm	University classes
5.00–7.30pm	Training at river Weights sessions 3/week following rowing
8.00pm	Early nights—arrives at the university dining hall just in time for late meal sitting: Meat/fish/chicken—large serves (often 2 meals) Rice or potatoes—sometimes pasta Vegies or salad Bread Jelly/fruit salad/rice pudding/icecream
	Late nights—misses the official meal time. Makes jam sandwiches—sometimes almost a loaf of bread. Probably eats too much, but what else can he do?
9.00–10.30pm	Study Bed

• Terry was often caught between eating too little or aggravating his heartburn problems with a huge meal.

The solution lay in making practical changes to increase food opportunities and to change the bulkiness of the meals. Terry was right about the problem of eating too much food at one sitting—however, with a pattern of six or seven meals and snacks a day, and with the clever use of nutritious drinks (low-bulk and high-energy) he could eat a high-energy intake without causing gastrointestinal distress.

Firstly, Terry needed to have increased access to food. The dietitian met with the chef at the university dining hall and negotiated a plan for his special needs. The chef was happy to provide Terry with some food for his room—all rooms were provided with a small fridge and tea-making facilities. Terry would receive some supplies of breakfast cereal, milk, canned fruit, and muesli bars. And he was encouraged to order two 'lunch bags' for each day—one to be eaten as a morning tea and lunch, and one to be kept as a snack between rowing and the weight session at night. Sandwiches, buns and fruit were easily eaten in the back of class, so he could divide the one meal bag into two sittings, and avoid the discomfort of a single big lunch.

As for the evening meal, the chef made plans to keep a meal waiting on the nights that he was late. Having already had a snack, this would top up his night intake.

Next item on the agenda was to learn how to make nutritious high-energy drinks. Terry was encouraged to invest in a Bamix to mix up delicious concoctions of Sustagen powder, milk, fruit, and low-fat yoghurt or icecream. He could afford to cut down the size of his dinner and breakfast meals and then boost energy intake with 500–1000ml of an action-packed drink. This left him able to have a mid-morning and late-evening snack without feeling sick, and his lunch bag or the supplies in his room were available for this purpose.

Exceed Sports Meal supplement, a ready-to-go version of his high-energy drink, was purchased for an afternoon snack in class. This left him relatively light and empty for the afternoon training session, yet continued to pour in the fuel. Lastly a sports drink was added, to drink in the boat and as soon as the session was over. While he was rehydrating he might as well pump in a little extra carbohydrate. Being able to consume this straight after training was an added bonus for recovery of muscle glycogen stores.

With consistent practice of this plan, Terry gradually began to regain the kilos and find new vigour at training. The heartburn and bloatedness after meals was also greatly reduced, making him feel better in the boat. It was sometimes a nuisance having to be so organised, and unless he kept varying his drink concoctions he became bored with the same thing three times a day. But while he remained one jump ahead of himself, he remained streets ahead in performance.

PROFILE: MAREE
Rowing lightweight

Maree tried out for selection in the state rowing squad as a light-weight single sculler. She did well in the physiological testing, and was assessed as having a good stroke technique. Inevitably the scales poked their way into the assessment, and the news was discouraging. At 63.5kg she was nearly five kilograms over the competition weight limit of 59kg. Some of the other girls were even worse off than this— two were up to nearly 69kg. One of these girls had collapsed in her last race, clearly exhausted and dehydrated, and she had had to go to the medical tent for intravenous rehydration.

Maree's own battle with the scales was gradually becoming a losing struggle. When she started rowing four years ago she hovered around 60–61kg, and needed only a small push in competition week to make the weight limit. At first the whole business had seemed exciting and mystical. She had watched the pairs and fours carrying out the weight-loss rituals as a team, and thought that it would bond their spirit together. Later down the track, though, it had become harder and harder to get the weight off, and she had realised that weeks of starv-ing, and days of sitting in saunas or running in thick tracksuits, made teams irritable and squabbling rather than close and cohesive. The crews were allowed to average their weights, so there was always niggling within the team about who should lose more weight and who was letting the others down.

Maree's weight thoughts were now no longer confined to the week leading up to competition, but had become a full-time obsession. She was constantly trying to shed the kilos, and the more she tried the harder it became. If worry was supposed to make you lose weight, then she shouldn't have a problem. Thoughts of food and the scales filled her every waking hour, but all to no avail. The frustration took any of the former enjoyment out of her sport.

She didn't tell this to the selection coach, but then she didn't need to. The trials and tribulations of lightweight rowing were well known to him. He was well aware of the constant dieting, and of the dangerous techniques of sweating and fasting that occurred in competition. He ex-plained to Maree that he was not prepared to support this system, and was only interested in recruiting girls who could safely and healthily row in the lightweight division. While it might be cruel to turn people away, he did not want to be part of the misery and the damage.

The coach looked at Maree's skinfold levels—a sum of 81mm over seven sites. This was higher than it needed to be, giving Maree a real chance to lose weight. He also took into consideration that she had not yet had a mishap during competition. Maree had always rowed well, and could truthfully say that she had never resorted to the more severe weight loss practices of diuretics, laxatives and vomiting. The final decision was to award Maree a temporary scholarship—to be revised in ten weeks. The conditions were that she would see a sports dietitian, and would reduce her training weight to 60–61kg, with a measurable loss from her skinfold levels.

Maree agreed to this trial, but wondered about the usefulness of seeing a dietitian. She wondered what the dietitian could tell her about weight loss that she didn't already know—Maree felt that she had been there, done that when it came to diets. Nevertheless, she kept to her side of the bargain.

The dietitian listened to Maree's story of constant dieting, and her state of learned metabolic efficiency. She certainly seemed to have depressed her energy requirements through years of restricted kilojoule intake and yo-yo weight loss. Her daily eating patterns were described as follows:

A day in the life of Maree—lightweight sculler

6.00–8.00am	Rowing training
8.30am	2 green apples on the way to work
9.00–12.30pm	Work—numerous cups of black tea
12.30pm	Run at lunch time Salad sandwich—no margarine no meat or cheese
1.30–4.30pm	More tea at work
5.00–7.30pm	Rowing training and weights
8.00pm	Tea at home: Plate of steamed vegetables 1–2/week piece of meat or chicken
9.00pm	Green apple
Every couple of days—splurges with a block of chocolate	

The dietitian assessed the daily plan as low in kilojoules, and inadequate in protein, iron, calcium and other minerals. It was a wonder that she was able to keep up her training load with such a small intake of carbohydrate and energy. She suggested that Maree was probably not always aware of the extent of her splurges—and would be surprised to see how her total energy intake fluctuated.

With a 'nothing else to lose' attitude, Maree agreed to try the dietitian's meal plan which included:

- improved intake of protein, carbohydrate and minerals to support training and health requirements;
- a small treat each week;
- a low-dose broad-range vitamin/mineral tablet each day to ensure that all nutrient RDIs were met;

- foods chosen to fit with portable lifestyle—e.g. a breakfast that can be eaten on the way to work (see summary below);
- the minimum level of kilojoule intake that could be regarded as healthy and unlikely to cause metabolic adaptations. As was suggested in section 3.4, she was to try an energy intake of about 4320kJ + energy cost of training.

Training = 8 sessions a week @ 60 minutes
Energy cost of training (assume rowing energy expenditure is equal to moderate running @ 50kJ per minute)
    = 24 000kJ/week or 3430kJ/day
Therefore, suggested energy intake
    = 7748kJ/day (1850 kcal/day)

She warned that Maree's greatest need was to begin to let go of her fears and worries, and to think more positively about her food and weight. With confidence and a happier outlook, she would be less likely to get out of control and splurge. This would need a lot of self-talk and support—after all she would need to reverse years of misery and frustration. She scheduled a weekly appointment for Maree to

Maree's new eating plan

Training sessions:	Sports drink (equal to about 500ml per day) Water
After training:	Carton of non-fat fruit yoghurt 1 breakfast bar or muesli bar Small carton of fruit salad
Lunch:	Salad sandwich (no marg.) Lean meat/chicken/low-fat cheese slice/salmon + thick salad filling Piece of fruit Low-joule drinks or water
Training sessions:	Sports drink Water
Dinner:	100g serve (cooked weight) of lean meat, fish or chicken Large potato or cup of rice or pasta 3–4 different cooked vegies or salad—large serves 1 thick slice bread (no marg.) Water
Supper:	Bowl of cereal + 200ml low-fat milk
Twice a week:	Chocolate frog
Analysis:	Energy = 7500kJ (1800 Cal) CHO = 305g (= 65% of energy) Protein = 100g Iron = 19mg Calcium = 920mg Vitamins meet RDI intake. For extra insurance a multivitamin/mineral supplement can be taken.

come and talk about her progress, and promised her that no scales would appear during that time. The emphasis would be on how Maree was feeling and coping.

Progress was slow but sure. Maree needed a lot of encouragement to change her old way of thinking. She agreed that she was happy with the meal plan, but needed to remind herself that a small treat was OK on occasions, and that she didn't need to watch the scales or have all the weight off within a week.

The first weight and skinfold check-in was after a month. The results were encouraging—weight was 62kg and skinfolds were 65mm. At the end of the second month, there was further progress—weight was 61kg and skinfolds 55mm. She met with the coach a fortnight later with a big smile on her face, and weighed in at 60.5kg. With a little fine-tuning before competition, and the nerves that went with big races, she would be well able to meet event limits. The rewards for her effort were not only a full rowing scholarship, but a totally changed outlook on her life and her sport.

Australian
Rules
Football

Australian Rules Football is played predominantly by males, with the major league, the Australian Football League, having developed into a national competition. It is played from primary school upwards, at a variety of levels both amateur and professional.

A game is made up of four 20-minute quarters, with time-on (usually five to ten minutes) added for the time that the ball is out of play. The first and third quarters are separated by a short break, with a longer break at half-time. Each team consists of eighteen players on the ground, with another three 'interchange' players who may be swapped at any time for other players on the field.

The traditional line-up sees five lines of three players spread from one end of the ground (backs) to the other (forwards), with the other three players set to follow the play. However, as the game has evolved into a more mobile style of play, these traditional lines have lost much of their former meaning. In addition to running, players must leap to mark or punch the ball. Heavy physical contact and tackling also increase the demands on players.

Training

The football year can be divided into three sections: pre-season, season, and off-season. The length of each section will vary with the level of competition. A typical outline might be:

- Off-season: 1–3 months from October–January—little or no scheduled training. Often a time where body fat increases.
- Pre-season: 2–4 months—training may start as early as November with 3 to 5 sessions per week. Individual players are often selected for specific programs according to the requirements of their position or their individual weaknesses. In general, training revolves around a running program, building up an aerobic base and then anaerobic speed and endurance. Weight training is built into the program—especially for players who need to build up bulk and strength. Other sports such as boxing or swimming may also be included. Skills training is introduced as pre-season progresses, with practice matches leading into the season.
- Competitive season: There are roughly six days between matches. Most clubs schedule three or four training sessions between these games, with a heavy session mid-week, and lighter skill-oriented sessions later in the week.

Most training sessions are held in the late afternoon to fit in with work schedules.

Competition

The AFL season consists of 20–25 games, one played each weekend from March to August, with finals being held in September. Most games are played on Saturday or Sunday afternoons with the under-age and reserve matches preceding the main game. The national competition now involves interstate travel, with some games being played at night under lights. A supplementary night competition and pre-season practice matches generally start in early February and may add another six matches to the year's tally.

An Australian Rules Football match lasts about two hours, with the physiological demands varying considerably between field positions. On-ball players may run between twelve and twenty kilometres each match, with a fairly even proportion of aerobic and anaerobic activities and a high total-fuel requirement. Typically players run at top speed for 10–50 metres, followed by a walk or jog back to position.

Full-forwards and full-backs perform very short, high-intensity sprints with almost purely anaerobic requirements and lower total energy demands.

The repeated physical contact and the resulting damage to muscle fibres must be taken into consideration in the recovery between matches.

Physical characteristics

The Australian Rules Football team has been introduced as a mixed bag of field positions and playing skills. It should come as no surprise that the physical profile of the Australian Rules Football player is varied—from 200cm rucks to 170cm rovers. Lower body-fat levels are expected amongst running players. Greater height and muscle mass are expected in key positions where players directly contest each other for the ball.

Typical physique (elite Australian Rules Football player)

	Ruck	Running player	Key position player
Height	200cm	174cm	189cm
Weight	99kg	75kg	94kg
Skinfold sum	55mm	56mm	59mm

Other comments

Tradition has played a strong role in the development of Australian Rules football. Many competition and training practices have persisted long after they have become outdated by scientific thinking—often because players become coaches or trainers and pass on the old methods. Fortunately, accredited courses for coaches and trainers are gradually causing the death of many old wives' tales.

Another characteristic which has helped to retain tradition is the close-knit environment of the team and the persuasive power of peer influence. Attitudes and behaviour are shared, and because 'everybody' does something, it is regarded as normal, even when the practice is not normal outside the football club, or for that matter, a sensible and healthy practice.

Despite this, Australian Rules Football has changed dramatically in the past twenty years and now requires greater commitment and professionalism from players. Today's footballers play a different style of game to that played by their childhood heroes. The new game is faster, and requires players to be fitter both in terms of speed and endurance. Players must also look more closely at recovery—both within and after the game, then through the week's training to the next match. Although there has been some progress in the scientific basis of training and match preparation, there are still many areas that are yet to be refined.

Common nutrition issues

General nutrition knowledge and cooking skills

The top football leagues begin to recruit new players as young as fifteen or sixteen years. This sometimes means relocating young players to a new city. Accommodation is often found with families, however many young recruits and indeed older players share houses in which no-one has any real nutrition knowledge or cooking skills.

Even at the professional level, many footballers have full-time employment. When the heavy commitment of training, matches and other club activities are added to work hours, there may be little time for food shopping and preparation. A pattern of skipped meals and reliance on take-away foods is common.

Australian Rules Football players should be screened to find those at risk. Basic nutrition education and cooking lessons can be a valuable tool in improving the dietary intake of these players.

Take-aways and restaurants

Take-away foods are typical fare for weekends (after the game) and may become the staple of footballers who can't cook for themselves. Upgraded cooking skills should enable quick and easy meals to be made at home. However, players should also be educated about good choices with take-aways, and how to eat well in restaurants. It is inevitable that these opportunities will continue to contribute to food intake, but with careful selection they should also be able to contribute to total nutrition goals. See the section on take-aways in the Basketball chapter.

Weight control—or more importantly, control of body fat

Many players start pre-season or come back from injury heavier than their usual playing weight. In football circles, the traditional emphasis has been on total body weight rather than an understanding of muscle mass versus body fat. Ideally, clubs should arrange for someone on their sports medicine/fitness staff to be trained to take skinfold measurements. Body-fat levels should be monitored at strategic times of the football year and individual targets set for each player. Chapter 3 explains how body-fat measurements are taken and how body-fat goals are set. Footballers are notorious for using crash and fad diets to achieve weight loss. For a better approach to steady and permanent loss of body fat, read Chapter 3.3. Rodney's story below shows how this can work in real-life.

Gaining muscle mass

At the other end of the spectrum is the young slightly-built recruit who wishes to gain weight to withstand the physical contact of the game. In fact, it is a gain of muscle mass and strength that is required. As outlined in Chapters 3.6 and 3.7, bulking up requires an appropriate weights program, a high-energy diet and realistic expectations. In addition, specialist coaching may help slender players to adopt body-positioning and game skills that overcome many of the problems of being pushed around.

Alcohol intake

The alcohol intake of many footballers is a good example of the power of peer group behaviour over principles of peak training nutrition— and even plain commonsense. The typical drinking patterns of Australian Rules Football players are examined in the account at the end of this chapter. Although football players rationalise that this is normal, poor use of alcohol will prevent optimum performance from being reached in a number of ways. A better approach to alcohol in sport is presented in Chapter 1.6.

Recovery and muscle glycogen

Traditionally, football players have considered carbohydrate only on the eve of the match. The sentiment has been to eat protein at the beginning of the week, carbohydrate at the end. Yet recovery from a match, and between each training session, requires a high carbohydrate intake *every* day. It is likely that the game combined with long training nights will draw heavily on muscle glycogen stores particularly for running players. Muscle damage and injury, caused for example by body contact and tackling, will increase carbohydrate requirements for glycogen restoration.

Active recovery should begin as soon as each exercise session finishes. The study reported below shows that elite footballers are not aware of this. They eat a typical Australian training diet rather than the high-carbohydrate diet needed to promote muscle glycogen refuelling. And the most crucial period for active recovery—immediately after the game—is probably the time that nutritional needs are most neglected.

Read Chapter 5 on active recovery and then organise your post-match activities to look after fluid and carbohydrate replacement. Perhaps your club can organise a suitable post-match function to encourage this as a team priority. Daily recovery of fuel stores will require a high carbohydrate intake all week round, starting straight after each training session. Read Chapters 1.3 and 2.2 for hints on everyday use of carbohydrate foods. The ability to bounce back immediately from each match and training session should give you edge over your opponents, and save you from that end-of-the-week fatigue.

Preparation for the match

When footballers started thinking about their diets, they initially focused on what to eat on match morning. Later this was expanded to what to eat on the night before. If you have paid the proper attention to recovery, then preparation for the match is, for the most part, already taken care of. Building up muscle glycogen stores for the game happens as soon as the last training session finishes, starting Thursday night rather than Friday night in most cases. In Chapter 4.1 you will see that a further 24–36 hours of rest on a high-carbohydrate intake will top up your muscle fuel stores to see you through the game.

One note of caution—make sure that you can identify real carbohydrate sources both in everyday and pre-match settings. The foods that many footballers choose on Friday nights—chocolate, fish and chips, and oily lasagne, to name a few—are often higher in fat than carbohydrate.

The pre-game meal

The pre-game meal has been a great point of tradition and superstition over the years, with the old guard proposing that steak and eggs were a 'real man's' meal. Although a high-fat meal like this may not seem an obvious disadvantage to all players, today's science advocates that a low-fat high-carbohydrate meal be on the pre-game menu. Read Chapter 4.3 for suggestions. If you have an afternoon or evening game you may be able to eat a bigger meal earlier in the day and finish with a ligher snack two hours before the match. Experiment to find the meal arrangement that suits you.

Fluid intake during training and matches

With the lengthening of seasons and the inclusion of non-Victorian teams (and grounds) in the national competition, training sessions and pre-season matches are now conducted in warm to hot weather. But even in winter, players should be on guard against dehydration. Football tradition has seen fluid and electrolyte practices that are now known to be quite wrong—and even dangerous. Hopefully there are few football clubs in these enlightened times that promote salt tablets to prevent cramp, or think that training without fluid intake 'toughens up' players. Water bottles should always be on hand during training sessions and matches. The breaks between quarters provide more opportunities to take in fluid during the game. Read Chapter 4.4 to remind yourself of good fluid intake practices.

Extra benefits to performance may accrue from using a carbohydrate-based drink during a match. For running players this may supplement depleted muscle glycogen stores towards the end of the match, and keep blood glucose levels steady for optimum central nervous system function. Cordial or a sports drink is commonly provided by many football clubs between quarters, and in sufficient quantities these can meet both fluid and carbohydrate opportunities. We look forward to studies of carbohydrate intake during a real-life game to see if a performance boost can be detected.

PROFILE
Drinking to your sports success

Alcohol intake was studied among players from a top club in the Australian Football League. The information was collected in a number of ways to provide support for the results. Fifty-four players took part in a large dietary study which required them to keep an accurate food record over a typical seven-day period during the season. This record included all alcohol consumed during this time, and players were instructed to eat (and drink) as normal. The players were then interviewed in person and questioned about their usual drinking patterns. Finally, since people often under-report or over-exaggerate their alcohol intake on questionnaires, an independent assessment was devised. Blood alcohol was measured in blood samples taken from 41 players at a Sunday morning training session between 9–10am. The readings were used to gauge the alcohol consumed on the previous evening, after the match.

The football club policy encouraged that no alcohol be drunk during the week. Most players reported that they abided by this rule and drank on weekends only, on Saturday nights after the game and Sundays. However, they made up for the week's abstinence on these occasions, claiming that heavy alcohol intake was part of team bonding and unwinding after the game. During the off-season, without the club policy in effect, the frequency of alcohol binges would increase. Only five of the footballers interviewed described themselves as non-drinkers.

From the food records it was calculated that an average of 20g of alcohol was consumed by each player per day, amounting to 3.5 per cent of their total energy intake. While this sounds moderate on paper, the 'average' figure covers up for the heavy drinking on weekends. Players who consumed alcohol on the Saturday night, drank an average of 120g or twelve standard drinks (see Figure 1.6). Individual intakes ranged from 37g of alcohol to 368g—almost 40 standard drinks. In an extreme case alcohol provided 43 per cent of the kilojoules consumed that day, but on average supplied almost one-fifth of total energy intake on the Saturday.

The results of the blood alcohol readings support the Saturday night binge story. Fourteen players were recorded with positive blood alcohol readings at 10am the next morning, ranging from 0.001 to 0.113g/100ml. Four players had blood alcohol readings that were over

'.05' (0.05g/100ml)—the legal limit for driving a car in the State of Victoria. Clearly, a lot of alcohol had been consumed by some players over the previous evening.

You might ask how professional athletes, paid to perform at their best, could have such an unprofessional attitude to alcohol misuse. The major problems are football tradition and peer group influence that support these practices. And the major obstacle to change is the 'everybody does it' excuse—a poor rationalisation at best.

Other illogical rationalisations include: 'I only do it once a week'; 'it's part of cultivating team spirit'; 'beer is good for carbos'; and 'I can sweat it out the next day'. Read Chapter 1.6 for the facts about alcohol and sports performance. In football, the most serious outcomes of binge drinking are:

Short-term: dehydrates players who are possibly already dehydrated; exacerbates soft tissue and bruising injuries, a big part of a contact sport

Long-term: adds to weight problems, not only by adding its own kilojoules, but by causing players to relax their attitude to other nutritional matters over the weekend.

If you spend enough time around a football club you will hear the stories about players who have missed important matches because of the lethal combination of a 'corked thigh' and a 'few' celebratory drinks after the previous match, and the players who return from the end-of-season trip seven kilograms over their playing weight.

Just because it is difficult to shift ground doesn't mean that individual players and football clubs can't push towards a more sensible approach to alcohol use. For a start:

- change the club policy on alcohol to remove the 'all or none' principle. It would be better for players to learn to drink a glass or two daily, rather than save it up for a weekend binge. Demystify the practice!

- make sure that all club functions and activities provide low alcohol and non-alcoholic drinks.

- create good role-models. Emphasise good players who have a moderate and healthy approach to alcohol intake—it is not necessary to give up alcohol altogether.

The results will be worth the effort!

PROFILE: RODNEY
Losing kilos and gaining metres

At 29 years, Rodney was one of the oldest players at his top league club. He had enjoyed a successful career and been part of a number of premierships. However, in the past year Rodney had become slow, even for a backline player. At least some of this was due to a gain of body fat, a stubborn increase of four or five kilograms over his best playing weight. In the middle of pre-season, the club fitness adviser brought some scales and skinfold calipers to training. Rod clocked in at 90kg and a total skinfold sum of 93mm (not a good position to be in when your contract has yet to be renewed!).

Rod consulted the club dietitian who instructed him to keep an accurate record of all food and drinks consumed during the next seven-day period. His average daily intake of energy and nutrients was estimated (see the 'Before' column in the following table).

The dietitian focused on fat and alcohol as expendable energy sources for achieving weight loss. She explained the importance of carbohydrate foods in promoting recovery between training sessions and advised Rod to actually increase his present carbohydrate intake. Rod admitted that the hard training sessions already left him tired, and was pleased that he could lose body fat without adding to this fatigue.

A meal plan was organised to cut back fat and oil intake. Rod's wife was enthusiastic to include all the family in this plan. Ideas included:

- switching to a lower-fat milk
- cooking with a minimum of fat or oil
- using a lighter spread of margarine on toast and bread
- choosing the leanest cuts of meat and chicken, and removing all fat and skin
- cutting the protein serve at dinner to two-thirds the old size, and having one slice of meat or cheese in each sandwich at lunch instead of thick layers of both
- when having take-aways at the weekend, choosing lower-fat types and having a small serve only.

Extra carbohydrate foods were added, including a generous serve of rice, pasta or potatoes at the evening meal. Snacks now came in the form of fresh fruit or from cakes and slices made with low-fat recipes. Rod made a great effort with his alcohol intake, limiting his drinking to a couple of cans of beer at the weekends. He often managed to make this a lower alcohol beer as well.

The results were immediate. Within six weeks, Rod had lost the five kilograms he desired. As proof of his long-term commitment to this healthy eating plan, another food record was kept six months later. His new diet showed a complete change in energy and nutrient intake (see the 'After' column in the table). Rod's body weight was remeasured at 85kg and his skinfold sum at 59mm. He reported feeling full of energy and with an extra 'metre' of pace in the games. His family

Rod's healthy weight loss diet—average daily intake

		Before	After
Energy	kilojoules	15 500	13 000
	Calories	3 705	3 115
Protein	grams	117	116
	% of energy	12.5%	15%
Fat	grams	154	91
	% of energy	40%	27%
Carbohydrate	grams	291	430
	% of energy	31.5%	56%
Alcohol	grams	86	11
	% of energy	16%	2%
Vitamins and minerals		All above RDI levels	All above RDI levels and greater than before

Comparison of footballers' (low-carbohydrate) diet and triathletes' (high-carbohydrate) food selections

Food group	Footballers (serves/day)	Triathletes (serves/day)
Bread and cereals	Equivalent to 8.5 slices of bread (mostly white)	Equivalent to 18 slices of bread (mostly wholemeal)
Meats and protein foods	Equivalent to 300g	Equivalent to 150g
Dairy products	Equivalent to 600ml of milk (mostly high-fat types)	Equivalent to 800ml of milk (mostly low-fat types)
Added fats and oils	Equivalent to 65g	Equivalent to 20g
Fruit and starchy vegetables	Equivalent to 5 pieces	Equivalent to 12 pieces

are now pleased to spend Sundays together, without him nursing a headache from the night before. As for the club, they are expecting a few good years out of him yet!

Carbohydrate all week round

Ideally, footballers should face the daily challenge of recovery from each match or training session by eating a high-carbohydrate diet all week round. Does this happen in real life? The dietary survey of the top league football club mentioned before, says no. Fifty-four players kept accurate food records for a typical seven-day period during the season. The average energy and nutrient intake of a footballer was estimated from these records with the average daily energy intake being 14 200 kilojoules (3395 Cals).

Carbohydrate provided an average of 44 per cent of total energy intake with fat providing another 37 per cent. These proportions are identical to the typical Australian diet. Not only is fat intake higher than nutrition experts recommend for good health, but it is providing energy intake at the expense of carbohydrate foods, and depriving the footballer of the opportunity to replenish fuel stores each day.

A similar study conducted on a group of elite triathletes found that these athletes chose their foods quite differently to provide 60 per cent of their total energy intake from carbohydrate foods. A quick summary of the two groups shows the differences in food patterns— see the preceding table. While both groups ate foods from each of the major food categories, the success of the triathletes was due to:

- emphasising the serve size of the carbohydrate food rather than the protein food
- choosing the low-fat versions of foods, and preparing meals with the minimum of added fats and oils.

Footballers could learn from these patterns!

Rugby League

Rugby League is the most popular football code in New South Wales and Queensland, with Australia's largest competition, the Australian Rugby League being expanded to a national competition, including a team from New Zealand. International competition is also available, and there are plans afoot to create a Super League competition. Competition starts at the school level, with modified rules in place to prevent injuries during scrums.

A Rugby League team consists of 13 players, six forming the forward pack and the rest making up the backline. In most leagues two reserves are allowed, but once a substitution takes place no further replacements can be made. The game, dominated by short bursts of running and heavy tackling, is basically a game of strength, skill and speed. A game takes place over two halves lasting forty minutes each.

Training

Like Australian Rules Football, the Rugby League year is broken into three phases: pre-season, competition and off-season. Again, the length of these phases will depend on the competition level, with the top professional teams following this typical pattern:

- Off-season: may be as short as a month. There is usually a break from all team training during this time, although some players may do their own conditioning work. At lower levels, a prolonged off-season can be a time of loss of fitness and gain of body fat.

- Pre-season: can start in late November-early December. Includes running and weights, often specifically set for each player or each playing position. Four to six practice matches may be played in January and February, often in the form of a pre-season competition prior to the main league.

- Competition season: March to September. Typically four to five training sessions are scheduled for the six days between games. Some sessions are devoted to strength training, while others will involve running, drills and other skill work. Training is held in the late afternoon, typically after work, since most players also work in full-time employment. Sessions may last from 1–2½ hours.

Competition

The Australian Rugby League season runs from March to August with the final series being held in September. Each team plays one game each weekend, with Saturday and Sunday afternoons being the traditional game time. Some games are played on Monday and Friday nights. With the supplementary pre-season competition, and the 'State of Origin' series that runs in mid-season, some players compete in almost 30 matches each year.

Periodically, an international tour may be organised, sending an Australian representative side to play games against English and French teams. This poses a great challenge to the elite players involved, requiring them to extend their competition peak right through two domestic seasons.

Rugby League, being a game of short bursts of play, is not demanding in terms of energy considerations. Fuel stores are not expected to be depleted during a game, provided that muscle glycogen levels have been successfully restored since the previous game, and maintained over the week of training. However, the game is physically challenging due to injuries, soft tissue damage and bruising, caused by heavy body contact and tackling.

Physical characteristics

Rugby League forwards are built to run the ball offensively and to tackle. The typical forward is heavy—with large muscle mass and a higher body-fat level than his backline counterpart. Backs are typically 10–20kg lighter, and in keeping with the running requirements of their game, have lower body-fat levels.

It is interesting to compare the typical physical characteristics of players in different football codes. In general, the average Rugby League player is heavier but shorter than an Australian Rules Football player, and both heavier and taller than a soccer player—reflecting the importance of muscle bulk and strength in the game of Rugby. Body-fat levels of the Rugby League player are generally higher than that of soccer players and Australian Rules Footballers, since greater aerobic fitness and mobility is required in the latter football codes.

Other comments

Many of the comments made about Australian Rules Football apply equally to Rugby League. Until recently, tradition has played a stronger part in determining training and competition practices than have sports science principles. Peer influence and mateship have also played a strong role in this code. Hopefully, the continued development of professionalism and science-based coaching amongst Rugby teams will increase the interest in better eating—and drinking—practices amongst players.

Common nutrition issues

Rugby League and Australian Rules Football share many nutrition concerns. Read the Australian Rules Football chapter, and the common nutrition issues (1–9) that are presented there. Special attention should be paid to the discussions concerning alcohol intake, and general nutrition knowledge and cooking skills.

In general, single players living outside a family situation are at high risk of poor nutrition. Lack of nutrition knowledge and cooking skills can be compounded by lack of time and post-training fatigue, making irregular meals and fast foods an easy pattern to fall into. As in the case of Tim below, dietary counselling can help players to find their way around the supermarket and kitchen. An astute football club will screen its team to identify players in need of nutrition education and support. Why waste talent simply because of poor eating habits?

Nutritional tradition or folklore in Rugby League is similar to Australian Rules Football, with many players still believing in high protein intakes during the week and some players continuing with pre-match meals of steak and eggs. Even more enlightened players still think of carbohydrate as a pre-game or night-before concern. Read the Australian Rules chapter, and for more detailed information about the optimum training diet, refer to Chapters 1 and 2 in Part I.

Although the fuel requirements of a Rugby League game are less than that of Australian Rules Football, optimum carbohydrate intake for training and competing in Rugby League may not be provided in a typical Australian diet—both in terms of amount and timing of intake.

As in Australian Rules Football, eating carbohydrate immediately following a game or heavy training session can help to promote recovery. When muscle damage has occurred—a feature to be expected in such a heavy body contact sport—even higher carbohydrate intake is required to help refill muscle fuel stores. Carbohydrate eaten soon after the finish of exercise is better stored as muscle glycogen than carbohydrate in later meals (see Chapter 5.2).

Another issue of importance in Rugby League as well as Australian Rules Football is:

Fluid intake during the game and training

The extended Rugby season and the inclusion of teams from tropical climates means that training sessions and matches may be held in hot weather. With large muscle mass, and perhaps a relatively high body-fat level, Rugby League players might be expected to have poorer heat tolerance than other athletes. Heavy jumpers and/or padding can also trap heat and add to heat stress problems.

While some players still need to improve their drinking practices during the game, training often presents the greater threat for dehydration and heat stress. In summer particularly, teams may conduct prolonged and intense training sessions in the hot afternoon sun, with little regard for sweat losses. Even in winter, fluid losses should be taken into account: the tradition of toughening players by withholding fluids during training is both unscientific and unsafe. Changing to good fluid intake habits may require the updating of attitudes of players and coaching staff, as well as practical arrangements at training to make drinks available during and after training as well as games.

The match fuel requirements of Rugby League may be met by well-stocked body stores. However, for some players, and in situations where good preparation is not possible, extra fuel during the game or training may delay fatigue and boost performance. Therefore sports drinks or cordial may be a good choice, although water will suffice when fluid needs are the only concern. After an exhausting game or training session, these carbohydrate drinks will come into their own by providing both for fluid and fuel recovery needs.

Issues that warrant additional comment for Rugby League are as follows:

Bulking-up

Muscle mass and strength play a greater role in Rugby League than in Australian Rules Football and soccer, and bulking-up may be a priority of training and eating goals. Some teams assign a playing weight for their players and considerable effort may be required during pre-season to live up to this expectation. Read Chapters 3.6 and 3.7 for hints on bulking-up. You will need to be committed to a high energy intake from nutritious foods. This might sound great, but it is often hard work to fit frequent meals and snacks into a busy lifestyle of work and training.

Nutrition during injury

At some stage in their sports career, most athletes suffer an injury that restricts or stops their training or competition for some time. Injuries are double-sided in body contact sports such as Rugby League—it is not just what you do to yourself in training or a game, but what other players inflict on you as well.

Nutritional considerations during injury and rehabilitation can vary between situations and individuals. Firstly, changes in energy expenditure need to be taken into account, particularly if the lay-off off exercise is extended. An injured athlete may not automatically reduce food intake to match the sudden drop in exercise level. This can result in a significant increase in body-fat levels, making the job of rehabilitation and return to form more difficult.

Muscle mass will be lost when strength-training athletes take time off weights work, or when surgery requires body parts to be immobilised. In the latter situation, muscle atrophy can become quite pronounced. Bulking-up principles of training and eating may be needed during rehabilitation (see Chapters 3.6 and 3.7). In any case, it is important to eat nutritiously while recovering from injury. Severe injury or extensive surgery will significantly increase requirements for energy, protein and other nutrients—and inadequate nutritional support will delay recovery.

Even with the best of intentions, many injured athletes find it difficult to look after their nutritional needs. Limited mobility can interfere with normal shopping and cooking activities. Injuries to the head and neck can also directly interfere with food intake, particularly if chewing and swallowing are restricted. A fractured jaw poses a special challenge—to achieve nutritional needs while eating through a straw for six to eight weeks. Liquid meal supplements and nutritious milk drinks play a crucial role under these circumstances, and in other situations when eating or preparing solid food is difficult. See a sports dietitian for specialised help.

PROFILE: TIM
Learning to cook in four easy steps

Tim was in his second year at a top Rugby League team. Being recruited from a country zone meant relocating to the city, a move made easier in the first year by boarding with a family. The next year however, Tim moved into a house with a friend from work, and an ideal domestic situation it was not. Tim had been too well looked after by his Mum, and then his housemother, and his only household experience to date had been to make his bed.

After six weeks of pre-season training, it was clear that something was amiss. Tim had lost 4kg, was well under his normal playing weight, and his training performances were sluggish. The club doctor sent him to a sports dietitian to see where the problem lay.

It was only after her assessment that the full picture of Tim's eating pattern—or perhaps more correctly the lack of an eating pattern—became apparent. The first problem to be discovered was a lack of food in the house. Tim and his housemate had not organised regular shopping expeditions. Instead, they made sporadic trips to the supermarket when motivated and midnight trips to the 7-Eleven when desperate. With no schedule of food buying, Tim would often confront the breakfast table to find no milk, no bread and Weetbix dust in the bottom of the packet.

Thus breakfast was often eaten from the vending machine in the lobby at work, or from the biscuit barrel in the tea room. In order to leave work early for training, Tim had only a half-hour break for lunch. This was well-spent in the sandwich bar next to work, but there was a limit to how much could be chewed in 30 minutes.

The next opportunity to eat was after training, and Tim admitted to often being too tired to eat, let alone cook. He estimated that it was only twice a week that he found the food and the energy to cook a real meal. His cooking repertoire was, in his own words, 'nothing flash'— sausages, steak or chops, with mashed potatoes and peas. On other nights he made toasted sandwiches or opened a tin of soup. From the financial viewpoint he tried to limit take-aways to weekends, and kept the dial-a-pizza number beside the telephone for these occasions.

'Pretty disorganised' was Tim's own comment, followed by 'How can I learn to cook?'.

The dietitian agreed that Tim's food intake was hit and miss, and that it was missing his nutritional needs in terms of total kilojoules and carbohydrate, and possibly other nutrients as well. The following plan was offered—not just to improve Tim's cooking skills but to work on his domestic organisation. Even if you are a culinary genius, it is difficult to cook a meal when your food pantry resembles that of old Mother Hubbard.

STEPS TO QUICK AND HEALTHY COOKING

Step 1: shop well

- Organise regular shopping expeditions. Non-perishable items may only need to be stocked up every now and again, but plan for a weekly trip to buy perishable foods.
- Shop from a list to ensure that you spend your time and money efficiently. It can be useful to keep a checklist of supplies inside the pantry door, to prompt you as you make your shopping list. The table on the following page provides some ideas, including a list of handy foods that can be stored for long periods and re-stocked periodically. These foods provide a great start for quick and nutritious meals.

Step 2: learn a couple of meal ideas and vary the themes

Quick and easy high-carbohydrate meals include the following themes:

Traditional 'meat and three vegies'

- Make these meals lower in fat by choosing lean and trimmed cuts of meat, fish or chicken. Cook with the minimum of added fats or oils.
- Break tradition by keeping to a medium serve of these protein foods, and bumping up your carbohydrate intake with a generous serve of oven- or microwave-baked potatoes, corn-on-the-cob, or side serves of rice or quick-cook noodles.
- Frozen vegies are a great time saver—no preparation, no wastage and no worries about them spoiling in the fridge before you can eat them. Not only do they come in individual varieties, but new 'mixed vegetable' combinations can add plenty of colour and nutritional variety to meals. Use fresh or frozen vegies to suit your needs.

Versatile all-in-one-pot sauces

- Take a base sauce—a commercial pasta sauce, or add your own herbs and spices to tinned tomatoes or tomato puree.
- Add some protein—diced lean meat or chicken, tinned fish and seafood, or beans (brown the meat or chicken pieces before adding to the sauce).
- Complete by adding vegies—fresh or frozen, chopped or diced.
- Make it chunky, like a casserole and serve with rice or noodles.
- Less chunky, it can be used as a sauce for pasta or a filling for giant baked potatoes.
- Experiment with the various combinations of ingredients.

Stir-fries
- Take the vegetable and protein combinations as above, and cut them into quick-cooking size pieces. Dry fry in a wok or large frying pan.
- Add a commercial sauce or flavour sachet for a short cut, or add your own herbs and spices as you grow confident.
- Lastly, add noodles or rice that have been cooked and drained.

Home-made pizza
- High-carbohydrate pizza bases can be purchased from many supermarket delis, or pita or Lebanese bread can be used to make your own.
- Spread with tomato paste or commercial pasta sauces and add your own low fat toppings, such as vegies, a little lean meat, chicken or seafood.
- Spinkle cheese lightly over the top—reduced-fat mozzarellas are available.

Step 3: use healthy eating recipes to add to your repertoire
- Use healthy nutrition recipe books to expand your cooking horizons. The box on p. 295 lists some recipe books that cater for high-carbohydrate, low-fat meals—some are even specifically written for athletes.
- If you have the time and the right ingredients, you may wish to follow a recipe right through. Alternatively, just by reading through recipe books you may pick up ideas to jazz up your own cooking —particularly to learn about herbs, spices and other flavourings.

Step 4: put time-saving tricks into practice
- In a group household it makes sense to share the cooking and shopping duties amongst similarly motivated housemates.
- If you are living alone or looking after your own meals, it pays to take some cooking short-cuts—particularly for nights when you arrive home late and tired.
  - use the less busy times of the week to catch up on cooking— e.g. nights off training or quiet times on weekends. It may be possible to prepare the week's meals at one go—refrigerating or freezing the food until you need it.
  - Many recipes—especially casseroles, soups and sauces—lend themselves to leftovers. It can be just as quick to cook up a double batch. What you don't eat on one night can be reheated the following night(s), or frozen into 'single serve' portions for a rainy day.

CHECKLIST FOR A WELL-STOCKED PANTRY AND FRIDGE

Handy foods for long-life storage
  Skim milk powder
  Wholegrain breakfast cereals
  Rolled oats
  Canned beans—baked beans, bean mix, kidney beans etc.
  Packets of beans and lentils
  Two-minute noodles
  Wholemeal rice
  Pasta and noodle varieties
  Canned salmon and tuna (in water/brine)
  Canned seafood—crab meat, mixed seafood etc.
  Pasta sauces
  Canned soups—especially low salt and main meal varieties
  Canned tomatoes, tomato puree, tomato paste
  Canned corn and champignons
  Rice cakes
  Sustagen or Exceed Sports Meal
  Herbs and spices

Medium-term freezer storage
  Frozen vegetables—single varieties and mixed vegetable
    combinations
  Bread
  Skim and low-fat milk
  Low-fat icecream
  Meat, fish, poultry
  Pizza bases
  Fresh pasta

Perishable food items for short storage
  Fruit juice
  Skim and low-fat milk
  Bread
  Fresh fruit
  Fresh vegies
  Meat, fish, poultry
  Eggs
  Low-fat yoghurt
  Cottage cheese
  Reduced-fat cheese
  Margarine or butter (shouldn't need to be replaced often)

RECIPE BOOKS BASED ON HIGH-CARBOHYDRATE, LOW-FAT EATING

Nancy Clark *The Athlete's Kitchen* (Bantam Books)
Gabriel Gaté *Family Food* (Anne O'Donovan)
Gabriel Gaté *Good Food Fast* (Anne O'Donovan)
Gabriel Gaté *Smart Food* (Anne O'Donovan)
Karen Inge and Chris Roberts *Food for Sport Cookbook* (Simon & Schuster)
National Heart Foundation *Guide to Healthy Eating* Vols 1 and 2
Helen O'Connor and Donna Hay *The Taste of Fitness* (Better Living Collections)
Suzanne Porter *It's only Natural* (Viking O'Neil)
Suzanne Porter *Simply Healthy* (Greenhouse)
Julie Stafford *Taste of Life* (Greenhouse and Viking O'Neil)
Rosemary Stanton *Eating for Life* (Murdoch Books)
Rosemary Stanton *The Health and Energy Cookbook* (Murdoch Books)

Soccer and field hockey

Soccer and field hockey are team games played on rectangular fields—the soccer field being slightly larger than a hockey field—with the usual playing surface being grass or artificial turf. They share a common link in having eleven players on a team (ten mobile players and a goal-keeper) and in being high-intensity intermittent exercise. Games are played in two halves of 45 minutes (soccer) and 35 minutes (hockey) with a short break between halves.

While there are both male and female competitions in each sport, the male competition dominates in soccer with both Olympic and World Cup status. Hockey is represented by both male and female competitions at the Olympic Games and conducts World Championships/Cups for both sexes.

Training

With games played in seasons, training will vary between the off-season, pre-season and competition itself. The Australian soccer scene now sees year-round play, with the National League being conducted over the summer months and State/club competitions continuing as winter sports. Hockey is predominantly played as a winter sport.

At low levels of competition in both sports, players may have extensive off-season lay-offs and relatively short pre-season preparation.

Body-fat levels may be considerably higher at the beginning of each season, due to prolonged periods of inactivity. Even at the elite level, many players may return to pre-season training with significant losses in both fitness and body condition.

As in the other football codes covered in this book, pre-season training in both hockey and soccer will involve general conditioning work, weight training and skill practice. Concentration on skills and match practice will increase as the season approaches. During the season, two to four training sessions are generally scheduled between matches, with mid-week sessions involving lengthy match practice, and the end of the week seeing a gradual easing-off in training load to prepare for the next match.

Competition

The competition season generally provides a weekly match, with the national competition in soccer also involving team travel, and some mid-week and double-header fixtures. Soccer and hockey may also be played in tournaments of one to several weeks, with a heavy schedule of matches. At the international level, extensive travel may also be involved in competition tours.

Hockey and soccer are played as fast games of intensive play, with light activity between bursts. While rules restrict the amount of tackling and body contact that is permitted, both games can have a significant component of physical contact, with the potential for contact injuries. Time-motion studies of soccer have determined that the average distance covered per match by national and international level players is about ten kilometres. This of course will vary between positions on the field, as well as the level of competition. However, studies have also reported that the main difference between players of different levels is not in the total distance covered, but in the speed of play, the length of maximal bursts and the number of tackles and headings. Goalkeepers have been estimated to cover about four kilometres in the course of a match, with this activity level partly accounted for by the necessity to maintain arousal.

Games that are played under hot conditions, as well as drawing heavily on fuel stores, will challenge the fluid stores of players. While 1–2kg fluid losses have been reported during standard soccer games, under hot humid conditions sweat losses have been reported at double this level.

Physical characteristics

Hockey and soccer players, as well as being skilled, must be agile and fast. Players vary widely in body size, and differences in physical characteristics may not so much limit performance, as determine position on the field or style of play. While most players tend to be well-muscled, regardless of height and weight characteristics, a low body-fat level is also an advantage for speed and agility.

Typical physique (elite hockey players)

	Male	Female
Height	175–186cm	161–171cm
Weight	71–80kg	55–69kg
Skinfold sum	40–60mm	59–83mm

Typical physique (elite soccer players)

	Male
Height	176–187cm
Weight	72–87kg
Skinfold sum	43–58mm

Common nutrition issues

Body-fat levels

So you have the skill to be a good hockey or soccer player, but you're lacking a little in speed and stamina. Could it be that you are carrying extra weight that you don't need? Perhaps after a good rest over the off-season you have returned almost twice the player you used to be. Or perhaps, as in the case of Michael below, an injury has kept you inactive and in energy imbalance. At some time in your playing career you may find yourself battling the bulge.

For healthy and permanent fat-loss methods, read Chapter 3. And for year-round weight control, be aware of changes in your energy requirements. At the end of the season, you may need to significantly reduce your food intake to match the decrease in training output—or alternatively you may choose to keep up some activity to give you a head-start on next season.

The training diet—week-round recovery

Recovery between matches is difficult when a heavy training load is carried out on the intervening days. A soccer study has reported that muscle glycogen levels of players recovered very slowly in the days after the match, due to a combination of inadequate carbohydrate intake and continued training. Damage to muscle fibres arising from the match may also slow down the rate of glycogen storage.

The traditional approach of 'carbohydrates at the end of the week' is no longer appropriate for hockey and soccer players, who need a daily intake of carbohydrates to continually replenish their muscle stores. Read Chapters 1 and 2 for an overview of all aspects of the training diet, but pay special attention to the idea of a high-carbohydrate intake every day. This will keep you in constant recovery mode—avoiding mid-week slumps and progressive fatigue over the season. When you are in heavy training, it makes sense to start recovery nutrition tactics immediately after each session. Read Chapter 5 for guidelines.

Match preparation

With a good recovery diet in week-round practice, muscle fuel stores should gradually increase over the week. Light training at the end of the week, and the continuation of high-carbohydrate meals, will top-up muscle and liver glycogen stores as much as possible. Read Chapter 4.2 for general ideas, and make sure that your carbohydrate meals are as high in carbohydrate as you think. Chapters 1.3 and 2.2 provide practical ideas about carbohydrate foods.

The pre-match meal is eaten to top up carbohydrate stores on the day of the event and to make sure that fluid levels are looked after. You should experiment with the type, timing and amount of food that suits your game schedule and individual preferences. Don't let match nerves and travel requirements interfere with what you need, and if a certain meal suits you—regardless of how 'scientific' it seems—then stick to what you like. Most players have adopted high-carbohydrate low-fat meals but for others the tradition of the high-protein (and high-fat) meal dies hard. The most important aspect of the pre-event meal is that you feel comfortable and confident with your choice.

See Chapter 4.4 for more details, and see how Leon successfully solved his match day food later in this chapter.

Match considerations

Soccer and hockey matches place reasonable demands on both the fluid and carbohydrate stores of its players, particularly when there is a carry-over effect from matches played in close proximity (e.g. a tournament or mid-week fixture). Soccer studies have reported low muscle glycogen levels in players after a match—sometimes with significant depletion occurring by half time. Low muscle glycogen levels are likely to interfere with both endurance and high intensity exercise capacity—and indeed in these studies, players with depleted muscle glycogen stores had a slower average speed and covered less ground than their team-mates in the second half of the match.

Measurements on first-class soccer players have also shown that at least some players finish the game with low blood-sugar levels. It has been speculated that such a condition could impair the speed and accuracy of mental processing—and thus skill level.

In accordance with these results, some soccer studies have reported an improvement in match performance when carbohydrate is consumed just prior to the game as well as during half-time. The effect has been attributed to both an improvement in movement during the second half of the game (better muscle carbohydrate availability) as well as better skills/less mistakes during this period (prevention of central nervous system fatigue).

Sweat losses during matches can be significant—especially when competitions or tournaments are held in hot weather. Only soccer matches have been studied in detail, with various studies reporting sweat losses of 1.0–2.5 litres per 90 minute game in cool to moderate conditions, and approximately 4 litres during a match in a hot environment. However, the reported fluid intake of players was less than half of the sweat rate. In cool to warm weather some soccer players reported little or no fluid intake at all.

It appears that some players lack an awareness of sweat losses or have a poor appreciation of the disadvantages of dehydration. Restricted access to fluids is also likely to be a cause of poor fluid intake. In some cases the actual rules of the code or the competition/tournament may make good hydration practices impossible. For example, current FIFA guidelines prevent trainers or players carrying drinks onto the playing field. Therefore, fluid can only be consumed at half-time breaks (after 45 minutes), or whenever players are off the field. Yet dehydration can pose a serious threat to performance and health, as shown in the 1988 USA Youth Soccer Cup, held in very hot conditions, when 34 players collapsed from heat exhaustion.

In such situations it is good to see some modifications of the rules being negotiated by competition organisers and coaches—for example, a short drink break after 15–20 minutes of play. Bottles can also be left at strategic points around the perimeter of the field, so that players can take advantage of a small break in play following a goal, injury or rule infraction, to run over and grab a drink.

Sports drinks may be of value to hockey or soccer players—looking after fluid and carbohydrate needs simultaneously, both during and after the game. If you are a running player you may find both areas challenged. The studies that have reported better soccer performance with carbohydrate intake during matches have generally used a sports drink to provide this additional fuel supply. Fluid and carbohydrate losses may be compounded during tournament situations, requiring more aggressive strategies both during each match and in the recovery period between. Read about learning to gauge fluid needs in Chapter 1.5, and the special merits of sports drinks in Chapter 4.8.

Post-match recovery

Recovery should begin straight after the match—a time that is most often swallowed up in celebrations, commiserations or general relaxation, rather than careful attention to nutritional needs. But with the next match a maximum of six days away, and a training session scheduled in 24–48 hours, carbohydrate and fluid losses need immediate attention (see Chapter 5 for an explanation of the role of timing in recovery after exhaustive exercise).

Organise to have suitable drinks and snacks available after the match as a team activity so that everyone can enjoy the benefits. A post-match spread of sandwiches, fruit, soup and carbohydrate drinks in the club, or a box of supplies in the bus on the way back from 'away' matches can get recovery off to a good start. Players can make their own decisions about the rest of the evening's activities—whether it be discos or take-aways—hopefully taking heed of the club lesson on priorities.

Alcohol intake

There is a tendency in team sports to celebrate matches with alcohol intake—and unfortunately more alcohol intake than is good for sports performance. Read Chapter 1.6 to learn about the sensible use of alcohol in sport, particularly in post-match recovery. There is no need to be a teetotaller, but neither can excessive intake (even once a week with 'everyone' doing it) be condoned as professional behaviour. Take special care with bruising and soft tissue injuries that occur in a match or match practice. A good dose of alcohol will significantly increase the damage and prolong the time for recovery and rehabilitation.

Tournaments and travelling

Hockey and soccer tournaments may involve many games in quick succession, placing great importance on the recovery strategies already discussed. The plan, in a nutshell, is to recover as quickly after a match as possible, to continue to rebuild muscle glycogen stores between matches, and to supply additional fluid and carbohydrates during matches. Each of these strategies will take on greater importance as the tournament continues.

Of course, when the competition means being away from home or travelling on a tour, the challenge becomes greater and being organised becomes imperative. For help as a travelling athlete, read the account in the Tennis chapter.

PROFILE: MICHAEL
Injury—frustration and fat gain

Michael couldn't believe that in three months his hockey career had turned from bright to uncertain, and his body from trim and taut to, well, cuddly. The irony was that he had spent most of his teen years

301

as a bean pole, able to put anything into his mouth and never gain a gram. It was only in recent years of heavy training and weight work that his body had filled out. Then, in the past ten weeks while nursing a tibial stress fracture, his skinfolds had climbed from 47mm to 81mm, and his weight had rocketed by 7kg.

At his latest medical check, the doctor had ordered him to see the clinic dietitian, warning that the extra weight was not only bad for his game but that it put extra load on his weakened leg. It was likely that this had already delayed his recovery. After the usual six-week rest he had attempted to resume light training, only to suffer a recurrence of tibial pain.

Michael explained his plight to the dietitian, complaining that he had never had to worry about his weight or food intake before. Why was there suddenly a problem?

After a full assessment of the situation, the dietitian offered a simple explanation—'energy in' was greater than 'energy out': and a number of factors were operating to cause this:

- A change in metabolic rate with age. As an adolescent, Michael had burnt up many thousands of kilojoules each day to cope with the needs of growth and training. Now that this had slowed down, he needed to be a bit more careful of the 'bottomless pit' eating habits that he had learned.

- Drastic change of activity level. Playing both state and club level hockey had kept Michael busy with training or matches every day of the week. A sudden standstill in his exercise program was a major change to his lifestyle and to energy requirements. Michael admitted that he had taken things a little too easy in his rehabilitation. Although the physiotherapist had suggested swimming and cycling as alternative exercise modes, Michael had not enjoyed either and had let the program slide.

- Poor general dietary habits. Michael had always thought that if your weight was OK, then you must be eating well—and never having had to worry about his skinfold levels before, he had kept himself insulated from any advice about good nutrition practices. The dietitian assessed Michael's diet to be high in fat—deadly for kilojoule intake.

- Boredom eating and drinking. Being injured leaves a lot of time to sit around the house, feeling sorry for yourself and becoming bored. Not used to being home straight after work—usually he went to training—Michael had begun new habits of afternoon snacks and a beer after work. In fact, thinking about it, there had been quite a few commiseration sessions spent with friends at the pub. The alcohol and 'comfort foods' were sneaking in far more kilojoules than he had realised.

Michael committed himself to a full plan of rehabilitation—both for his leg and for his abdominal skinfolds. It was time to take stock of his new energy requirements, and to change his energy balance in favour of body-fat loss—at least until he could resume full training. A proper plan of swimming, upper-body weight work and cycling was organised. Not only did this burn up some kilojoules, but it kept him out of the house (and the fridge) and gave him a focus of encouragement and goal-setting. A dietary plan was written, limiting food quantities in general, and fat and oil intake in particular. A weekly quota of light beer was negotiated, although Michael suggested that he was happy to go 'on the wagon' for the rest of the season, or at least until his body fat was below 50mm again.

Within six weeks, the bulk of the body fat had been lost and Michael was back in half-training. Food quantities were adjusted as energy requirements and body-fat goals changed. The dietitian promised Michael that his food patterns were not only good for weight control, now and in the future, but with his new concentration on carbohydrate intake, he could expect action-packed training and matches. Michael can't wait to put it to the test in his first game back in two to three weeks' time.

PROFILE: LEON
The pre-event meal

When Leon moved up into the senior team at his soccer club, his father gave him some advice: 'You'll need a lot of stamina at this level son, especially with the game kicking off at 3.00pm. When I used to play I always had a big breakfast for energy—steak, eggs and toast. I'll get your mother onto it.'

The next Sunday, Leon sat down to his father's tried and true pre-match meal. At one o'clock when they left for the ground his stomach was full of food and butterflies. In the first half he felt sick, at half-time he was sick, and in the second half he wandered around the field feeling empty and a bit tired.

The following week Leon went back to the breakfast he had eaten in his junior league days—a couple of pieces of toast and honey and some fruit juice. This was light and compact and had served him well in an 11.00am match. However eaten at 9.00am in the morning it didn't seem substantial enough to get him through an afternoon match. By midday he was feeling hungry again and by match-time it was hard to concentrate on his game above the rumbling of his stomach.

He asked the coach for some advice, and found that a sports dietitian had been organised to come to the club to talk about this very topic. With a revamped and expanded league this season, the coach was worried about having to face some new match-day conditions.

The inclusion of some new clubs would mean a four-hour bus trip to some of the 'away' matches. He wondered whether he should organise a team breakfast along the road to break up the trip, or whether they should take some food supplies on the bus. Later in the year, the team might play in a country league tournament with matches at various times of the day over a week or so of competition. Should his players eat differently for morning matches to evening matches? Time for some expert advice!

The dietitian explained that the role of the pre-match meal was to tie up the loose ends of the weekly eating efforts—not to be a magic wand for performance. She asked the players to nominate whether they were happy with their present pre-match meal routines, or whether they thought there was room for improvement. About a third of the team admitted they had experienced problems at some time. Some, like Leon, had difficulties with knowing how much and at what time to eat. Others suffered with pre-game nerves to the extent that they were unable to eat anything.

The dietitian compiled a list of the types of foods chosen by the players for their pre-event meal, and presented it for discussion. There was a wide range of meal patterns, ranging from two small meals to a late-morning brunch, and from cooked breakfasts to a piece of toast. The first thing that was obvious to the players, was that each person had an individual approach to his needs—and that different plans suited different players.

The goals of the pre-event meal were outlined:

- to top-up liver and perhaps muscle glycogen stores;

- to top-up fluid levels;

- to feel comfortable (neither too full nor too hungry), and to avoid foods that disagree; and

- to feel confident and ready for action.

The most obvious way to fulfil these goals was with a high-carbohydrate meal, and the dietitian listed some suitable food combinations—from typical breakfast fare such as cereal, toast and fruit to more elaborate meals such as rice pudding, pancakes and syrup and pasta with tomato sauces. She also discussed low-carbohydrate or high-fat foods that athletes often ate as pre-event meals—including steak, bacon and eggs, and oily lasagnes.

Were these foods bad, the dietitian was asked? She agreed they fitted the tradition rather than the scientific theory of an ideal pregame meal, but suggested that for some players they didn't seem to cause ill-effects. She recounted the tale of an American swimmer who had eaten an amazing spread of hamburgers and cookies before swimming to a gold medal, and concluded that many of the effects of the last meal were psychological as well as nutritional. It was obviously important to believe in what you had done.

Most players were interested in experimenting with the low-fat high-carbohydrate menu plans, although a couple of die-hards decided to stick to their 'lucky steaks' (eaten no doubt with their 'lucky' knives and forks). The dietitian advised that the amount and timing of meals on match morning was an individual preference also, and suggested that each player began by working from his everyday breakfast routine to find a pre-match plan. For example, someone who usually ate a hearty breakfast of cereal and six rounds of toast might need a bigger meal than someone who was satisfied with a muffin and fruit juice.

Whatever time the match was played, at least two hours pre-event was the eating schedule to work back from. For afternoon matches, the choice between a single (larger) meal and an early breakfast followed by a later snack would rest on individual comfort as well as the match travel arrangements. For home games it may not be necessary to leave for the ground until the early afternoon, whereas many of the 'away' games may mean an early departure from home. The dietitian suggested that for long trips to matches, an organised meal-stop en route could be good for team morale as well as nutrition. She suggested that a regular venue be chosen and supplied with a menu, and that a buffet format would enable players to better cater for their individual likes and needs.

What about players who needed a small top-up to breakfast, either at the ground or at home? Light snacks could include sandwiches, fruit, or a liquid meal supplement such as Sustagen Sport, Gator-Pro or Exceed Sports Meal, with the liquid meals being handy for those unable to keep down any solid food. The final item to remember was fluid intake, including special attention on hot and humid days. With all players trained to drink during their stretching and warm-up to the match, hydration needs seemed to be well-looked after.

Rehydration during and after training sessions is also important. Studies of junior elite soccer players at the AIS have shown that sweat losses approximated nearly a litre per hour of training in warm conditions, with players usually replacing less than half of these fluid losses. Better hydration means better training—see chapter 1.5 for practical ways to improve your drinking strategies.

The players at Leon's club now eat their own 'secret weapon' breakfasts, and occasionally tease each other about their special pancakes or their Sustagen Sport rituals. Nevertheless, they all know that once they take to the field they are ready for anything, with the pre-event meal being the icing on the cake of a good week's training and nutrition.

Basketball and netball

Basketball and netball are team ball games, played both on indoor and outdoor courts. While basketball is played at a high level by both males and females, netball is predominantly a female participation sport. Strong international competition exists for both sports, with basketball being an Olympic sport.

Basketball is played by teams of up to ten players, with five players appearing on the court at one time. Each player has a specific role to play on the court, but all players are mobile—covering the whole court and being involved in both offensive and defensive plays. Players are continually substituted from the bench throughout the game. A basketball game can be played in four 12-minute quarters, or in two 20-minute halves, with a break of 10–15 minutes at half-time. Since the timing clock stops when the ball is out of play, the actual time elapsed for each game is considerably more.

A netball team is composed of seven players, each in a specific position with a defined role and a defined court space. Reserve players are allowed, but once a substitution is made a benched player cannot return to the court unless replacing an injured team-mate. A netball game can be played as a game of 15-minute quarters or two 20-minute halves, again with a short break at the half-way point.

At the elite level, both netball and basketball are fast-paced and skilled, and are both physical games, in spite of rules against direct contact between components. Considerable demands are placed upon anaerobic energy systems, with aerobic fitness assisting recovery between bursts of play.

Training

Basketball and netball are generally played in competition seasons with national leagues existing in both sports. The competition season for the National Basketball League spreads from March to September, with the play-offs for the finals in October. Training for the next season may start soon after Christmas, leaving only a short break in between seasons. Most players at this level will remain active for the whole year, indulging in personal training when the team does not hold official practice. At lower levels, players may have longer breaks between seasons, and find themselves at risk for weight gain and loss of fitness during this time.

Elite players train on a daily basis, and in some cases—for example, training camps for national teams—twice daily sessions may be undertaken. In pre-season, the emphasis is on building a fitness base, with training involving greater amounts of running and strength work than at other times of the year. Skills work and practice matches, where set plays are developed, are practised all year round and are the dominant mode of training.

The number of training sessions undertaken each week will vary with the number of games played. The team will normally meet for three or four sessions per week, and players may train individually or in small groups at other sessions, concentrating on weaknesses and specific tasks relevant to their roles on court.

At a non-elite level, training loads vary. Many basketball and netball players simply train individually to keep fit and to practise skills, and then play in a weekly competition with perhaps one or two team training sessions a week.

Competition

For national league competition, it is practical to divide the program into home games, and games played on tour. Home games are usually played on a Friday or Saturday night, with a single game each weekend. Tours may involve playing two or three games (Friday night, Saturday night and Sunday afternoon), often in different cities. This presents a great challenge, both in terms of recovery between games, as well as the interruption to sleep, diet and training caused by travelling.

Even at a sub-elite and recreational level, many players enjoy playing for a number of teams, or in a number of competitions, and may find themselves with a weekly commitment of two or three matches.

This may pose a similar challenge of recovery against the background of a less than ideal lifestyle.

Tournament competitions, over weekends or weeks, present an even more difficult routine. Depending on the size of the competition, teams may be organised into a draw, with the winners of each zone or pool meeting in a final series.

Physical characteristics

Height is the most noticeable physical characteristic in these ball-games—particularly in basketball, and particularly for centres and forwards. In netball, there is greater allowance for shorter players in some positions, particularly where the ball is played close to the ground. However, netball players are generally above-average height.

Lower body-fat levels are an advantage in improving agility and speed, and with assisting movement off the ground. The body-fat levels of elite players may be relatively low, reflecting both the training load as well as the advantages of being lean, however, they do not usually drop as low as those of endurance athletes. At lower levels of play it is possible to be skilled but less trim and fit.

Typical physique (elite basketball players)

	Male	Female
Height	190–208cm	170–184cm
Weight	87–112kg	62–82kg
Skinfold sum	53–81mm	58–85mm

Typical physique (elite netball players)

	Female
Height	171–180cm
Weight	63–76kg
Skinfold sum	73–116mm

Common nutrition issues

The training diet—being organised

Energy requirements in basketball and netball can be high, but reflect the size and growth needs of some players more than energy expenditure from exercise. Training and matches, while a lengthy part of the day, are generally not as energy-intensive as they might appear, due to the emphasis on skill practice, and stop-start play.

A single game of netball or basketball does not provide a great threat to the fuel capabilities of a trained athlete. However, in many situations players struggle with their recovery, due to the carry-over effects of a daily schedule of training and matches. It is not just that special nutritional needs are created, such as the need for a high daily carbohydrate intake, but rather that players can find it hard to set an organised meal plan, because of their hectic and unpredictable lifestyle. The majority of training sessions and matches are generally carried out at night—and often late into the night. For those with full-time jobs, or even those who are full-time athletes, this can mean a busy day.

How do you spread your food over the day to fit exercise needs—such as not eating too close to a game—as well as fit in with the general schedule of meal-times followed by your family or the rest of the world? Juggled meals can often mean disorganised nutrition. An evening game may finish late at night, leaving the player unmotivated to cook, unable to find somewhere to eat out, or uncomfortable about eating a big meal before going to bed. Since the player may have been reluctant or unable to eat a planned meal before the game, the whole day may become a series of grabbed snacks—often poor in nutritional quality. If this is the pattern for the week, overall nutritional status can be jeopardised. Busy players may find, between games, training and basketball meetings that they only get to eat a cooked meal once a week.

The principles of training nutrition are explained in Chapters 1 and 2. The major task of most players will be to organise a meal routine that allows all goals to be met. You may need to use nights at home to catch up with cooking for the week, thus providing quick meals for game nights. You may need to experiment with the pre-game meal plan, to split your food into a pre-event snack and a post-event top-up. Snacks can be nutritious if well-planned. You might even like to switch the focus of the day to make your lunch the main meal, and have lighter meals for the rest of the day.

Losing body fat

The beginning of the season may see you needing to lose body fat, or perhaps you are coming back from an injury. For some female players it is a constant struggle to reach an ideal playing weight. See Chapter 3 for safe and sensible ideas, and read the account of Vicki below.

Iron status

Low iron status may be a problem for female players and some male players. Contact and impact events—hitting other players or landing hard on the floor—may increase iron losses through increased red-blood-cell destruction. In any case, female athletes and athletes on weight-loss diets are at risk of iron deficiency due to a low iron intake. See Chapter 2.5 for a discussion of iron requirements and ways to ensure a high iron intake.

Match preparation—the pre-event meal

In theory, the pre-event meal should be a light, high-carbohydrate meal eaten at least two hours before the match. Experiment to find something that suits you. Since it is likely that you will play matches at various times of the day or night, you may need to be versatile with meal ideas to suit a number of occasions. See Chapter 4.4.

Match and training fluids

If you are working hard, and the stadium is hot, it is possible to lose a significant amount of fluid through sweating. Look after fluid levels by drinking before training or matches, and for hot, lengthy sessions, take a water bottle to the court. And of course, rehydrate well after you have finished—especially if you have another session or match coming up soon. Water may be adequate, but a sports drink may promote better performance in situations where fuel stores can't recover between sessions. Tournament schedules and heavy training sessions can challenge fuel recovery. See Chapter 4.7.

Tournament nutrition

Tournament schedules are often challenging, setting you to play a number of matches over a short period. Travelling may also be part of the deal. As soon as you know your likely schedule of matches, begin to plan a meal routine. You will need to take into account suitable pre-event meals (Chapter 4.4), and post-event recovery strategies (Chapter 5). If you are on the move, or playing in foreign parts, then the notes on the travelling athlete will be of help (see Tennis chapter).

On the road again

Being on the road for the weekend is tough work. Not only is there disruption to your normal eating, sleeping and training schedule, but you may be required to play two or three games over three days. This will challenge your skills of recovery and organisation. See the account of the Travelling Athlete in the Tennis chapter to learn a three-pronged plan of attack:

- Know your nutrition goals, including recovery (Chapter 5), pre-event meals (Chapter 4.4), and the general principles of training nutrition (Chapters 1 and 2).
- Plan ahead. You may be able to find restaurants to eat at or make some plans with your hotel to cater for the meals that you need at the time that you need them. (Remember, your pre-event and post-event meal schedule may not fit in with their normal dining room times.)

- Be assertive and make things happen the way that you want them to.

Some teams leave a lot of this to be organised by a team manager or the team captain, and eat most of their meals as a team. In other clubs, players are responsible for most of their own eating and are given a *per diem*, or daily allowance, for their food. For financial and practical reasons (where else can you eat late at night) take-aways and fast foods can make up a big part of the weekend's eating. Take-aways have a bad reputation—nutritionally speaking—that is not always deserved. Read the account below to learn about fitting them into your lifestyle and your nutrition goals.

PROFILE: VICKI
Lose body fat, once and for all!

In one year, Vicki had lost over 20kg—that is to say, that she had lost the same two kilograms over and over. She certainly had the desire and motivation to lose weight. Her netball coach at school had rated her as a potential state-level player, but a centre cannot afford to carry extra body-fat. At sixteen, Vicki had stopped growing up, and had started to grow 'out'. Now, in Year 12, she was four kilograms heavier than at the end of last year, and she was beginning to feel and show it on the court. Her self-initiated dieting was not going anywhere. After grapefruit breakfasts and green apple lunches she would lose 1–2kg, only to put it back on in the next week. The coach insisted that a more healthy and long-term weight control program be found.

A round-table conference was held with her parents to discuss a plan of attack. Vicki's mother was enthusiastic and decided that the whole family would watch their food intake. They bought a copy of a healthy nutrition recipe book and followed the directions. Skim milk was introduced, non-fat cooking methods became the order of the day, and take-aways were banished to a monthly treat.

But even without the skin on the chicken and the chocolate biscuits, Vicki's weight remained high. It didn't seem fair—the team trained three nights a week and played on weekends, and Vicki ran for a half hour on the other days. Her best friend didn't exercise at all, ate McDonalds twice a week, and didn't have an ounce of excess fat on her body.

Vicki and her Mum eventually took the problem to a sports dietitian and were congratulated on their progress so far. The dietitian consoled Vicki that her energy needs did seem to be lower than others, but said that comparing herself to other girls would not solve the problem. Instead, she had to look at her own situation carefully, and find ways to increase energy expenditure and/or decrease energy intake from food.

311

The demands of school and homework did not leave much time for extra training, although Vicki agreed that she could step up her runs to 40 or 50 minutes. This meant the major solution had to come from changes in food intake. Vicki described her usual meal patterns to the dietitian, and it appeared that the family food plan already provided the right types of food. Vicki's mother questioned this carefully, saying that in her day carbohydrate foods were considered fattening and she couldn't believe the amount of bread and potatoes that the new dietary principles encouraged.

The dietitian reinforced the nutrition messages from the healthy nutrition book, and agreed that the attitude to carbohydrate had changed. She reminded them that carbohydrate foods provided the most important fuel for exercise and therefore could not be neglected. She was puzzled, though, that Vicki's serve sizes did not seem extraordinary or unreasonably large—so where was the difficulty in losing weight? Vicki was sent home to keep a food record, and that's when the problem emerged.

Even Vicki was surprised to see the number of snacks she had eaten, but the food record had captured it in black and white. The hours spent in the evenings, cramming in homework before she went to bed, were also spent in and out of the kitchen. Weekends and afternoons free from training were worse, with frequent bowls of cereal and sandwiches. Between her study and training commitments, Vicki didn't have much time for leisure, so she used food to break the boredom. It wasn't so much the types of foods that she snacked on—they were all high carbohydrate and low-fat—but that the extra kilojoules were being consumed in the name of entertainment rather than need.

The dietitian helped Vicki to reorganise her homework schedule to include blocks of study, rewarded with some real 'time out'. A list of enjoyable activities was written to give her alternatives to eating when she became bored. In addition, she was allowed to have a weekly treat—a small portion of her favourite food.

The plan worked well. Within six weeks she had lost most of the excess weight, and the dietitian was able to show her that her skinfolds had dropped by 25mm. Because she knows how she achieved these goals, and has reorganised her eating behaviour to sustain the effort, Vicki should not have any further difficulties with this weight 'finding' her again.

PROFILE
Take-aways—fast food doesn't need to be junk food!

When you live life in the fast lane, it is inevitable that fast food will be part of it. For athletes, take-aways may provide a quick meal after a late training session or match, or they may be part of the travelling diet when cooking facilities are not available and restaurants are out of the budget range. Maybe after a hard week of work and training, you just want a day when you don't have to exert yourself with domestic duties.

Despite their convenience, fast foods and take-aways do not generally have a good reputation. 'Junk food' is a frequent description for these foods, although that doesn't stop people from eating (or liking) them. Most people feel a little guilty about making take-aways a big part of their diet, and some people feel guilty about eating them at all. Is the reputation warranted?

Fast foods generally go against the principles of healthy nutrition and the optimum training diet. A nutritional assessment of popular take-away foods—for example, the menus at the big hamburger chains and fried chicken outlets—finds that they are high in fat, salt, sugar and kilojoules, and low in fibre and some vitamins, particularly vitamins A and C. For an athlete, many take-aways may lack sufficient carbohydrate to meet fuel needs. From the financial point of view, take-aways are more expensive than a home prepared meal, though you may not notice this on a once-off occasion. However, they are less expensive than general restaurant eating.

Thus it is likely that indiscriminate use of take-aways may prevent the athlete from achieving nutritional goals. However, this does not have to be the case. With planning and good nutrition knowledge, it is possible to let take-aways play a useful role in your diet. Use the following strategies as an overall guide.

- Limit the number of times that you eat take-aways—make use of their convenience when you really need it.
- Be selective in making your order. It is possible to make selections or modify choices so that they are more in line with the healthy nutrition guidelines.
- Have a small portion only and make up the rest of your meal with other foods. Alternatively, eat just what you need, rather than the full menu.
- Make sure that the rest of your meals compensate for mismatched nutritional goals from your fast-food meals.
- Think wider than the well-known chains. There are some 'healthy' take-away outlets being set up, and a sandwich is the quintessential healthy fast food which you can buy almost anywhere.

As a rule of thumb, choose foods that are based on carbohydrate—either bread, rice, potato or pasta. Avoid batters and deep-fried foods, and be aware that pastry is high in fat (unless it is filo pastry). Make up fillings with vegetables and salads rather than lots of protein (and fat). The following table compares some good food choices with foods that fail to meet the dietary guidelines.

313

A GUIDE TO TAKE-AWAYS

High-carbohydrate/low-fat choices	High-fat choices
Roll or sandwich—no margarine. Lean meat/chicken/salmon/cottage cheese/ cheese (medium serve). Plenty of salad.	Toasted ham and cheese sandwiches dripping with margarine
Pizza—thick crust (especially whole-meal). Vegetarian, lean meat, chicken or seafood topping. Ask for less cheese.	Pizza with the lot— especially the 'meat-lovers' special' with extra cheese
Salad hamburger—one rissole, plenty of salad and wholemeal roll if possible. Watch the mayonnaise or dressings.	The Quarter-Pounder with the lot
Steak sandwich—as for hamburger	Crumbed schnitzel
Souvlaki—another version of the hamburger or other low-fat filling (bread with meat plus salad)	Pies, pasties, sausage rolls etc.
Baked potato with a little cheese and coleslaw or other low-fat filling (avoid butter or sour cream)	Chips (and fried fish etc.)
Chicken roll with coleslaw and corn on the cob	Deep fried chicken or chicken nuggets
Fruit juice	
Low-fat fruit smoothies (low-fat milk, icecream or yoghurt and fruit)	Thickshake
Low fat frozen yoghurt, Gisé or Vitari	Icecream—especially extra creamy types

Tennis

Tennis is played by both men and women, in singles and in doubles competition (same-sex and mixed-sex pairs), and at levels varying from a 'social hit' to the lucrative international circuit. Other variables in the game include the court surface, and whether it is located indoor or outdoors.

At an elite level, tennis is a fast and mobile game, characterised by bursts of intense exercise against a background of quiet movement. The average tennis point lasts eight seconds, with the longest points, even at the world class level, rarely lasting more than half a minute. Thus the game itself is highly reliant on anaerobic energy systems, although a developed aerobic capacity is an advantage in terms of recovery between points, stamina and tolerance to heat.

Tennis is a game of skill, speed, agility and concentration—and often, endurance. Men's matches at international tournaments are often marathon efforts of four or five hours, with long rallies for each point and many sets going to tie-breakers. While the exercise is not continuous for this duration, such a game is likely to challenge the carbohydrate fuel stores of the athlete, and require great discipline to maintain concentration.

Training

For professional players, tennis is a full-time job. Between tournaments, 20–40 hours per week may be spent in training—with the majority of this devoted to on-court practice. Most players will supplement this with about an hour per day of off-court conditioning work, such as running, weight training and agility work. This work may vary according to different stages of preparation, and the specific weaknesses in a player's game.

Further down the competition level, tennis players will not have the luxury of hours to spend on training. Nevertheless, the balance of time available will again be spent on court practice.

Competition

Most competitive tennis in Australia is played in the form of graded pennant competitions, with teams (four members) meeting each other in a weekly draw. A final series amongst the top finishing teams then determines the pennant winner.

The other form of tennis competition, particularly at the elite level, is tournament tennis. This begins at the sub-elite level with weekend tournaments, and continues from satellite tournaments to the elite circuit of Grand Prix and Grand Slam events. The length of the tournament varies with the number of player entries, being run as a 'cut-throat' competition where losing players are eliminated, while winners continue to the next round. The standard Grand Prix tournament, beginning with 32 or 64 entries, is held over a week, with the winner needing to win four to six matches to take out the trophy.

A tennis match is played over the best of three or five sets for men, and the best of three sets for women. The length of a match varies greatly, from 30 minutes to three hours for a three-set match, and from 80 minutes to more than five hours for a five-set competition. The fuel and fluid demands of a match will vary accordingly. However, in tournament tennis, the nutritional focus is not so much on the effects of a single match, but on the carry-over effects from playing so many matches in succession.

Tournament tennis sets an extremely tough schedule for players, requiring many to play in a single and doubles match each day—with perhaps only one rest day—until their outcome is decided. While muscle glycogen levels may survive one match, the continual daily schedule will challenge the athlete to fully recover fuel stores between matches. Depleted muscle glycogen levels will interfere with both sprint and endurance components of performance, and limit the player's ability to perform at an optimum level.

For elite tennis players, life is a continual program of tournaments and exhibition matches, with most taking only short breaks between each venture onto the circuit to recover and prepare for the next. On average, an elite player participates in twenty tournaments each year.

Physical characteristics

Some general physical characteristics that are of value to a tennis player include long arms and a relatively low centre of gravity (short legs in proportion to the trunk). These features should assist a player, with extra reach for playing strokes and height for serving, and with greater mobility around the court.

Other physical characteristics do not so much limit performance as help determine the style of game a player can play well. For example, tall muscular players might best use their height and power with an aggressive serve and volley game, while shorter, agile players may do better with a mobile court-covering game.

In general, the body-fat levels of tennis players are relatively low, since excess body fat can reduce both stamina and heat tolerance. In women's tennis, this feature hasn't always been so. In earlier times, many top females were skilled but relatively fat and lacking in aerobic fitness. Martina Navratilova set a trend in women's tennis, by trimming her body-fat level and developing great strength and fitness, to become almost invincible during the 1980s.

Typical physique (elite junior tennis player)

	Male	Female
Height	168–182cm	159–171cm
Weight	55–75kg	45–61kg
Skinfold sum	40–59mm	66–114mm

Common nutrition issues

Training nutrition

During the 1980s Ivan Lendl and Martina Navratilova publicised the importance of nutrition in their game preparation. Martina featured in Robert Haas' book *Eat to Win*, extolling the virtues of her new style of eating. Although some aspects of the *Eat to Win* diet run contrary to the advice in this book, the essential shared element is the encouragement to boost carbohydrate intake to fuel exercise needs, and to reduce the characteristic fat, salt and sugar intakes of the Western diet.

The testimony of these champions has influenced tennis players of all levels to consider their nutrition more carefully. The optimum training diet will not make you a Wimbledon champion—unless you've got the shots. However, when training and playing become a serious part of your life, you must meet the special nutritional needs that are created before your tennis skills can be fully developed and showcased.

The training and playing schedules of many elite players set up large energy and carbohydrate requirements. At a lower level of play, carbohydrate needs may not be as great, but may still be beyond the level supplied in the typical Australian diet. See Chapters 1 and 2 for a full account of the optimum training diet.

Body-fat levels

Many players, especially females, do not automatically arrive at the body-fat level that does them justice on the court. Being overweight will reduce your speed and stamina, and increase your suffering during hot days on the court. If you need to lose body fat, read Chapter 3 for advice on setting suitable goals and adopting a healthy plan of eating and exercise.

Fluid intake during matches and training

Tennis is often played in sweltering conditions. Court surface temperatures of 50 degrees Celsius have been reported from centre court during the Australian Open—and some of the concrete outer courts may be even hotter! When matches drag out to three hours or more, and rallies are long and intense, players can amass large sweat losses. To reduce the risk of dehydration and heat injury, players should follow a plan of fluid intake before, during and after matches to keep reasonable pace with sweat losses.

Be aware of your sweat losses during a match, and be especially aggressive on hot and humid days. Keep a supply of cool and refreshing fluids court-side and grab a drink as appropriate—both in terms of your needs as well as opportunities during the match. On some days it may be sufficient to drink between sets, but it is probably good practice to grab a quick drink as you change ends after every second game. After the match, the remaining fluid deficit needs to be replaced—hopefully before the next match—to prevent problems of chronic dehydration.

Don't forget about good hydration practices during training either, particularly if you are out in the heat of the day for long periods. Not only will this look after your training performance, but it will give you the opportunity to practise some match strategies, including your choice of drinks.

While water is adequate to replace fluid losses, there may be additional advantages in providing carbohydrate during long intense matches, especially if you are gradually becoming glycogen-depleted over a long week of tournament matches. Carbohydrate intake during the match may help to boost flagging fuel stores and delay the fatigue of muscle and brain. A sports drink—or alternatively, cordial or diluted fruit juice and soft drinks—may provide carbohydrate and fluid needs simultaneously. Read more in Chapters 4.6 and 4.7.

Life on the circuit

Elite tennis players can look forward to a life of travelling—around Australia and around the world. While this can be exciting, it can also be stressful. It is often hard to meet nutritional needs in unfamiliar surroundings, especially when time and finances are limited. Read the accounts below for practical advice on travelling nutrition. The first article provides general strategies for life on the run, while the story of Sue further illustrates the problems faced by a touring tennis player.

Tournament tennis

Tournament tennis is challenging from many nutritional viewpoints. Apart from the considerations of being away from home—even for a weekend tournament—the tournament schedule places great demands on nutritional strategies for recovery, and on a player's flexibility and ingenuity. Not only must a player be committed to looking after fluid and carbohydrate needs between matches, but they must do so without a definite time-table of their day's activities.

Since each day's match draw is determined by the results of the previous day's play, players receive short notice about their daily schedule. Forward planning is also made difficult by the loose nature of the daily timetable. While the starting time for the first match of each session can be set, all other matches simply follow in succession. Given the great range in the duration of matches, it is often difficult for a player to predict accurately the time of their matches.

As in the case of Sue below, tournament players must learn to be adaptable with their eating plans—having a clear idea of the goals of competition nutrition, but being prepared to handle all possible outcomes in a day's play.

PROFILE
The travelling athlete—an accidental tourist

Take a modern athlete and you have probably also got a seasoned traveller, both within Australia and overseas. At the elite level, frequent international competition is demanded by both the economics and performance standards of many sports. In addition to big events such as World Championships and the Olympic and Commonwealth Games, many top athletes undertake regular training/competition tours overseas, in search of better weather during Southern Hemisphere winters, specialised training such as altitude training, or general fame and fortune on the competition circuit.

National competitions and championships have opened up domestic travelling. In some sports this is no longer an annual national title, but a week-by-week requirement to go on the road. Even recreational-level athletes can be caught up in this mobile world. Who hasn't travelled away to a basketball tournament, triathlon or tennis competition? Some athletes even choose to combine an overseas event with their recreational or business travel—for example, for their annual holiday they might go to New York to run the marathon, or do a triathlon in Fiji.

While travel provides its own rewards and opportunities, for the athlete with special nutritional goals it can also pose some challenges. Some of the food related problems you may face as a travelling athlete are:

- being in a foreign country with a different food supply and different eating customs. As a result, it may be difficult to obtain the types of foods that you like, and that you know will meet your dietary goals. The local food customs may not assist with your nutritional needs as an athlete, and it can be hard to find out the composition of foods and dishes, especially if you don't speak the language. For example, many an athlete with a fussy palate has lost weight because they did not find the local fare to their liking, while others have struggled to find enough carbohydrate sources to load up for an endurance event.

- food safety and hygiene. Many countries have lower standards of hygiene and food quality control than you enjoy at home. Finding safe foods and drinks, in particular, can use up most of your resources, patience and time. The consequences can be gastrointestinal upsets—ranging in seriousness from a nuisance to a disaster.

- being unable to prepare your own foods—needing to rely on restaurants and take-aways. Often when you are travelling for short periods you will be staying in a hotel or other accommodation that provides minimal facilities for food preparation or storage. Not only is it expensive to buy all your meals individually, but you are often compromised by the type of food outlets available and the times that you can be served.

- communal eating. So, you are staying in a Games Village or on campus in an institution. You might be lucky enough to be provided with unlimited access to a menu designed for athletes. Foolproof?—unfortunately not. There are many pitfalls to eating in a communal setting, including being mesmerised by the quantities and varieties of food, and being distracted by the eating habits of those around you.

- distraction. Sometimes, just being away from home creates a holiday atmosphere. Indeed for some athletes the trip may actually be doubling as a vacation. As a result, many athletes find that their trips away are sabotaged by a 'let's just enjoy ourselves' spirit.

320

- travelling itself. Food intake and nutritional goals can become separated when you are actually on the move. Travelling can be stressful, involving long hours, changes in your body clock, and disruption to your training schedule.

It is easy to see how an athlete will not eat—and thus compete or train—at an optimal level under these circumstances.

Eating well as a travelling athlete requires a three-pronged attack:

1 Be clear about your nutritional goals, and how these might change at various times in training and competition. Read through the appropriate sections in Part I of this book.
2 Plan ahead and prepare for your trip. It is often possible to organise food opportunities to suit your needs ahead of time.
3 While you are away, be assertive about handling nutrition decisions to make sure that your nutritional goals are achieved.

HINTS FOR THE TRAVELLING ATHLETE

Prepare ahead
- Find out what to expect at your travel destination(s) and what challenges your training or competition schedule will throw out. Good sources of information are other athletes who have blazed the trail ahead of you, and the organisers of the events you plan to do. Other athletes can usually give you a lengthy account of what to do and what not to do—usually from bitter experience.
- Plan your accommodation with meals in mind. If you are planning to stay in the same place for a long period, or if you have special nutritional needs that may be hard to meet by conventional arrangements (e.g. unusual meal times), then you might be best to find lodgings that provide full cooking facilities. Even facilities for minimal food preparation and storage—e.g. a fridge in your hotel room—can promote better flexibility and possibilities for food intake. Another consideration is to choose an area that is close to shops or restaurants, especially if you will have limited means of transport. For long trips when you are continually on the move, a mobile home or caravan may be an alternative to a succession of hotels.
- Pre-arrange meals where appropriate. Looking over your travel arrangements, you should consider the meals that will be professionally catered—whether by an airline, a restaurant or a hotel. Often it is possible and useful to contact these people ahead of time and arrange to have special meals organised. The hospitality industry does not always do justice to the special needs of athletes.

Don't leave yourself open to problems such as inadequate carbohydrate intake, excess fat and kilojoules for those with lower energy needs, and nouvelle cuisine for a pack of hungry high-energy consumers. This can also help to reduce waiting time, and make meal times less confusing when travelling with a large group.

Give the airline or caterers ample notice, and where possible a menu outline. Airlines often have alternative menus, such as 'vegetarian', 'low-fat/high fibre' or 'Pritikin-style', and will be pleased to supply extra bread and fruit for hungry carbohydrate-eaters. It may pay to check what the airline means by its special diet classification—for example, their 'low-fat' diet may simply be a bland diet suitable for someone with gastrointestinal disorders.

- Take a food supply with you. Depending on where you are going and how long you will be away, you may decide to bring some or all of your own food requirements. For example, if you are driving interstate, an Esky may allow you to bring many of your meals or food items for a couple of days. Even if you are travelling overseas for extended times, an emergency food supply can be of great value.

  What you should take will depend on the difficulties that you anticipate with the food supply at your travel destination(s)—for example, whether food items will simply be unavailable there, whether you may not have suitable time and access to go shopping, or whether your travel budget will not spread far. In some Asian and Eastern Bloc countries one or all of these barriers may apply.

  Food items that are sturdy, non-perishable, and require no cooking may be of great value on an overseas trip. See the table on the following page for ideas. These supplies can be supplemented with fresh foods such as bread, fruit, low-fat milk and yoghurts once you have settled in a spot. Keep a food stash for emergencies such as missing a meal, or for times when you need to supplement the meals that have been organised for you. For example, you may come home from a sponsor's dinner at a fancy restaurant feeling that you are still hungry and that your legs will require extra carbohydrate for tomorrow's exercise challenge.

  A low-dose broad-range multivitamin and mineral supplement may be in order if you are unsure of the quality of the food supply or your opportunities to set up a consistent eating pattern.

On the trip: assert yourself

- Look after yourself while actually on the move. Realise that travelling can be extremely boring for an athlete. It may be a time of enforced inactivity (and lower energy needs). Don't equate boredom with hunger and simply eat for entertainment. Eat to a plan, and if you have pre-arranged your meals—e.g. with the airline—stick to this schedule. Watch your fluid balance, especially when flying in pressurised air-cabins. Drink plenty of fruit juices or low-joule drinks, depending on your energy needs. Caffeine drinks (coffee, tea and cola drinks) may dehydrate you if drunk in large quantities, and alcohol is a problem for the same reason.

- Be careful with food safety. 'Traveller's Trots' and 'Delhi Belly' can make a mess of athletic performance. Don't take any risk with food poisoning in foreign countries. Heed the local warnings—you will be told where the water is safe to drink, where it is unwise to eat fresh produce, and which eating places are generally 'safe'.

- Make good choices in restaurants (see Golf Chapter) and with take-aways (see Basketball chapter). These may form a greater part of your diet when travelling than when you are at home.

- Eating well in a cafeteria-style dining hall, commonly part of an athlete's village or university accommodation, can be harder than it looks. Focus on what you need rather than what everybody else is eating (see Swimming chapter).

If you apply the same dietary commitment during your travels as you do while at home, then your trip should reward you with sporting success in addition to new stamps in your passport!

PROFILE: SUE
Tournament nutrition

Sue was sure that she knew her nutritional goals for competition, but turning theory into practice in tournament tennis was a difficult task. But she was convinced that it was a crucial part of sustaining her performance level over the week of competition. Too many times she had watched the final being fought out between players she should have beaten, while she had bowed out in dismal style in the middle of the tournament. Often she felt that she had eaten badly over the week and the effects had gradually taken their toll, leaving her tired and unable to play at anywhere near her best.

Of course, it wasn't always just food that caused problems. Life on the circuit often meant lack of sleep, homesickness, and more stress and challenge than was good for her game. It had been especially hard in the early days on the satellite circuit. Not only was the life-style new and bewildering, but conditions were harder for those struggling to make themselves known.

Being short of cash usually meant staying in cheap accommodation away from the tennis centre, and having to spend precious time travelling on public transport to get to and from matches. Access to food, at least the right sort of food, was limited by both time and money and often many days passed before a properly planned meal was managed. In these circumstances it was hard to keep coming up, day after day, particularly if the three or four days of the tournament were preceded by qualifying rounds.

Sue welcomed the improved conditions that accompanied her recent graduation to the Grand Prix circuit. She was now entitled to stay in good hotels situated close to the competition venues, and caterers provided a spread of food in the player facilities at the courts. With food being more accessible, the major challenges now lay in the unpredictable nature of the game of tennis itself.

Sue talked the situation over with a sports dietitian and they agreed that the main principles of tournament nutrition were:

- Maximise and speed-up recovery after each match—particularly long, gruelling battles—by beginning carbohydrate and fluid restoration immediately the match is over. Ideally, start with a carbohydrate snack and/or drink within 15–30 minutes of the end of play.
- When there is a long gap between matches—overnight or a rest day—continue to eat nutritiously, with the emphasis on carbohydrate intake.
- Eat before each match to feel comfortable and refuelled—ideally a light snack about two hours pre-match. Make sure that fluids are topped up on hot days.
- Experiment with a sports drink during matches, drinking to keep pace with fluid losses and carbohydrate needs. Long matches and hot days require extra vigilance.

Separated into its components like this it seemed easy to make a plan. However, Sue explained that difficulties arose because of the loose and unpredictable time-table of events. The day's match schedule was variable, crude and given at short notice. Unless you were drawn for the first match on each court, you could not be sure of the time you were playing. While you could predict an approximate time for the fourth match on court 1, there was never the certainty of a fixed time-table.

This made it difficult to time the pre-match meal or to know what to have between two matches (a singles then a doubles match) on the same day. Sue remembered back to some disastrous experiences, like the occasion when she was scheduled for the third match of the afternoon, and had eaten a reasonable lunch just before the start of the session. Not only was the first match a one-sided affair lasting 35 minutes, but the second match was forfeited after five minutes due to an ankle injury to one of the players. Suddenly, Sue found herself on the court, with a fuller stomach than she would have liked.

On another occasion, during a satellite tournament, Sue had eaten her packed lunch in anticipation of her match, only to find that a rain delay put matches back indefinitely. What was she to do then? Go hungry, or take a chance and eat a snack? And would the little tennis centre kiosk stock anything that passed for high-carbohydrate, low-fat food? Apart from anything else, the worry of making the right decision interfered with her game.

Post-match eating was still sometimes a problem, even with the courtside meals available for the players. When centre court matches stretched into the night, Sue found herself finishing after the caterers had gone home for the day. This left only restaurants (often too late to find one open) or hotel room service (often unsuitable menus). And of course, with late games, sleep sometimes took priority over eating.

The dietitian suggested that two philosophies were needed to handle the situation. First was the idea of flexibility. It would be good to plan the ideal way of tackling a nutritional goal, but it would be better to have a 'plan B' up her sleeve for sudden changes of schedule.

For example, the ideal match preparation would be a light meal about 2–2$\frac{1}{2}$ hours pre-match, followed by a warm-up hit and perhaps a top-up with extra fluids (water) before the match. Matches set to a definite schedule, such as the first match in a session, could be tackled in this fashion.

However, with an uncertain time-table, additional or alternative snacks would be needed at hand. Ready-to-go liquid meal supplements—for example, Exceed Sports Meal—would be particularly versatile in helping to fill in the gaps and handle emergencies. Being liquid and easy to digest, they could supply a nutritious, carbohydrate-based meal without the discomfort of solid food. This would be handy between two matches close together, or as a top-up to an earlier meal when the next match was running late. They could also be a quick no-preparation snack after the game, or a boost to turn a sandwich snack into a more filling meal. With a bit of experimentation, there should be many other food ideas for this trouble-shooting role.

Being self-reliant is the other helpful philosophy. Even at the big tournaments where hotels and court catering are provided, many players choose to organise their own apartments with cooking facilities. This allows them to be more in control, cooking the meals they want at the times they want—although they can fall back on the other food facilities when they want a break. In addition, after weeks on the circuit, it is often nice to have some home cooking rather than restaurant fare. Sometimes, it makes the difference between succumbing to homesickness/travel fatigue or not.

NON-PERISHABLE FOOD SUPPLIES FOR THE TRAVELLING ATHLETE

- Liquid meal preparations: Powder type (e.g. Sustagen Sport) if you need to conserve space

  Liquid ready-to-go types (e.g. Exceed Sports Meal) for times when you do not have food preparation facilities or when the local water supply is unsafe.

- Breakfast cereals and powdered low-fat milk
- Dried fruit, fruit juice packs, and canned fruit (comes in plastic 'snack packs' if you need to save on weight)
- Quick cook noodle and pasta varieties
- Muesli bars and slices (preferably not the chocolate-coated types)
- Dried biscuits or rice cakes with jam or honey

  (or Vegemite if you are going to be homesick!)
- Low-dose broad-range multivitamin mineral supplement (if you are unsure of the consistency and the quality of your food intake)

At the lower rungs of the circuit, where the lifestyle isn't so rich and famous, being self-reliant is even more important. If you can afford to stay in a unit, perhaps sharing costs in a group, then with some organisation you may be able to supply the bulk of your own meals. Even in billet or hotel accommodation, you can organise some of your supplies—a travelling food kit can be a great help (see story and table above). Having your own food and drinks at the court can be important in making your tournament nutrition happen as planned—again, what you want, when you want it.

Poor nutrition will undoubtedly put your tennis performance below par, through gradual muscle fuel depletion and dehydration in the short-term, and perhaps nutritional deficiencies and weight problems over a long tour. With better planning, not only can you avoid all these physiological traps, but you can go into matches with the confidence boost of knowing you are at your best. There is every chance that you will meet an opponent, even someone with more talent than yourself, who has not prepared for their nutritional needs as well. Your commitment may well mean their loss.

Golf

Golf is a sport of many levels. At one end of the spectrum are the thousands of Australians who enjoy a social round of nine or eighteen holes on weekends. At the other are some of the highest paid sportspeople in this country—for example, of the top twenty earners in Australian sport for 1990, fourteen were golf players.

Golf is basically a game of skill. A handicapping system operates to level the golfing ability of beginners, and for many recreational players the fun and incentive of golf is not only to play against others but to lower personal handicap scores.

Competitive golf is played at both amateur and professional levels. State and national amateur titles are conducted, with the players involved often struggling to support themselves while practising and playing golf for the requisite hours each day. Golfers can turn professional either through an apprenticeship or by attending Player's School. Under both schemes, potential pro-golfers undertake business studies as well as learning golf skills. While some professional golfers become attached to golf clubs and concentrate on providing golf tuition and running golf shops, others look to making their mark on the professional competitive circuit in Australia, and perhaps overseas.

Training

Recreational golfers may practise their golf game by simply playing. At the other end of the spectrum, professional competition golfers can spend up to eight hours a day on the golf course, practising specific skills, playing practice rounds or playing in actual competitions.

Even during a competition, many players will conduct a practice session at the end of the day's play.

Some players also include general fitness training in their competition preparation—for example, weight training or aerobic activities such as running and swimming. While this training may not directly improve golf skills, some players believe that improved fitness will reduce the deterioration in skills caused by fatigue, and that improved strength may help in the transference of power to the ball.

Competition

A round of competition golf is played over 18 holes, with golf tournaments being conducted either as a single round on one day, or as multi-day competitions of two or four rounds on consecutive days. In a tournament, there are usually two tee-off times—a morning group starting between 7.00 and 9.00am, and an afternoon group beginning between 11.00am and 1.00pm. A round typically takes three to five hours to play, depending on the skill level of the player and the number of other players on the course. The average golf course is seven kilometres from first to last hole, although a player may walk 10–20 kilometres in a game depending on the accuracy of their shots.

In Australia, winter is the pro-am competition season and professional players typically travel on a circuit between club tournaments. During this season a pro-golfer could play in ten tournaments, for a total of fifteen days of competition, each month. The major international tournaments in Australia are played from January to March and from October to December, flanking the major season overseas. Australian golfers may launch themselves on the international circuit, with either an American or European tour from April to October. The world's best golfers are almost continually on tour, with players such as Greg Norman spending only a few months at home each year.

Physical characteristics

Golf is a game of skill rather than physical fitness and physical attributes. Therefore top golfers come in many shapes and sizes, with Brett Ogle and Chris Patton showing the extremes among current players. In general, since most players do not undertake intense daily exercise the average body-fat levels of top golfers are higher than aerobically-trained athletes.

Typical physique (elite Australian Amateur golfers)

	Male	Female
Height	175–186cm	161–168cm
Weight	72–81kg	58–62kg
Skinfolds	85–118mm	96–135mm

Common nutrition issues

Is overweight a handicap?

Players such as American pro-golfer Chris Patton, weighing in at around 140kg, raise the question of whether high body-fat levels affect golf performance. Certainly, being significantly overweight is not an ideal situation in terms of general health. In terms of direct golf skill, we might speculate that a large girth could reduce the flexibility of a player's swing, but equally, that being heavier could provide greater momentum to transfer to the ball.

Theoretically, overweight might also handicap a golfer by reducing general fitness levels and making the player more prone to physical fatigue—and thus more likely to suffer loss of skill and mental concentration. Since body fat works as an insulator, an overweight golfer would also be expected to suffer greater heat intolerance in hot conditions. In both cases, fatigue could cause a drop in skill level over the course of the round and over the days of a tournament.

Of course, these are all theoretical concepts and there is no scientific evidence to support the belief that all overweight players will improve their golfing game by losing body fat. In fact, Craig Stadler, another heavyweight American golfer, reputedly lost body fat only to find that his golf swing was disrupted. To be fair, the blame might equally be placed on his emotional/psychological adjustment to weight loss as well as the direct physical changes.

The best advice is to find a body weight and body-fat level that is healthy and comfortable for you, and to remember that a sport like golf will allow a greater range of tolerance with its ideal physical characteristics. If you do feel that your health and fitness could be improved by loss of body fat, read Chapter 3 for safe and sensible advice to achieve it. By achieving weight loss gradually with a healthy diet and exercise program, you should improve your self-confidence as well as your physical condition. Both effects could be good for your game.

Training nutrition

The principles of optimum training nutrition are essentially those of a healthy eating plan, and apply to golfers who play on weekends as well as those who spend eight hours a day on the golf course. Of course as energy expenditure increases with increased training loads, so do requirements for energy and carbohydrate. Read Chapters 1 and 2 for details of the optimum training diet.

Tournament nutrition

A top golfer must strive to maintain skills and concentration over three to five hours, perhaps for days on end. Once physical fatigue sets in, deterioration in such skills can be expected. Although a golfer is not faced with the level of strenuous exercise faced by other athletes, prolonged moderate-level activity accompanied by the stress of competition and often inclement weather conditions, can take its toll. Both dehydration and low blood-sugar levels are possible physical hazards to face during competition, and each would be expected to impair golfing performance.

Sweat losses may be considerable when tournaments are played in hot and windy environments or even when high adrenalin levels combine with moderate conditions. Although many golf courses provide drink stations for players, they may be at infrequent intervals and not a significant source of fluid replacement during a game. Since players will usually miss a meal while playing a round, they may be faced with no carbohydrate intake for five or six hours. Combined with exercise and nervous stress, this situation may cause a drop in blood-sugar levels in susceptible individuals, affecting brain function and skill.

When tournaments are held over several days the situation may be compounded, particularly with respect to inadequate fluid replacement. Does your weight drop markedly over the tournament, a sign of chronic dehydration? If you find yourself eating only two meals a day (before and after the day's competition), insufficient kilojoule intake can be another cause of weight loss, and inadequate carbohydrate can add to fatigue levels.

The careful golfer leaves nothing to chance, taking provisions out onto the course to meet the nutritional needs that will arise in competition. There is no need to miss meals or to dehydrate. The plan may vary with individuals and with competition settings, but you should decide for yourself how much fluid you are likely to lose through sweating and how important it is for you to keep up carbohydrate levels during a round. Experiment in practice rounds under simulated competition conditions to determine both your needs and the best way to meet them.

Carbohydrate drinks such as sports drinks, fruit juice and soft drink provide a simple way of consuming fluids and carbohydrates. Work out a schedule of intake that keeps you feeling comfortable. Aim for frequent intake of small amounts—say 150ml every twenty minutes, and keep drinks cool. Food such as sandwiches, fruit or muesli bars can provide additional or alternate forms of carbohydrate intake, and unless you are extremely nervous, these are not likely to cause gastric discomfort. See Chapters 4.6 and 4.7 for more details.

Despite the stress of competition, the golfer should aim to eat well before and after the day's competition. See Chapter 4.4 for discussion about suitable pre-event meals, and be prepared to promote recovery after each round by looking out for fluid and carbohydrate needs as soon as you have finished. This might mean a snack before you go back out onto the practice fairways.

Life on the circuit

When you are travelling on the golf circuit, both within the country or overseas, meeting your nutritional needs can be a challenge. Whether you are eating in restaurants or catering for yourself, it is often difficult to get what you want at the right time. And to be at your best, both in spirit and in physical form, you need to be on top of your nutrition goals. Read the Tennis chapter for advice about travelling nutrition, and find handy hints for restaurant eating in the guide below.

Alcohol intake

A golf game traditionally finishes at the 'nineteenth hole'—the bar in the clubrooms. It is also traditional to share a round with your golf partners. Of course this does not necessarily have to mean alcohol intake, but in most cases it probably does.

Read the comments about alcohol in Chapter 1.6. While there may be no harm in having a couple of drinks, it is easy to slip into a pattern of drinking more than you realise or need. It is probably better to avoid alcohol intake during tournaments—after all, you need all the skills and concentration that your brain can muster.

PROFILE
Waiter—a healthy meal please!

Most people eat at restaurants occasionally—and for that matter, on special occasions. Under these circumstances it is usual to relax everyday nutritional goals and enjoy a special meal, or even to have a total dietary splurge. However, for athletes on the circuit, continually travelling and relying on hotel accommodation, eating out becomes the way of life.

When restaurants become the major source of your food intake, it is important to know how to make your nutritional requirements turn up on your plate. This is even more crucial when your nutritional requirements are skewed by strenuous exercise—for example, if you are training intensely or competing in heavy competition. In the competition setting, of course, the right food intake is crucial to let you achieve your optimum performance.

The food provided in restaurants generally typifies Australian or Western tastes, and is perhaps a little more exotic than home cooking. Therefore, it can be higher in fat, salt and sugar, and lower in carbohydrate and fibre than the optimum training diet discussed in Chapter 1. This provides an immediate problem in that an athlete may not easily achieve daily carbohydrate requirements. Weight gain may also result because of the temptation to overeat total quantities of food and to over-consume fat in particular.

HINTS FOR EATING WELL IN A RESTAURANT

- Set nutritional goals for a restaurant meal, according to its importance in the overall scheme of your performance. If it is a special or unusual occasion you may decide to take a more relaxed attitude. However if this is a crucial time in training or competition, or eating out is your way of life, then choose food for its nutritional contribution rather than its taste appeal alone.

- It helps to be familiar with a restaurant. If you are in an unfamiliar area, ask advice—especially from other athletes.

  When you travel to a new place, scout around to see what restaurants are available. Being armed with some knowledge lets you plan in advance where you will eat. If you wait until you are tired and desperately hungry to look or decide on a place, you will probably make a compromised decision. Also, remember that many restaurants are run as a franchise or chain—if you find a good place in one city, you may be able to make use of its equivalents on your travels.

- Remember that restaurants are a hospitality industry, and by rights should be pleased to provide the service that you request. Don't be afraid to arrange for your special needs—whether it be meal timing, or the type of food you would like.

- There may be occasions when it is important to eat straight away, to promote rapid recovery or to conserve precious sleep time. To avoid long waits in a restaurant, try 'phoning the restaurant ahead of time and organise your order. This can be especially useful if you are in a large group.

- Smorgasbord restaurants generally offer a speedier service, plus more freedom of choice over what you eat. However, you may need to use greater skills to avoid the distraction of quantities and types of food that are not on your menu.

- If saving money is a priority, you may be able to make up your own breakfast and lunch meals from easy-to-prepare foods that you can buy or keep in your room. Make the most of dinner in a restaurant to maintain variety and make up for any nutritional shortfalls in the other meals. (Of course, depending on your schedule, you may like to make lunch the main meal of the day.)

Of course, it is not always the fault of the restaurant or its food. Many athletes cause their own problems by eating completely out of character—forgetting their nutritional goals and their usual meal patterns. Those who are normally happy with cereal and toast for breakfast suddenly get distracted by the Eggs Benedict on the menu. And three-course hot lunches begin to replace the customary sandwiches and fruit.

Meal timing can also be a problem. Restaurant hours may not always suit your training or competition schedule. You may finish late at night, or need to start early in the morning, and find that you are out of step with the hospitality industry. Even if you appreciate that recovery will be enhanced after a strenuous session by eating carbohydrate immediately, getting those carbohydrates could be another thing. You may find a restaurant open, but then be stymied by the long delay before your order is taken and the food appears in front of you.

And then there is the matter of money. Unless you are a very successful athlete, or the restaurant is included in the circuit hospitality, you may find yourself making food decisions on the basis of financial considerations rather than nutritional concerns.

For general considerations about eating on the circuit, see the Tennis chapter for an account of the travelling athlete. Meanwhile the following hints may help you to cope well with restaurant eating— whether it be a one-off occasion or your everyday life. The table on pp. 334–9 summarises some specific tips for choosing well in particular restaurants, focusing on special tactics to ensure adequate carbohydrate intake, as well as skills to prevent excessive kilojoule intake for those at risk.

HOW TO MEET YOUR NUTRITIONAL GOALS IN A RESTAURANT

Situation	Tips to increase carbohydrate intake	Tips to avoid excess kilojoule intake
General comments	Be aware that you will be working against the Western trend to eat protein (and fat) with carbohydrate foods as an accompaniment. Either choose a dish that is based on carbohydrate, or order a smaller serve of a protein based meal (meat, fish, chicken, egg, cheese, etc.), and add generous side-serves of carbohydrate foods (fruit/juice, bread, potato, rice, noodles, etc.)	Choose only as much as you need—limit the number of courses or ask for smaller serves. If all else fails, leave what you don't require. Be vigilant about limiting fat intake, and watch the added extras with meals—e.g. garlic bread, french fries, and high-kilojoule drinks (alcohol especially). Look for bulky low-joule foods or low-joule drinks to fill up with instead. Take extra care with buffet or smorgasbord type meals, especially with regard to coming back for seconds.
Breakfast	Breakfast is perhaps the easiest meal to cater for. Nutritious carbohydrate foods include juice, fruit, cereals, toast, muffins and crumpets. If you would like something warm try porridge, pancakes, baked beans or spaghetti.	Limit fat intake by asking for low-fat milk on your cereal and by being a miser with the butter/margarine on breads. Your main enemies are croissants, and high-fat cooked meals such as bacon and eggs.
Lunch	Meals based on breads—rolls or sandwiches—are quick and nutritious. Have a thick layer of bread and	Watch the spreads on your bread and oily dressings. Otherwise, fill up the meal with salads. Low-joule drinks

Situation	Tips to increase carbohydrate intake	Tips to avoid excess kilojoule intake
	fill with a little protein and lots of salad. Other variations include hearty soups with bread, baked potatoes with a filling, and gourmet hamburgers. If you need extra kilojoules, finish up with scones, muffins or a healthy cake. Fruit or fruit salad, and low-fat icecream or yoghurt are other high-carbohydrate foods. Drinks include juices, soft drinks and sports drinks—or if you really need to push the kilojoules and carbohydrates, ask for a low-fat fruit smoothie.	include iced water (ask for a jug), plain mineral water and diet soft drinks. You may be able to afford a dessert, but save 'fat' kilojoules by removing cream or cream cheese icing. What about a low-fat yoghurt, or a soft-serve of the same? Vitari and Gisé are other low-fat 'icecreams'. Fruit is always a good choice.
General restaurant/ French restaurant	The usual choice of an entree and main course based on protein foods blocks out room for the carbos. If you need an entree, try thick vegie soup with bread. For a main course, choose a main or entree-size protein meal (consider it a side-dish) and order extra serves of potatoes, rice or noodles as well as your vegies. Stick to non-fat cooking methods (see next column). High-carbohydrate, low-fat desserts include fruit salad, low-fat icecreams,	Apart from the total quantity of food you eat (see general comments above), your main concern is your fat intake. Choose lean cuts of meat/fish/chicken (e.g. avoid processed meats, fatty mince meats and high-fat duck). Ask for non-fat cooking methods—grilling, stewing, dry baking. A large baked potato has plenty of carbos for less kilojoules than small roast potatoes or chips. Watch sauces and gravies that are based on butter or cream, or

Situation	Tips to increase carbohydrate intake	Tips to avoid excess kilojoule intake
	sorbets and yoghurts, rice pudding and fruit crumble. Bread and high-carbohydrate drinks (see lunch ideas) can also boost total carbohydrate intake.	oil and butter brushed on your vegies. Don't hesitate to request that your meal is served without the sauces, or with the sauces on the side (to use sparingly). Ask for plain bread rather than oily herb or garlic breads, and for salads that are left plain or with low-oil dressings. You can decide to go without dessert altogether or perhaps share one with someone else. If you would like something sweet try some fruit, a little low-fat icecream/yoghurt/sorbet—or perhaps a single chocolate with your tea/coffee.
Italian	Pasta is a great carbohydrate food, but be aware that many pasta dishes are not what they seem. Lasagnes and cannelloni, for example, may be more filling than pasta, and the fillings may be high in fat—oil, fatty meat and cheese. High-fat sauces based on cream and oil can also make a spaghetti dish high in fat rather than carbohydrate. Order well—a vegetable or	Order an entree course of pasta for your main meal and be extra careful to choose a low-fat sauce—even if that means making a special request. If the sauce arrives in greater quantities or with more oil than you expected, try to eat only a little to make the pasta tasty.

Situation	Tips to increase carbohydrate intake	Tips to avoid excess kilojoule intake
	tomato-based sauce is usually best. Meat, chicken and bolognaise sauces can be fine, if the meat is lean and oil is used sparingly. See general restaurant comments for other ideas.	
Chinese Malaysian Thai	Rice and noodles are the Malaysian mainstay of Asian cuisine. Your best bet is to order stirfried meat and vegetable dishes, adding these as a topping to bowls of steamed rice or noodles. Watch the traps that add lots of fat to a meal so that you can concentrate on the carbohydrates. (see next column)	Since most dishes are based on small amounts of meat/fish/chicken, most of the fat in Asian cooking comes from oil added in cooking. Avoid dishes that have been battered or deep fried, and request that stirfries are cooked with minimum oil. Base meals on plain rice or noodles rather than special fried rices— there is already plenty of flavour in the dishes you will add to the rice/noodle base. Avoid banquets with numerous courses and lots of spring rolls and deep-fried finger-foods. If you are sharing courses in a group, make a conscious decision about what you will eat —e.g. how many times you will fill up your bowl. It is tempting to keep picking, and refilling your bowl, without judging how much you have eaten.

Situation	Tips to increase carbohydrate intake	Tips to avoid excess kilojoule intake
Indian	As for Chinese above— use steamed rice as a base for the rest of the meal. Other good carbohydrate foods are lentils, chickpeas, and Indian bread— preferably the non-fried varieties.	As for Chinese, ask for dishes cooked with little oil, and avoid fried and battered foods, including samosas and fried breads. Small serves of curries eaten on rice can be a great meal—but make sure that you quench your thirst with low-joule drinks after a hot spicy meal!
Mexican	Rice, beans and Mexican flat bread (tortillas) are all good carbohydrate foods. Try not to fill up on too much cheese, meat and sour cream—you may not have enough room for the foods you really need. In some ways it can help to order individual items from the menu rather than set main courses. You can put together some tostadas, beans, rice and extra tortillas, for example, rather than a plate full of high-fat items. 'Fajitas' are usually a good choice combining salsa, rice, salad and char-grilled beef or chicken strips, all wrapped in tortilla bread.	Be wary of the giant main courses that are legendary in Mexican restaurants and of the high-fat dishes. As suggested in the Carbohydrate column, you may be better to order à-la-carte to choose just what you need. Corn chips are made with oil and are therefore high in kilojoules, so it is a mistake to sit with a pile of nachos smothered in cheese and sour cream in front of you.

Pritikin and health restaurants	Many restaurants now cater for high-carbohydrate low-fat meals. Be a little wary of restaurants labelled 'health food'—there may still be plenty of high-fat ingredients used, such as pastry, oil and cheese. Nevertheless, many restaurants meet the challenge well, providing dishes that meet the guidelines for healthy nutrition as well as appealing to gourmet tastebuds. If you need to watch your kilojoule intake, be careful about the total quantity that you eat—it is still possible to eat too much of a good thing.
Alcohol	Most people associate restaurants with 'wining and dining', and a couple of glasses of alcohol can be a pleasant part of a healthy meal and an enjoyable night. However, think carefully about the effect of alcohol on your performance. You may decide to forego alcohol when dining out in the midst of competition or strenuous training, or leave it for special occasions rather than every time you eat in a restaurant.

Cricket

Cricket is a game of skill and tradition that touches the lives of most Australians each summer. Teams of eleven play against each other, with slightly different rules governing the limited-over (one-day) games compared to those based on two innings for each side (four or five day games). While both men's and women's competitions exist, it is the men's scene that dominates with lucrative professional and international competition. It is hard to progress though the ranks of district and state (Sheffield Shield) level cricket to this level. Most cricket in Australia is played at a social and recreational level with many leagues and competitions carrying grades down to 'F' level.

Roughly speaking, a cricket team is broken into specialist batsmen, specialist bowlers and a wicket-keeper. Theoretically, all team members get to bat and to field, while usually only the specialists are required to undertake the task of bowling. The game is based on skill, and only at a high level of play and only in recent years, has there been a requirement for reasonable aerobic fitness. Even so, there are many top-level cricketers who are better titled as sportsmen rather than athletes, and whose off-field activities create as many stories and legends as their on-field exploits.

Training

Cricket is a summer sport, with the season beginning at the end of October and progressing through to a final series in March–April. At the top level, some cricketers play all year round, playing in international tours during the northern hemisphere summer, or travelling to England to play in their county cricket season. Alternatively, a few cricketers at the top level will continue to train, or at least to remain fit, over winter. However, the usual pattern is to stop playing once the season is over, and unless the cricketer gets involved in another sport over winter—perhaps football—fitness levels may be very poor by the beginning of the next season.

At first-grade cricket level, pre-season training begins around June, most often in the form of general fitness work, and is often unsupervised or left to the individual player. As the season draws closer, organised team training takes over and the component of skills practice is increased.

During the season at a top club, three team training sessions are organised each week between matches. Each session lasts 2–2^1/$_2$ hours and involves batting and bowling practice, fielding skills and drills, and perhaps some general running or fitness work. Some individual players at the top level may be motivated to organise their own fitness program in addition to this, and may undertake additional aerobic training and perhaps weights.

In low-grade competition there may be little or no organised training.

Competition

District cricket is played on weekends with many grades or levels of competition. This may be in the form of two-day fixtures and/or limited over (one-day) competition, with these competitions often happening simultaneously. The state-level cricket competition (Sheffield Shield) is organised into four-day matches (Friday to Monday) and often interrupts the district level season for those who are chosen to play.

Summer is a busy time for international cricket in Australia. The program usually includes a test series (five-day matches) and a World Series Cup (one-day, limited-over matches) played against touring teams from other cricket-playing nations. Between matches, the cricketers may go back to their state level competition, and may train with their state teams or district clubs. When an overseas tour is organised, the Australian team will travel together for a period of time, and may include team training sessions between matches.

The physical requirements of a cricket game vary with the format of the match (multi-day versus limited-over game), and with the player's position in the team. Test games are played at 'gentleman's hours'—six hours of match play plus breaks, between 11.00am and 6.00pm. The limited-over series may also involve day–night matches and a slightly different time-table of play.

Games played in the middle to end of summer are often played in very hot conditions, requiring players to stand for many hours in the sun. Those at most risk of heat stress are those standing out the longest (e.g. the fielding team) and the fast bowlers who may work intensely in short spells over the day. Batsmen who stay in for a long innings may also have to run repeatedly in this heat.

Physical characteristics

Cricketers come in all shapes and sizes—even at the top level. It has only been in recent years that cricket coaches have demanded that body fat be kept at a reasonable level to accompany the increased fitness level expected of players. A healthier level of body fat would theoretically improve speed, stamina and heat tolerance. Speed becomes important at a high level of play, particularly in the limited-over matches, since skilled fielding and running between wickets is helpful for success. Many fast bowlers have been singled out as deserving of lower body-fat levels and improved fitness, in the belief that this will improve their speed and therefore their delivery, as well as increasing their stamina to bowl and field over the day. Wicket-keepers must be strong as well as agile—in an average day of keeping, the equivalent of 600 squats may be done.

Typical physique (elite cricket players)

	Male	Female
Height	176–192cm	165–175cm
Weight	78–94kg	60–72kg
Skinfold sum	54–100mm	71–110mm

Common nutrition issues

Body-fat levels

If you feel that your life would be healthier, your cricket game faster, and your captain happier by shedding some weight, then opt for a fat-loss program that is based on sensible and long-term principles. Many male (and female) cricketers find themselves wanting to lose weight but not knowing how to do it—nutrition and fitness may never have been a big consideration in their lives. The cricketing lifestyle may not help the cause either, being made up of low-exercise levels, and too much of the good life. Read the account of Duncan below, and Chapter 3 for ideas on healthy fat loss.

Training nutrition

Cricketers are among the last group of sportspeople to warm to the idea of a healthy nutrition lifestyle. For most, the rewards will be improved health and vitality, and better weight control. However, for the new breed of cricketers who undertake an organised fitness and training schedule, the special dietary needs of daily training will be met by these same nutrition principles. Read Chapters 1 and 2 for an outline of the optimum diet for health and training.

Match day nutrition

Match day nutrition is run on tradition rather than science, even at the top level. Players may rise late, especially if there was a celebration the night before (see the comments on alcohol below), and pre-event meals are variable in quantity and type. Test players staying in hotels may even start the day with a hearty (high-fat) cooked breakfast.

Matches are generally played with a drink break every hour, and a set break for lunch (40 minutes) and tea (20 minutes). A meal is usually eaten in the lunch break, and great tradition prevails in its organisation. At elite-level cricket, meals are catered by the ground social club and can range from a light snack to a heavy meal of roast or fried fish. The legendary 'cricketer's salad' generally consists of cold meats, salads and bread, but may also be high in fat (due to the dressings, added margarine and processed meats) and relatively low in carbohydrate.

Further down the competition scale, the tradition of a 'social' lunch also applies, with the home team responsible for providing the food. Wives and girlfriends may organise a roster or organise for everyone to bring a plate. The time-table varies a little with the schedule of one-day matches, but the tradition remains essentially the same.

After reading Chapter 4, you will see that very few of the state-of-the-art competition nutrition ideas have found their way into cricket. And indeed, it might be argued that with a game of skill, there is less need for such scientific concerns. Nevertheless, cricketers might consider updating some of their competition practices. In terms of comfort and topping up carbohydrate stores, light, high-carbohydrate meals would be more appropriate as pre-match and lunch-time meals.

Combating dehydration is an important issue, and cricketers should drink at least 250–500ml of fluid at each drink break to replace sweat losses on hot days (see the case history below). For those players who are actually working—the batsmen, bowlers and wicket-keeper—the provision of carbohydrate in these drinks may be of additional benefit. Experiment with cordial or a sports drink. Lastly, post-match strategies should promote recovery, especially when in the midst of a multi-day match. Recovery practices include fluid, carbohydrate and rest—not always a priority of cricketers (see comments on alcohol).

Alcohol intake

Alcohol intake is heavily interwoven in the cricketer's lifestyle. Cricketing traditions include having a beer with the opposition team at the end of the day, or in the case of international cricket (where team tactics frown on being too friendly with the competition) having a beer with your own team-mates. Even during a multi-day match and even at high levels of play, it is acceptable behaviour to go out wining and dining, or drinking and dancing until late into the night. And of course, when the match is over, or the test series has been decided, it is almost mandatory that newspapers carry a picture of the winning team in their locker rooms celebrating heartily with some alcoholic drinks.

Not only is alcohol intake an expected part of the game, but heavy drinking is also glorified and becomes the stuff of legends. Not only do cricketing afficionados know how many half-centuries were made by an international cricketer on a tour of England, but also the number of cans of beer he drank on the flight home.

Clearly such drinking practices go against the principles of healthy nutrition and optimum performance. Read Chapter 1.6 for a discussion of the role of alcohol in sport. As in other male-dominated team sports, it will take time and a change of attitude before healthier practices become widespread in cricket. It is hoped that the emerging group of first-class cricketers will include sensible drinking practices among their ideas of professionalism—not only looking after their own lives and sporting careers, but providing a role model for thousands of young cricket players.

Travelling on tour or abroad

Cricketers on tour live out of hotels and suitcases, and in the case of many overseas tours, they may be constantly on the move for a number of months. Standing in the way of optimum nutrition are the usual problems associated with being a travelling athlete, as well as the strong traditions associated with being a cricketer on tour. Remind yourself of your nutrition priorities (Chapters 1 and 2), and for specific advice on travelling nutrition read the sections in the Tennis chapter (the travelling athlete) and the Golf chapter (eating in restaurants).

PROFILE: DUNCAN
Lose weight or lose match payments!

There was a new order in at Duncan's cricket club and Duncan was worried. Duncan was a fast bowler, with the potential to be a very fast bowler if he wasn't so fat. The new captain-coach called the team together at the beginning of pre-season training and explained his ideas for a new, fit team that would blast the opposition with speed and professionalism as well as skill. Each player was interviewed separately, and Duncan was given instructions to lose nine kilos—or face fines. A fitness program was drawn up and an appointment set in a fortnight for Duncan to report in on his progress with the weight loss.

Duncan had heard talk like this before. Last year they had told him to lose weight also—the same old nine kilograms. But Duncan had dodged his way through the season, laughing to the club officials that he had carefully developed a life of 'organised sloth'. The weight had stayed put, but his season's figures were moderately successful so no-one had really bothered to pursue the matter.

This year was different, however. The new captain-coach didn't look like he would stand any nonsense, and a new fast-bowler had been recruited. If Duncan wanted to hold his position, it looked like he would have to make some changes. How could he lose the weight?

Duncan tried the 'Israeli Army diet', and after a week achieved nothing except a dislike for green apples. One of his mates told him about the 'Drinking Man's diet'. This sounded like his kind of diet, but they were unable to find a copy. Duncan attended his first fortnightly weigh-in with the captain-coach and found himself fined $200 dollars for the lack of progress. That really hurt! However, the coach then explained that the money would be used to pay for a series of consultations with a sports dietitian.

Duncan was surprised when the dietitian didn't immediately give him a diet sheet. However, she explained that rigid dietary plans were usually only successful in the short-term. If Duncan wanted to go to the trouble of losing weight, he might as well do it properly and lose it forever—by learning a new, healthier lifestyle. The dietitian likened this to the help that he received from the specialist bowling coach at the club. This coach carefully examined Duncan's bowling style, picking out the faults and weaknesses and helping him to remodel and improve his deliveries.

Duncan's typical daily diet was discussed and assessed. The dietitian learned that he lived at home, but was rarely there to eat meals. Nevertheless, it was a potential source of food, and Duncan explained that his mother had become pretty careful about her cooking since his father's heart attack, four years ago. The typical intake for his day is summarised in the table on the following page.

The dietitian was honest in her assessment, telling Duncan that his diet was high in fat and that his alcohol intake was inconsistent with a trim waistline and good performance. The uneven spread of energy over the day—skipped meals and heavy intake late at night—also worked against his weight control. She explained the principles of healthy training nutrition to him (see Chapter 1) and together they negotiated an eating plan that fitted this mould.

Food for sports performance

Duncan's diet—before and after

	Original diet—a typical day	Healthy weight loss diet—a new daily plan
Breakfast	none (late for work)	bowl of wholegrain cereal with low fat milk, fruit juice
Lunch	pies/sausage rolls, flavoured milk 1/week: counter lunch with 2–3 beers	salad sandwich with cheese/ham/chicken/tuna/beef medium serve of fresh fruit salad
After training	two or three times/week: 4–5 beers at the pub	2 light beers (2 per cent alcohol)
Dinner	fried fish, chips, salad at the pub	Restaurant or home meal: grilled meat/fish/chicken, medium serve, all fat trimmed. 2 bread rolls or large potato, or cup rice/pasta pizza made on large pita bread base with reduced-fat cheese, tomato paste, vegetables, and perhaps diced meat/chicken/seafood. 1 stubbie of light beer or Diet Coke.
Later in night	corn chips and Coke while watching TV, or a medium pizza with the lot plus a litre of Coke or couple of stubbies	TV snacks—homemade popcorn (minimum oil), Diet Coke

Important changes included:

- no more skipping breakfast. With less late nights, Duncan would aim to get up in plenty of time for a healthy breakfast before work.

- a sandwich-based lunch to replace high-fat take-aways. Duncan wasn't too keen on eating fruit, but liked the look of the fresh fruit salad in the shop next to work.

- either a better chosen (low-fat) restaurant meal, or home to some of Mum's healthy cooking. Some serving sizes were given.

- instead of calling out for pizza on late training nights, the dietitian gave Duncan a recipe for a quick, low-fat version, using low-fat cheese and vegetables on pita bread.

- switching to light alcohol beer—and rationing himself to one stubbie a night. Duncan was a bit reluctant, but realised that many of his mates were already moving to this trend because of drink-driving laws.

- replacing Coke with low-joule drinks.

When the plans were laid out side-by-side, Duncan was surprised to see how much food he could now eat. The dietitian assured him that the new diet contained far less kilojoules and far more carbohydrate and vitamins/minerals than his old diet. He tackled the new plan with gusto, and with his fitness program and new attitude felt a new man. Duncan's success exceeded even his own expectations. The weight was lost within two months, and a month later Duncan reached what he considered his new 'fighting weight'. Being fit and motivated, his game became more aggressive and confident. Not only did he keep his place at the club, but he was recently selected to train with the state side.

PROFILE
The twelfth man—carrying the drinks is an undervalued role!

Despite the shake-up provided by World Series Cricket and the limited-overs game format, cricket remains a game of tradition. Cricket evolved in the moderate climate of England, and the rules that govern its play sometimes still reflect those days and those conditions. According to a recent study undertaken by Dr Chris Gore from the Australian Institute of Sport, these rules may not be suited to the sometimes fiery summers experienced in Australia—or indeed many of the other cricket-playing countries such as Pakistan, India, Sri Lanka, the West Indies and South Africa.

Not only are many cricketers required to take the field in weather exceeding 40°C, but many of them undertake intense activity for a number of hours in these conditions—particularly the fast bowlers. Running between wickets or fielding may also involve a prolonged and heavy work rate during some games. The clothing worn by cricketers, including the protective equipment worn while batting, may add to thermal stress by retarding heat loss. Clearly, sweat losses may be high in extreme conditions and yet the rules of cricket may interfere with adequate rehydration. According to the rules, drink breaks are held each hour, with the 'twelfth man' carrying drinks out onto the field. In very hot weather, drink breaks may be held every forty minutes. However, these official breaks and the luncheon and tea intervals provide the only sanctioned opportunities for fluid intake.

To test the relevance of these practices, Dr Chris Gore recently completed a study of sweat rates, temperature control and fluid intakes in 20 first-class cricket players. Measurements were taken during a real match, and some simulated matches, in weather conditions that were designated as cool (forecast temperature 22°), warm (forecast temperature 30°) and hot (forecast temperature 38°). The games were played under the rules of first-class games; the first session played from 11.00–13.00, the second session from 13.40–15.40, and the last session from 16.00–18.00. Water was available according to the normal rules—before the match, every hour during the cool and warm matches, every forty minutes during the hot match, and during luncheon and tea breaks. Players were able to drink as much as they desired.

The results showed that the weather significantly affected the sweat losses of players. On the cool day, the average sweat loss over the day was 540ml per hour—470ml/hour for the batsmen and 710ml/hour for the bowlers. On the warm day, the average sweat loss was 670ml/hr—600ml/hr for the batsmen and 690ml/hr for the bowlers. It was also noted that on the warm day, sweat rates were greater during the second and third sessions of play than during the opening session. Only bowlers were monitored on the hot day—recording sweat losses of 1670ml/hr for the first session, and 1070ml/hr for the second. There was no third session of play because these bowlers were successful in bowling the opposition team out by the tea break.

Fluid intake on the cool and warm days managed to keep pace with sweat losses. The cricket players drank about 500ml of fluid during each hourly break on the cool day, and 600–700ml on the warm day. Fluid intake during the luncheon break averaged about 900–1000ml on both days, and at the tea break 400ml and 600ml of fluid were consumed on the cool and warm day respectively. At the conclusion of play the total fluid balance of the players was a negligible to slight level of dehydration— –.3 per cent on the cool day and 1.2 per cent on the warm day.

The hot day gave different results. Drink breaks were taken each 40 minutes in response to the weather, and an average of 300–600ml of fluid was consumed on each occasion. By the end of the first session of play the bowlers were significantly dehydrated, showing a 3.8 per cent fluid deficit. During the luncheon break they showered in an attempt to cool down, and drank an average of 960ml. Despite this and further drink breaks during the second session, by the end of this (final) session of play the average level of dehydration was 4.3 per cent of body weight.

It appears that there is a maximum comfortable level of fluid intake that can be managed in each of the breaks, regardless of the weather. In hot weather it appears that more opportunities to consume fluid are required if total fluid intake is to be increased to match sweat losses. The level of dehydration sustained by players on the hot day would have certainly reduced their performance—and made for an uncomfortable day of cricket. Luckily a third session of play was not warranted on this day! Dehydration is known to reduce work output, and more importantly in a game of skill like cricket, to impair mental performance. Concentration and visual motor skills are likely to suffer and sometimes, health and safety are under threat. There are some well-remembered occasions when cricketers have experienced severe dehydration in extreme conditions, requiring hospitalisation and intravenous fluid therapy.

After looking at his data, Dr Gore recommended that the present rules of cricket be amended in hot weather to allow players unlimited access to fluid during the day, rather than restrict opportunities to the organised drink breaks. Perhaps cricketers need to look at other sports to find creative ways to place drink bottles at strategic points of the ground, or to have trainers who can quickly bring a drink to players at an appropriate moment in play. Better hydration will produce greater enjoyment, better performance and greater safety in cricket.

Skiing

The ski season in Australia is limited to a few months and a few ski fields. Yet each winter thousands of Australians take to the ski slopes and trails to enjoy the thrills of downhill or cross-country skiing. In fact, a 1990 survey found that over 17 per cent of the population is involved in skiing, ranking it as one of the top 10 participatory sports in Australia. Not bad for a country normally recognised for its beaches! At the competitive level, Australia has enjoyed a small but enthusiastic participation in international winter sport competitions, including Winter Olympics and World Cup and Championship events. This chapter will confine itself to issues related to competitive alpine skiing, cross-country skiing and biathlon, and to recreational skiing.

Training and touring

Cross-country skiing involves the use of both arms and legs, and can be performed at high aerobic intensities; in fact, cross-country skiers are often claimed to be the 'fittest' athletes in the world, in recognition of the very high aerobic capacities reported for some elite cross-country skiers. At the elite level, training for this sport usually involves 1–3 sessions per day (perhaps 6–8 hours in total), with sessions varying in their emphasis on endurance, speed and strength work. Many skiers also use other aerobic activities in their training, such as running, cycling, paddling or roller skiing—especially during the off-season or when snow isn't available. Whereas cross-country skiing involves rhythmic activity for 1–3 hours, alpine skiing is much more intermittent, a consequence of the time it takes to get back up to the top of the mountain. Alpine skiers can also train for many hours. However, their competition performance requires speed and skill rather than endurance.

At the recreational level, ski enthusiasts in Australia tend to enjoy less frequent but more 'concentrated' skiing time—winter holidays or weekends at the snow—during which they try to spend as much time as possible out on the slopes. For some, this represents a major increase in the usual daily exercise load. Ski touring can involve a single day or a number of days of cross-country skiing, with skiers staying overnight in lodges or ski-huts at pre-determined stages on their route, or camping out with their own equipment. Again, energy turnover on these days may be unusually high. Hopefully these skiers have prepared adequately for tours by undertaking a good pre-tour fitness program and organising a sound nutrition plan and supplies.

Competition

World Cup events, World Championships and Winter Olympics represent the major competition in skiing. Alpine skiing events are based on competition against the clock over downhill, slalom, giant slalom and super giant slalom courses, top honours going to the skier who completes the course in the fastest time. In slalom events, speed and skill are required as the skier battles the slope and the 'gates'; the time for two runs are added to produce the final score.

Cross-country skiing is an older competitive sport, requiring competitors to race each other across a variety of terrain and distances. Standard races can be held over 10–50km for men and 5–30km for women, or as 4-member relay teams. In some competitions, the skiers are sent off at 30-second intervals. Other races and marathons are held as mass participation events of up to 90km distances, including famous events such as the Norwegian Birkebeiner 55 kilometre race, which is part of the World Loppet Series. Australia hosts the only southern hemisphere race in the 13-race Loppet series. The race, known as the Kangaroo Hoppet and held at Falls Creek, attracts a field of around 1400 people annually. Long-distance cross-country ski races are won by elite skiers at average speeds of 25–30km/hr (e.g. 1 hour 40 mins for a 42km event). Recreational skiers may take 4–6 hours to complete this same distance.

Biathlon combines the sports of cross-country skiing and rifle shooting, with competitors racing over 7.5 and 15km (women), and 10 and 20km (men), or in a 4-member relay. During the race, biathletes stop at a 50-metre rifle range, incurring time penalties (or a penalty loop) for missed shots. In order to excel in this sport, athletes need to match shooting skills with good skiing technique and a high aerobic capacity.

Physical characteristics

Cross-country skiers are lean—a low body-fat level is a performance advantage when moving over long distances, just as it is in other endurance sports.

Common nutrition issues

High energy and carbohydrate requirements

A full day's skiing, especially cross-country skiing, burns fuel and calories. This may require a caloric and carbohydrate adjustment for recreational skiers who are taking advantage of some days or weeks on the slopes. However, for professional and elite skiers, meeting fuel and energy requirements can be a day-to-day challenge. In one study, the daily energy cost of being an elite cross-country skier in normal training was estimated (using doubly-labelled water techniques) to be 25 400–34 900kJ (6050–8310 Cals) per day for the males, and 15 000–20 200kJ (3570–4820 Cals) per day for the females. Undereating energy needs can lead to too much weight loss, inability to refuel and recover each day, and general lethargy. Like most endurance-training athletes, skiers trying to eat such high-energy intakes will have to contend with the 'fillingness' of many high-carbohydrate foods, and lack of time in the day to eat (when you take out the time spent training, sleeping, drying and cleaning equipment and doing other daily chores).

A high-energy, high-carbohydrate diet requires good food knowledge and good time management. Read Chapters 1 and 2 to be sure that you are up-to-date with nutritious food choices. Increasing your energy and carbohydrate intake is simple once you know how to make foods compact and easy to consume, and how to get yourself organised to 'graze' over the day. Chapter 3.7 has extra hints.

Achieving low body-fat levels

Like most endurance or speed sports, skiing performance is assisted by low body-fat levels. The ideal is individual to the skier and to the type of skiing program. Many skiers, especially cross-country skiers, 'naturally' achieve a low body-fat level—that is, they seem to automatically arrive at a level that seems good for performance and health. This may occur as a result of genetics, heavy training, a good diet, or a combination of all three. Other skiers may need to sharpen up their act to achieve a lower and better body-fat level. This is typical of many female skiers, alpine skiers (who may not burn up as much energy in training as cross-country skiers), and skiers coming back from the off-season or injury. Even for recreational skiers, preparation for the ski season may require shedding some of the 'fat layer' stored during autumn. It would be a shame to waste time and reduce enjoyment on the slopes by struggling around in an unfit or unhealthy condition. Your knees won't like it either!

Losing body fat requires a long term commitment to rebalancing your energy intake and your energy expenditure. An assessment of your current situation will tell you what needs to change. From the dietary point of view, reducing fat intake, checking the suitability of food serve sizes, and reducing boredom/stress eating are the most effective strategies. This is discussed in more detail in Chapter 3.3.

Before you start thinking about the strategies however, make sure that you have set yourself a sensible goal. Trying to lose too much body fat, or too much too quickly, can cause problems rather than reap rewards. Some skiers, particularly females, attempt to reach body-fat levels that are unsuited to their natural body composition. The result—partially also the result of the efforts needed to get to this level—can cause problems such as inadequate nutrition, overtraining and disrupted hormone patterns (such as loss of menstrual periods in women). Eating disorders and eating problems can interfere with the performance, health and happiness of some skiers. Get some expert help from a sports dietitian if you are unsure of what is ideal for you and how to get there.

Iron status

Low iron levels are frequently reported in heavily-training athletes, and cross-country skiers are considered to be a 'high-risk group'. Females and adolescents are doubly at risk due to increased physiological needs for iron to cover growth and menstruation, as well as increased iron losses through training. Training may either draw on iron stores of skiers to produce new red blood cells, or it may simply alter blood measures that are commonly used to measure iron status. Being, or training, at high altitudes may also produce the same two effects.

In short, skiers may experience changes in blood measurements of iron status either as a result of normal body adaptations, or because the skier is becoming low in iron. In the former case there are no problems; in the latter situation the skier may experience fatigue and loss of performance. Read Chapter 2.5 to see that low iron status can result from inadequate iron intake. You'll find plenty of ways to include a regular iron boost in a high-carbohydrate training diet. If you are in a high-risk group for low iron stores, organise with your sports medicine doctor and dietitian to be regularly monitored. Iron supplements may be part of the treatment or prevention of low iron status, but should only be taken on the advice of these experts. There are often other more important factors to consider.

Looking after fluid needs

Many skiers underestimate their sweat and fluid losses out on the slopes. Many feel that because they are working in cold conditions, sweat losses will be minimal. Others may be aware that they become dehydrated as they ski, but don't find themselves close to a fluid stop. Or perhaps they worry that if they drink, they will soon need to empty some of it out at the other end—and that's a nuisance when you're rugged up in many layers and there's not a toilet in sight.

In fact, sweat losses can be quite significant during skiing. Skiing is hard work, especially if you are cross-country skiing in hilly conditions. What's more, the air around you is dry—which means that sweat evaporates quickly and you lose moisture every time you take a breath. Dehydration will affect your performance—whether you are skiing in a cross-country marathon, or just enjoying a day on the slopes. If you are in a race you may be lucky to have aid stations organised for you. Make the most of these (see section below on fluid and food needs while racing). When you are out on your own, training or touring, you will need to make your own fluid supplies available. Buy a 'bum bag' or belt that will allow you to take a drink bottle with you. Or plant your own drink stations and keep coming back to these for a top-up. Drinking small amounts regularly should keep you well hydrated as well as comfortable.

Many athletes have not developed habits that look after their fluid needs, whether in training, competition or throughout the day. Chapter 1.5 explores some of the problems and excuses—and provides some strategies for better hydration practices.

Recovery

Whether you are training once or more each day for an important competition, or just trying to make the most of your week at the snow, you will want to bounce back as quickly as possible after each session on the snow. Recovery after strenuous exercise is an active process and rapid refuelling and rehydrating are good recovery strategies. Read Chapter 5 for the low-down on eating and drinking soon after each session. Sometimes this is not practical—you feel too tired to eat, you've got to look after your equipment, or there aren't any suitable foods and drinks handy. Some skiers choose post-exercise eating and drinking strategies that interfere with rather than promote recovery (see the section on apres-ski below). Chapter 5 provides some ideas for snacks that are easy to grab when you come in from the slopes or trails.

Travelling—the competition ski season

If you are planning on a career in professional skiing, you can plan on having a well-used passport. Most elite skiers need to spend extended periods in the northern hemisphere—to follow the competition circuit or simply to find snow during our summer season. This can be a challenge to finances as well as to eating plans. Travelling to Northern America will not provide a major food culture shock, but you will probably find that people in Europe do not enjoy the same foods that we do. Planning ahead will allow you to organise accommodation with nutrition in mind (self-contained units/lodges will provide greater food flexibility as well as a more economical stay), and to pack a food supply to take with you (you may be pleased that you brought your favourite breakfast cereal with you when you find that breakfast in some European countries is cold eggs, ham and cheese). The tennis chapter provides more hints for the travelling athlete.

Competition preparation

Whatever your competition event, you need to be fuelled-up and comfortable when you approach the starting line or starting gates. Preparation strategies will vary according to the needs of the event and the time that you have to prepare. Chapter 4 outlines strategies for fuelling-up for short events, and extra 'carbo-loading' strategies for long races such as cross-country ski marathons, when you will need all the muscle glycogen that you can store.

The pre-race meal is also a time for last-minute fuelling and hydrating, but you need to choose foods that will keep you feeling comfortable throughout the race. A high-carbohydrate, low-fat meal is the best choice—it could be as simple as your usual breakfast or another meal from your everyday eating plan. Some skiers need to reduce the fibre content or the total amount of food eaten before competition to reduce the risk of gastrointestinal problems. Competition nerves can also be a challenge. Read Chapter 4 for some hints on pre-race meals.

Food and fluid needs during cross-country ski races

In a ski race of an hour or longer, your performance will be affected by fuel and hydration considerations. Good preparation will help you to start the race with optimal fluid and fuel stores, however topping up along the way will become important as the race increases in length or intensity, or in situations where you were unable to achieve an optimal preparation. You should attempt to stay as well-hydrated as possible, matching sweat losses with frequent drinks. Intake of carbohydrate foods and fluids will supply an additional fuel supply to extend glycogen stores. This is explained further in Chapter 4.6–4.8.

So, what type of foods and fluids can be used, and where will you find supplies? This varies according to the skier and the race—traditions vary in different countries and in different events. In some cross-country marathons, a network of aid-stations or feed-stations provides a large menu of high-carbohydrate foods and drinks to competitors. In the Kangaroo Hoppet race for example, six feed-stations offer jelly beans, chocolate bars, fruit buns, bananas and oranges. Sports drinks and water are also provided. Chapter 4.8 explains that sports drinks are an efficient way to look after fluid and carbohydrate needs simultaneously. Of course, it can be a nuisance in very cold conditions to find that your drink is frozen. For this reason, some skiers and feed-stations warm up their drinks.

Sports drinks are generally made up at a 5–7 per cent concentration to provide a ratio of fluid and carbohydrate delivery that suits a moderate climate. We have seen that in hot conditions, athletes might choose to make up their drinks at a weaker concentration—thus assisting stomach-emptying and making fluid delivery the priority. In cold conditions, it is likely that sweat losses will be smaller and that fluid requirements, although important, may be smaller than in other sports. Thus, some skiers drink sports drinks and other carbohydrate drinks at a higher-than-normal concentration—10 per cent or even more. In some races in the northern hemisphere, aid-stations serve thick sugary drinks and 'blueberry soup'—often up to 25 per cent in concentration. With practice, skiers seem to be able to tolerate these concentrations although they fall outside usual scientific recommendations. Hot drinks, such as hot coffee, are also often served at feed-stations, usually in the second half of a race, to provide a 'warm up' for competitors who have been moving slowly in the cold conditions.

Generally, feed-stations service the race needs of recreational competitors. Elite competitors are often so concerned with race pace that they have little time to stop for food or fluid. When they do, they need to be able to grab a drink or a snack quickly—hardly breaking a stride. Most of the time, elite competitors rely on carrying food/drinks in special belts or bum bags. The best time for drinking or eating is when they hit a downhill or easy part of the course. Many recreational competitors also carry food/drink bags so that they have access to supplies between aid-stations.

If you are doing a race that will be aided by fluid and food intake throughout, read Chapter 4.6–4.8 to form a plan. The ideal plan will depend on the length of the race and the amount of support offered by the race organisers. Make sure that you practice your strategies in training to fine-tune your strategies.

Nutrition for touring

Touring, like long distance racing, will require carbohydrate and fluid intake along the way. This time it will be up to the skier to provide their own supplies and compact carbohydrate choices are required. After all you don't want to be laden down any more than can be helped. Popular snacks include jelly beans, bagels and fruit buns, sports bars, fruit biscuits, chocolate and 'trail mix' (mixtures of dried fruit, nuts and seeds). Some of these choices are higher in fat and fibre than might be considered optimal for 'during exercise' eating. However, many skiers do not experience gastrointestinal problems even with higher fat snacks. This can be because skiing is a gliding type of exercise and less likely to 'joggle' up gut contents. Also, most touring skiers are usually working at a lower intensity over longer periods than racing skiers.

Fluid needs will also be important, and touring skiers will need to carry drinks. Of course, snow can always be melted to top up supplies.

Recreational skiing: Nutrition for a day on the slopes

A day on the slopes can be hard work. If maximum enjoyment, maximum performance, maximum value from your lift ticket and minimum risk of injury are your goals, then you will need to refuel and rehydrate well over the day. You may need to plan some snacks for constant topping-up over the day, and a good lunch to break up the morning and afternoon sessions.

Studies have shown that injuries and accidents in the snow occur more frequently in the afternoons—perhaps as a result of fatigued skiers still being out on the slopes, or insisting that they get one or two more runs for the day. Dehydration, muscle glycogen depletion and low blood-sugar levels can all contribute to fatigue.

Good carbohydrate and fluid snacks have been discussed in the touring and competition sections above. These can be carried in pockets in your ski suit, or in special belts and bum bags. If you don't want to be weighed down too much you may be able to plant a snack stop at a convenient point and return to this at regular intervals. It is good to continually top-up fluid and carbohydrate levels as you go instead of waiting until you feel fatigued. You can stop for a quick break or grab a snack as you are catching your next lift/chair/pommer etc.

Whether you are going back to your lodge or eating from the restaurants and bars in the ski village, a high-carbohydrate lunch should be high on your menu. Many of the offerings found in restaurants and takeaways may sound warm and filling, but they do not provide the nutrients that your body and muscles need. Pies, cheesy pastries and oily fast foods are high in fat. There are many high-carbohydrate alternatives that will appeal to your taste buds *and* your nutritional requirements—hearty soups, hot breads and scones, toasted sandwiches made with minimum margarine/butter, hot casseroles and chilli served with rice, pasta meals with lean meat or vegetable sauces and healthy pizzas. Or what could be more warming than a baked potato with a hot casserole or chilli filling? Cold choices include rolls and sandwiches, fruit salad with yoghurt or icecream, fruit smoothies, and fruit buns/scones. The choices are endless—and they shouldn't give your wallet too much of a fright, especially if you can do some or all of your own catering. A thermos may allow you to bring hot soup and casseroles with you. Or you can buy a hot drink to go with your packaged lunch.

Recreational skiing: Some words about après-ski

For some skiers, recreational and elite, the main attraction of life on the slopes is the après-ski. This includes drinking and discoing until late in the night, and then trying to 'sweat-out' or 'exercise-off' the effects of the alcohol the next day. Unfortunately, there is no simple way to get rid of excess alcohol intake and its effects. Of course, some problems also arise because of the associated activities—lack of sleep and little or poorly chosen food intake. While it might sound like a fun lifestyle to some, it is not conducive to good performance or good health. In fact, in some situations it can lead to tragedies in the snow.

Skiing with a moderate or significant blood alcohol level—courtesy of a few drinks over lunch between sessions or a large intake the night before—can cause several problems. Reduced competence on the skis coupled with impaired judgement can cause skiers to take risks, make mistakes, ski in a fatigued state and otherwise increase their risk of accidents and injury. What's more, temperature-regulation is also impaired under the influence of alcohol. Heat losses are greater, increasing the risk of hypothermia and cold exposure.

The best advice is to make après-ski a time of 'R & R'—recovery and relaxation, in that order. Recovery tactics include refuelling and rehydrating straight after your ski session. If a high-carbohydrate meal is not immediately available, then start with a refuelling snack—hot soup and bread, hot chocolate and scones, a fruit smoothie, muesli bars and fruit juice or sports drink. If you start drinking alcohol right off, a 'write-off' is what you'll be. Wait until your recovery tactics are well in place, then consume alcohol in moderation. Adequate fluid, fuel and sleep will see you back out on your skis tomorrow ready to take on the challenges of the day.

PROFILE
A fat load of good...

James is an up and coming cross-country skier, hoping to make his name on the international circuit. Recently he met an American winter sports enthusiast who competes in various sled races and aspires to the great Iditarod race. He told James about a new theory that some of his skiing friends were trying—fat-loading. He said that it was well-tried with racing sled dogs. In fact huskies and other snow dogs raced with increased stamina on diets containing more than 50 per cent of energy from fat. He assured James that scientific studies had shown that fat-loading was better than carbohydrate-loading—and more practical. After all, even the leanest athlete has sizeable fat stores compared to the fuel requirements of even the longest events, and compared to the potential of body carbohydrate stores. Wouldn't it be more efficient to train the athlete to become a better 'fat-burner', he argued? If the athlete could learn to burn more fat in the exercise–fuel mix, then carbohydrate stores (i.e. muscle glycogen) could be 'spared', allowing endurance time to be increased. This strategy might come in handy in marathon races over 45km or more.

James, understandably, was confused. Since the 1960s, exercise scientists had conducted hundreds of studies on endurance exercise, including research using muscle biopsy techniques to investigate the fuel status of the muscle. These studies had provided plenty of support for the importance of carbohydrate stores in performance of prolonged exercise: keep the muscle fuelled with carbohydrate and performance can be prolonged; deplete the body's carbohydrate stores and fatigue soon results.

Luckily James was attending a training camp at the AIS and had the opportunity to ask questions about it in a session with an exercise physiologist. The physiologist was up-to-date with the latest scientific research, and agreed that the idea of turning endurance athletes into 'fat-burners' sounded plausible. After all, exercise training itself causes muscle adaptations that produce increased oxidation of fat and 'carbohydrate-sparing' during exercise, compared to the untrained state. This is one of the key reasons why your hard work increases your endurance capacity. The increased fat-burning capacity is probably a result of many muscle changes—including an increased number of blood capillaries to the working muscle which provide it with a better oxygen supply, an increase in muscle enzymes that are involved in fat oxidation, and perhaps a more efficient system to transport fatty acids from the blood into the muscle. The muscle can oxidise fat from two sources—fatty acids in the blood, and triglycerides already stored within the muscle cell.

In fact, a recent review paper by exercise physiologists Drs John Hawley and Will Hopkins proposed that there are, in fact, four separate power systems in exercise metabolism. They argued that the aerobic metabolism of fats should be considered separately from aerobic metabolism of carbohydrate, since they are functionally distinct and can each be enhanced by separate dietary and training strategies.

However, the exercise physiologist told James and his group that even with the training changes that promote fatty acid burning, it is still relatively underutilised in humans. On the other hand, some animals such as rats and dogs can adapt better to fat fuel. This explained why some rat studies had reported success with fat-loading, and why some endurance animals like sled dogs in the Antarctic may be able to thrive on diets that are 50 per cent fat or more and less than 15 per cent carbohydrate.

The physiologist outlined a number of methods that had been used in studies to increase the oxidation of fats in the body, including intravenous infusion of fats, the consumption of a high-fat diet, and the use of some drugs such as heparin. Some studies had shown that these methods cause an increased fat-burning during exercise and a decrease in carbohydrate-utilisation. He also mentioned some new sports bars on the market (e.g. Eicotec Bar and PR-Bar) that claim that they increase fat-oxidation by manipulating hormone levels although these claims remain unproven.

What do the studies say about fat-loading and exercise performance? Unfortunately, some of the studies that have reported greater fat-burning and glycogen-sparing during exercise following 1–4 days of higher-fat/lower-carbohydrate eating have not actually measured the resultant effect on performance. It is unfair to speculate, but the physiologist told the group about the three studies which are generally promoted as sympathetic to the fat-loading theory.

The first study, known as the 'Phinney study', fed its subjects a very high-fat, low-carbohydrate diet for 4 weeks. It reported lower muscle-glycogen levels, but a lower glycogen-utilisation and no decrement to performance during an exercise trial at the end of this adaptation period. While there was no positive outcome from high-fat eating, this study might have surprised the experts who expected worse performance after low-carbohydrate eating. Being critical for a moment, the physiologist noted that the exercise test was conducted at a low intensity (65 per cent of VO_2 max). Not only is this intensity not representative of most competitive sports events, but it is generally considered a 'fat-burning' rather than 'carbohydrate-burning' intensity. More about that later. What's more, he noted, only five subjects took part in the study. One subject showed an amazing performance improvement (60%) which made a substantial and unrepresentative impact on the statistical analyses of the whole group. Finally, there was no control trial or control group used, so we don't know what would have happened after four weeks of high-carbohydrate eating.

The physiologist then described how the second study by Deborah Muoio and colleagues, reported in a recent issue of the *Medicine and Science in Sports and Exercise Science Journal*, had created sensational headlines in lay magazines: 'High fat diet improves exercise performance'. Yet when he scrutinised the article he could not find proof for these claims or indeed any evidence that this was how the authors themselves had interpreted the results. The project involved performance testing of six elite runners after 7 days on a 'normal' diet, 7 days on a 'high-fat diet', and 7 days on a 'high-carbohydrate diet'. The results showed a significantly improved time to exhaustion on the 'high-fat' diet compared to the other two diets.

However, the study suffered from some methodological drawbacks which made these results open to criticism. Unfortunately, because of practical problems in recruiting the runners, the study had to be carried out in an 'unscientific' manner—to be specific, each runner completed the diets in the same order. So we don't know if there was 'an order effect', or whether some other factor in the lives of the athletes (their training, the time of the season, etc.) affected the performance tests. A better designed study would have had each of the subjects assigned to each of the diets in a different order, cancelling out the order effect.

In any case, the diets used in this study probably weren't as extreme as their names suggested. For example, the 'high-fat' diet had an energy ratio of 50 per cent carbohydrate and 38 per cent fat, while the 'high-carbohydrate' was more extreme at 73 per cent carbos and 15 per cent fat. It would be fairer to say that the study tested a very high-carbohydrate diet against a moderate-carbohydrate diet, or a low-fat diet against a moderate-fat diet. While the authors discussed an apparent move towards greater-fat burning during their 'high-fat' diet (really a moderate-fat diet), this study did not really test the metabolic response to the dietary extremes proposed by the real 'fat-loading' theorists.

The final study, from South African researchers led by Dr Vicki Lambert, compared performance during 'high-intensity' exercise (90% VO_2 max) and 'moderate-intensity' exercise (60% VO_2 max) in subjects after 2 weeks of a high-fat (70% of energy) or high-carbohydrate (70% of energy) diet. They reported no change in performance in high-intensity exercise with the high-fat diet compared to the high-carbohydrate plan, but greater endurance (longer time to fatigue) at the moderate-exercise intensity. They described metabolic changes that suggested that the muscles had 'retooled' to increase fat-burning with the high-fat eating in the presence of low muscle glycogen stores.

The physiologist agreed that there is plenty of scope for more work before the decisions can be made on fat-loading. In the meantime, he summarised the following factors that might stand in the way of positive findings or a future recommendation for all athletes to consume high-fat diets:

- Fatty acids support most of the fuel needs of low-intensity exercise (<50 per cent VO_2 max) and a declining contribution towards exercise at the typical pace of endurance exercise (65–75 per cent VO_2 max). However, carbohydrate becomes the fuel of choice for exercise at 85 per cent VO_2 max and above. This is because carbohydrate oxidation is more efficient as an aerobically-oxidised substrate (it produces more ATP per unit of oxygen) and it can also be metabolised anaerobically (without oxygen). In other words, when the going gets tough, the body burns carbohydrate! Fat adaptation may therefore only be useful for athletes in ultra-endurance sports.

- Overconsumption of high-fat diets appears to be more likely to cause increases in body fat than overindulgence in high-carbohydrate eating. Excess caloric intake from fat appears to be more metabolically likely to be stored as body fat. And because fat is a more compact energy source (9 Cals/gram) than carbohydrate (4 Cals/gram), it will require smaller amounts of food to overindulge.
- The long-term consumption of high-fat diets may be associated with increased risks of certain diseases such as coronary heart disease and some cancers.

In summary, the physiologist suggested that the future would tell us if 'fat loading' would be useful to athletes, but that the applications were likely to be beneficial only to a small number of athletes, principally those in ultra-endurance events. He doubted that high-fat diets would ever be recommended, long-term, for any athlete. However, future studies may develop short-term strategies of high-fat eating, or fat intake during exercise, or special training sessions to promote better utilisation of fat in some exercise events. In other words, 'fat adaptation' rather than 'fat loading' may bring some good news, but only for some athletes. In the meantime, high-carbohydrate eating remains the tried and true formula and the long-term plan.

PROFILE
Kerryn Rim: A crack shot at skiing

Kerryn Rim, perhaps better known as Kerryn Pethybridge, has been one of Australia's best performing skiers, competing in the sport of biathlon. She has competed in two Winter Olympics—finishing 8th in the Lillehammer 15km event—and achieved three 4th placings in World Cup events in 1990, missing a bronze medal by 2 seconds! She began her biathlon career in 1983 when this event was introduced for women at the World Championships. Her background covered a number of endurance sports, including cross-country skiing. However in biathlon she discovered a talent in the combination of two unusually matched sports—cross-country skiing and shooting—finding that she was able to maintain her shooting skills even under the high heart-rates resulting from skiing.

Kerryn's life is divided into two parts. First there is her 'Australian life' where she juggles 4–5 days/week of nursing work, family life and a background training program of 1 session per day (1–1.5 hours). This can involve a number of activities such as running, kayaking, roller skiing and cycling. Things change dramatically when she heads overseas each year for 2–3 months of serious training and competition. Training is increased to 2–3 sessions per day of skiing, weights, shooting and other off-snow work-outs.

While good nutrition has always been part of her program, it becomes a major focus during this competition season. Germany, Italy and Austria are common travel destinations and Kerryn and her husband find accommodation in cheap apartments so that they are able to do their own cooking. This has major financial advantages as well as ensuring that Kerryn can eat exactly what she wants and needs. Bringing some food supplies from home is also an important factor in this plan, since many of Kerryn's food choices are either unavailable or excessively priced in the snow-fields of Europe. Handy foods include breakfast cereal, skim milk powder, home-dehydrated vegies, pasta sauces and fruit—and, of course, Vegemite. With skis, other equipment and food supplies, Kerryn's bags can be quite heavy!

Kerryn's meals are based around carbohydrate foods—breakfast cereal, bread, rice or pasta dishes and fruit—to which salads, vegies, and protein foods (e.g. meat, fish, chicken) are added. She takes extra care during this time to reduce her intake of fats and oils, and cuts out chocolate and alcohol to concentrate on 'quality foods'. Between training sessions and an afternoon sleep there is not a lot of time to prepare meals, so being organised and focused is important. She takes care to have a carbohydrate snack (e.g. fruit) at the end of a training session to enhance recovery, and is particularly vigilant about fluid intake. She prefers water during most training sessions, but uses a sports drink during lengthy exercise sessions (over 1.5 hours) when she knows that the additional carbohydrate will be of benefit.

Before a race Kerryn likes to have a lower-fibre breakfast than usual, and often uses carbohydrate drinks to top-up. Biathlon events are generally too short to require carbohydrate intake during the event itself. However, Kerryn is an enthusiast and master of many endurance sports and has often competed in 'enduro' events involving cycling, running and paddling—including some races which last over several days. These competitions definitely require fuel intake during the event, and jelly beans, sports bars, bananas and sports drinks have been useful.

Body-weight fluctuations have been an interesting factor in Kerryn's performances. Her body weight stays around 63–65kg in the off season, but she finds that she typically loses 3–4 kilograms in the first month or two of her European campaigns—a result of careful eating and increased training. This quickly settles to her 'racing weight' of 60kg. However, Kerryn is careful not to stay at this level for too long (or to keep up the factors that achieve it) since it appears to be too low and too strict for long-term health and life enjoyment. Whereas other elite athletes often use serial skinfold readings to check their progress, being away from Australia for long periods prevents regular access to these measurements. Kerryn must therefore rely on monitoring body weight, a good nutrition plan and commonsense to judge her ideal level of leanness. Between Winter Olympics she gained some weight—reaching a peak of 73kg in fact—but a healthy baby boy, Daniel, was involved in this phenomena. Regaining her pre-pregnancy 'shape'—in both fitness level and body characteristics—was a gradual process. Kerryn was able to breast-feed Daniel until 14 months (only stopped by logistical considerations during the next competition season), demonstrating both healthy nutrition and well-balanced lifestyle goals. Extra attention to hydration and to good eating played a key role in this success.

Due to her extensive travel needs, Kerryn often has to rely on her own judgement of her nutritional status, and on her own organisation of healthy food and fluid patterns. In an event in which Australians are perhaps disadvantaged by distance and limited exposure to snow and the culture of the sport, she has done us and herself proud.

Index

Page numbers in *italics* indicate references in case studies

acidic foods, *228*
adenosine tri phosphate (ATP), 79,
   131, 208, *215, 217*
adolescents, nutritional needs of,
   246–7, *259*, 266, 353
advertising, bodybuilding magazines,
   221–2
aerobic exercise: body-fat goals, 245;
   kilojoule requirements, 41
AFL *see* Australian Rules Football
airline food, 322, 323
alanine, 130
alcohol: àpres-ski, 358; Australian
   Rules players, 279, *281–2*;
   bingeing, 225; dehydration, 109,
   110, 117; effect on recovery,
   119, 301; golfers, 331; hockey
   players, 301; intake by
   cricketers, 344; Rugby League
   players, 288; sensible use of,
   33–6; soccer players, 301;
   team sports, 301; when dining,
   339
alternative diets, 177
amenorrhea, 55–6, 71, 143–4, 176,
   180, 247
amino acids, 46–7; bodybuilders,
   229; cost of supplements versus
   food, 133; inconclusive evidence
   of effects, 126, 129–30;
   weightlifters, *215, 217*
anabolic steroids, 213, 220, 226
anemia, 52, 176
anorexia nervosa, 175, 249
anti-oxidants, 129
appetite, lack of, 118
àpres-ski, 358
arginine, 129
ascorbic acid, 27, 51
Australian Institute of Sport, 63, 65,
   160
Australian Rules Football: case
   studies, *281–5*; competition,

276–7; nutrition issues, 278;
   overview, 275; physical
   characteristics, 277; training,
   276

Barry Sears diet, 154–5
basal metabolic rate, 37, 38, 40, 72
basketball: competition, 307–8;
   nutrition issues, 308–11;
   overview, 306–7; physical
   characteristics, 308; training, 307
bee pollen, 131
biathlon, 351, *363*
bicarbonate, as an ergogenic aid,
   126, 127–8
bidons, 145, 166, 167
bingeing, 225, *282*
Birkebeiner race, Norway, 351
blood glucose: as fuel for muscles,
   14, 80, 96, 112; 'bonking,' 166;
   effect of carbohydrates on,
   17–20; fatigue, 357; sugar prior
   to events, 90, 91
blood lipids, 212–13
blood sodium imbalance, 81
BMR, 37, 38, 40, 72
body fat: aerobic exercise, 245;
   archers, 61, 65; assessment of,
   62–5; ballet dancers, 65;
   basketball players, 308, 309;
   bodybuilders, 62, 218, 219, 224;
   boxers, 235, *239, 240*; cricketers,
   342; cyclists, 65, 73, 165, 166;
   desirable levels, 61–2; distance
   runners, 61, 173–4, 175, *180*;
   divers, 62, 65, 73, 244–5; eating
   plan to reduce, 67–8; energy
   balance, 42; figure skaters, 65,
   73; football players, 277, 278;
   golfers, 61, 65, 328, 329;
   gymnasts, 62, 65, 73, 244–5, *253*;
   hockey players, 297, 298, *301–3*;
   hurdlers, *204, 205*; jumpers, 200;

body fat (*continued*):
losing, 65–70; low-energy consumers, 70–5; middle distance runners, 190–1; netball players, 308, 309, *311–12*; rowers, 264–5; Rugby League players, 287–8; runners, 65, 73; skiers, 352–3, *363*; soccer players, 297, 298; sprinters, 200; strength sports, 61, 211–12, 213; swimmers, 73, 153, 156; tennis players, 317, 318; triathletes, 61, 65, 142, 143; wrestlers, 235
body image, 72
bodybuilding: case studies, *226–33*; competition, 219; nutrition issues, 220–6; overview, 218; physical characteristics, 219; training, 218–19; unique world of, 219–20
bone structure, and calcium, 54–6
bones, low density of, 143–4, *179–82*, 247
'bonking,' 80, 96, 166
boxing: case studies, *239–41*; competition, 235; making weight, 75, 236–7; nutrition issues, 236–7; overview, 234; physical characteristics, 235; training, 235
branched-chain amino acids, 130
breastfeeding, energy allowance for, 40
bulimia, 156, 175, 249
bulking-up: Australian Rules players, 279; bodybuilders, 222–4, *226–7*, *230–3*; requirements for, 76; Rugby League players, 289–90; strength sports, 210–11, *213–15*

caffeine: as an ergogenic aid, 126, 127, 136; diuretic action, 109, 110, 117
calcium, 54–8; distance runners, *179–82*; gymnasts, 247; sources, 57, 58; supplements, 125; vegetarian diets, *259*; weightlifters, *215*
cancer, and fat, 8, *362*
carbo-loading *see* carbohydrate loading
carbohydrate-electrolyte drinks *see* sports drinks

carbohydrate loading: alcohol no use for, 34; bodybuilders, 224–5; counting to ensure daily targets, 44; cyclists, 168; distance runners, 177, *185–8*; endurance events, 83–6; plan for, 86; skiers, 355; triathletes, 144–5
carbohydrate requirements, 43–4; Australian Rules players, 279, 280–1, *284–5*; bodybuilders, 222, *227*, *229*; cyclists, 97, 165, 167–8, *169–71*; distance runners, 97, 173, 174; golfers, 330; hockey players, 298–9, 299–300; hurdlers, 200–1, *205–6*; middle distance runners, 192; rowers, 265; Rugby League players, 288–9; skiers, 97, 352, 356–7, *361*, *363*; soccer players, 298–9, 299–300, *304*; sprinters, 200–1; swimmers, 154, 157, *158–9*; tennis players, 318; triathletes, 97, 145
carbohydrates: as a source of energy, 8; as a source of fibre, 20–1; classification, 23; consumption during events, 91, 96–7, 99–102; depletion, 80, 84; diversity, 16–17; eating for recovery, 110–19; effect of sugar on, 90–1; effect on blood glucose, 17–20; Glycemic Index of, 18–20; increasing intake, 14–26; low-fat versus high fat foods, *187–8*; mixing with protein, *228*; nutritional value, 17; pre-event meals, 88, 89–90; preparation for competition, 82; reducing fat to make way for, 9; repair of muscle damage, 115; replacing lost stores of glycogen, 111–15; sources, 20, 24–5, 45, 98–9, 114, 260; supplements, 124; vegetarian diets, 260–1; *see also* carbohydrate loading; carbohydrate requirements
carnitine, 131, 222, 224, *229*
central fatigue, 80
Chinese restaurants, 337
cholesterol, 11, 212, 225–6
chromium picolinate, 132, *217*
coenzyme Q10, 131

communal eating, 157–8, *159–62*, 320, 323
competition *see* competition nutrition; multi-event competitions; *specific sports*
competition nutrition, 79–106; adolescents, 246–7; basketball players, 310; carbohydrate loading, 83–6; cricketers, 343; cyclists, 168; distance runners, 177–8; divers, 248; eating to recover, 107–21; endurance events, 94–102; fatigue factors, 79–81; fluid intake during events, 92–4, 95; golf, 329–30; gymnasts, 248; hurdlers, 201–2, *203–7, 206*; jumpers, 201–2; middle distance runners, 192; multi-event competitions, 119–21; netball players, 310; planning strategies, 118–19; post-competition bingeing, 225; pre-event meals, 87–90, 91; preparation for competition, 81–3; rowers, 266–7; skiers, 355; sprinters, 201–2, *202–3*; swimmers, 157; tennis players, *323–6*; travelling to races, 179; triathletes, 144–5; *see also* sports drinks; training nutrition
complementing, of proteins, 47, 48
complex carbohydrates, 16–17, 23
controlled testing, of ergogenic aids, 135–6
cooking skills, 10–11, 278, 288, *290–1*, 292–5
Costill, Dave, 154, 174
coxswains, 268
Coyle, Ed, 109
creatine phosphate, 79, 126, 128–9, 208
cricket: case studies, *344–9*; competition, 341–2; nutrition issues, 342–4; overview, 340; physical characteristics, 342; training, 340–1
cricketer's salad, 343
cross-country skiing *see* skiing
cutting-up, bodybuilding, 218, 219, 224
cycling: case studies, *169–71*; competition, 164; endurance events, 168; nutrition issues, 165–9; overview, 163–4; physical characteristics, 164–5; training, 164

dairy foods, 10, 56–8
dehydration, 28–33; as a fatigue factor, 80; Australian Rules players, 280; basketball players, 310; bodybuilders, 225; calculating rate of, 108; caused by alcohol, 34; cricketers, 343, *347–9*; effect on performance, 92–3; endurance events, 96, 97, 99–100, 101; fatigue, 357; fluid intake during events, 92–4, 95; forced, to make weight, *238*; golfers, 330; hockey players, 300; netball players, 310; relation to diarrhea, *193*; restoring fluid loss after exercise, 107–10; Rugby League players, 289; soccer players, 300, *305*; tennis players, 318
desserts and sweets, 11
diarrhea, during exercise, *192–4*
Diet for Runners, 194, 195
dietary extremism, 142, 175, *195–6*
dietary supplements, 122–5; bodybuilders, 221–2, *229–30*; strength sports, 211, *215–17*; triathletes, 145
diets: alternative, 177; dietician's assessment of, *203–7*; high-energy, 76–8, *213–15*; high-protein, 222–3; moderation in, 5, 7; nutrition experts, 220–1; Pritikin, 177, *194–7*; recovery from daily exercise, 111; study of weightlifters' diet, *215–17*; vegetarian, 177, *257–62*; *see also* competition nutrition; dietary extremism; dietary supplements; fat; training nutrition
digestive enzymes, *228*
discus *see* strength sports
distance running: blood sodium levels, 81; case studies, *179–88*; competition, 173; nutrition issues, 174–9; overview, 172; physical characteristics, 173–4; training, 172–3
diuretics, 93, 109, 156, 224

diving: case studies, *256–62*;
    competition, 244; nutrition
    issues, 244–8; overview, 242–3;
    physical characteristics, 244;
    training, 243
doubly-labelled water technique,
    71
drinking pouches, for cyclists, 145

Eat to Win, 317
eating disorders: dealing with, 252;
    divers, 248; female distance
    runners, 175; gymnasts, 248;
    'occupational,' 249; overview,
    248–51; swimmers, 156–7;
    symptoms, 250
Eicotec Bar, *360*
Eicotec diet, 154–5
electrolytes, 26–8, 102, 107–10, 225
empty calories, 21
empty kilojoules, 21
endurance events: food and fluid
    intake for, 94–102; protein
    requirements, 45, 46; *see also*
    specific sports
energy: energy balance, 39, 42, 72;
    expenditure, measurement of,
    70–2; high-energy diet, 76–8,
    213–15; high-energy drinks, *270*;
    percentage weight by, 14; sugar
    prior to events, 90–2
energy requirements *see* kilojoule
    requirements
ergogenic aids, nutritional *see*
    nutritional ergogenic aids
essential amino acids, 47, 115
estrogen, 55
extremism *see* dietary extremism

fast food, 278, 312–14
fat: calculating fat content of food,
    15; combined with sugar, 22;
    energy requirements, 8; 'fat
    burners,' 224, *359*; fat-loading,
    154–5, *358–62*; gain during
    injury, *301–3*; high intake of
    bodybuilders, 225; high intake
    of footballers, 280, 283, 285, 288;
    oxidation in the body, *359–60*;
    Pritikin diet, *195*; reducing,
    7–14, *282–4*; vegetarian diets,
    259, 260; *see also* body fat;
    percentage fat

fatigue: carbohydrate intake, 96;
    central, 130; checklist of factors,
    79–81; relation to iron
    deficiency, *184*; skiers, 357
ferritin, *183*
ferulic acid, 132
fibre, 20–1, 25, 77
field hockey *see* hockey
fluid requirements: Australian Rules
    players, 280–1; basketball
    players, 310; bodybuilders, 224;
    cricketers, *347–9*; cyclists, 93,
    166–7; distance runners, 178–9;
    endurance events, 94–102;
    general events, 92–4, 95; golfers,
    330; hockey players, 300;
    hurdlers, *201*; jumpers, *201*;
    netball players, 310; rowers,
    266; Rugby League players, 289;
    runners, in general, 93; skiers,
    93, 354, 355–6; soccer players,
    300; sprinters, *201*; swimmers,
    155; tennis players, 318;
    triathletes, 93, 144, 145
fluids: comparison of retention
    rates, 109–10; containing
    sodium, 109; monitoring balance
    of, 28–33; restoring loss, 107–10;
    see also sweat; fluid
    requirements
folate, 50
food: bingeing, 225; calculating fat
    content of, 15; combining food
    groups, 48, 54; food diaries, 39,
    68, 71, 72–3, 205, *214*, *281*, *312*;
    food pyramid, 7; 'good' and
    'bad,' 5, 13, 17, 142; personal
    likes, 20, 105, 106; variety in,
    4–7, 114, 142, *146–8*, 177, *228*,
    258, 260; *see also* diets; food
    requirements; meals
food requirements: cyclists, 166–7;
    distance runners, 178–9;
    endurance events, 94–102;
    hurdlers, *201*; jumpers, *201*;
    skiers, 355–6; sprinters, *201*;
    triathletes, 144, 145
football *see* Australian Rules
    Football; Rugby League; soccer
Frac, 132, *217*
free-form amino acids, 129, 222
free oxygen radicals, 129
French restaurants, 335–6

fructose, 113–14
'fullness,' 20, 33

gamma-oryzanol, 132, 222, *229*
gastrointestinal problems: caused by
    bicarbonate, 128; caused by
    carbohydrates, 97; dehydration,
    93, 99–100; distance runners,
    176–7; pre-event meals, 88–9,
    91, 92; rowers, *269, 270*; when
    travelling, 320
ginseng, 131, *215*
glucagon, 154
glucose, prior to events, 90
glucose polymers, 103–4
glutamine, 130
Glycemic Index, 18–20, 91, 114
glycogen *see* liver glycogen; muscle
    glycogen
golf: competition, 328; nutrition
    issues, 329–31; overview, 327;
    physical characteristics, 328;
    training, 327–8
Gore, Chris, *347*
Grand Prix circuits, 189, 190, 198,
    202
growth, energy allowance for, 40
growth hormone, 129–30
gymnastics: case studies, *251–6*;
    competition, 243–4; nutrition
    issues, 244–8; overview, 242–3;
    physical characteristics, 244;
    training, 243

hammer *see* strength sports
Hawley, John, *359*
HDL-cholesterol, 212, 225
health restaurants, 339
heart disease, and fat, 8, *362*
heat stress, 289, *347*
heme iron, 54
hemoglobin, 52
heparin, *360*
high-energy diets, 76–8, *213–15*
high-energy drinks, *270*
high jump *see* jumping
'hitting the wall,' 80, 111
hockey: case studies, *301–3*;
    competition, 297; nutrition
    issues, 298–301; overview, 296;
    physical characteristics, 297–8;
    training, 296–7
Hopkins, Will, *359*

horse racing, making weight, 75
hunger flat, 166, 167
hurdling: case studies, *203–7*;
    competition, 199–200; nutrition
    issues, 200–2; overview, 198;
    physical characteristics, 200;
    training, 199
hypoglycemia, 96
hyponatremia, 105
hypothermia, 34, 358
hypotonic to isotonic concentration,
    103

Indian restaurants, 338
injuries: effect of alcohol
    consumption, 34; fat gain,
    301–3; nutrition during, 290;
    recreational skiing, 357;
    repairing, 107; *see also* muscles,
    damage to
inosine, 131, *229*
insulin, 154
iron: requirements, 52–4; sources,
    54, 261; supplements, 125;
    vegetarian diets, 261; *see also*
    iron deficiency
iron deficiency: basketball players,
    309; cyclists, 165; distance
    runners, 176, *182–5*; female
    rowers, 266; netball players,
    309; skiers, 353; swimmers, 157;
    triathletes, 143; women on
    vegetarian diets, *259*
ISAK standards, skinfold
    measurements, 63, 65
isoleucine, 130
Israeli army diet, *345*
Italian restaurants, 336–7

javelin *see* strength sports
judo: kilojoule requirements, 41;
    making weight, 75
jumping: competition, 199–200;
    nutrition issues, 200–2; overview,
    198; physical characteristics,
    200; training, 199
junk foods, *186*, 313

kilojoule requirements, 37–43;
    badminton players, 41; ballroom
    dancers, 41; basketballers, 41;
    boxers, 41; by activity, 41;
    canoeists, 41; circuit training,

kilojoule requirements (*continued*):
41; cricketers, 41; cyclists, 41,
165, *169–71*; determining fat
intake, 8–9; golfers, 41;
gymnasts, 41; high-fat foods,
8–9, *256*; hockey players, 41;
judo, 41; low-energy consumers,
70–5, 143; rowers, 265, *268–70,
271–4*; runners, 41; skiers, 41,
352; squash players, 41;
strength sports, 211, *213–15*;
swimmers, 41, 156; table tennis
players, 41; tennis players, 41;
triathletes, 143; vegetarian diets,
260; volleyball players, 41;
walkers, 41; *see also specific
sports*
kilojoules, sources of, 260

lacto-ovo-vegetarians, *258*
lactose intolerance, 57
Lambert, Vicki, *361*
laxatives, 156, *238*, *239*
leucine, 130
lifestyle, in strength sports, 212
lightweight rowing, 267–8, *271–4*
liquid meal supplements: as a
source of carbohydrate, 33, 85;
as a source of energy, 78;
composition and uses, 124; cost,
133, 134; cyclists, 168; distance
runners, 176, 178, *187*; pre-event
meals, 90; recovery, 118;
rowers, 267; swimmers, *158*;
tennis players, *325*
liver glycogen, 14, 113–14, 299
long jump *see* jumping
low-energy consumers, 70–5

macronutrients, 154
Malay restaurants, 337
marathon running *see* distance
running
meals: communal eating, 157–8,
159–62, 320, 323; increasing
number of, *270*; on planes, 322,
323; timing of, 59–60, 113, *305*,
333; *see also* competition
nutrition; cooking skills; diets;
pre-event meals; restaurants;
training nutrition; travel
nutrition

menstruation: amenorrhea, 55–6, 71,
143–4, 176, *180*, 247; iron losses
during, 52
metabolism: aerobic and anaerobic,
79–80; low-energy consumers,
72; metabolic rate, 37, 38, 40,
48, 52; of exercise, *359–60*
Mexican restaurants, 338
middle distance running: case
studies, *192–7*; competition, 190;
nutrition issues, 191–2;
overview, 189; physical
characteristics, 190–1; training,
189–90
minerals: recovery, 115; sources,
261; supplements, 125;
vegetarian diets, *259*;
weightlifters' diet, *215–17*
moderation, in diet, 5, 7
MSG (monosodium glutamate), 27
multi-event competitions, 119–21
Muoio, Deborah, *360*
muscle glycogen: as a fuel source,
14, 79, 84; Australian Rules
players, 279–80, 281;
bodybuilders, 224, *228–9*;
carbohydrate loading, 44, 83;
carbohydrate–protein
combinations for recovery, 115;
cyclists, 165, 166, 167, 168;
depletion, 79, 80, 91, 96, 357;
distance runners, 173, 177, 178,
185–6; effect of type of
carbohydrate, 113–14; effects of
alcohol, 34; fat-loading, *359–60*;
fatigue, 357; hockey players,
299; hurdlers, 201; jumpers, 201;
middle distance runners, 192;
muscle damage, 115, 144, 192,
279, 289; preparation for
competition, 82–4, 87, 90;
recovery of stores in muscles,
18; replacing lost stores, 107,
110–15; Rugby League players,
289; skiers, 355; soccer players,
299; sprinters, 201; swimmers,
157; triathletes, 144–5
muscles: atrophy, 290; creatine in,
128; damage to, 114–15, 115,
117, 144, 192, 279, 289, 298;
effect of chromium picolinate,
132; fat as fuel, *359*; fatigue,
130, 357; preparation for

competition, 82–3; *see also*
muscle glycogen; muscles,
bulking-up of
muscles, bulking-up of: Australian
Rules players, 279;
bodybuilders, 222–4, *226–7,
230–3*; requirements for, 76;
Rugby League players, 289–90;
strength sports, 210–11, *213–15*
myoglobin, 52

National Basketball League, 307
netball: competition, 307–8; nutrition
issues, 308–11; overview, 306–7;
physical characteristics, 308;
training, 307
niacin, 50
nightwork, 212
Noakes, Tim, 174
non-heme iron, 54
nutrient analysis, of a hurdler's diet,
205–7
nutrients, and variety in food, 5
nutrition *see* competition nutrition;
diets; food; training nutrition;
travel nutrition
nutrition experts, 220–1
nutritional ergogenic aids:
bodybuilders, 221–2; deciding
whether to use, 127–32;
definition, 125; features, 126;
personal endorsements, 134–5;
placebo effect, 135, 136; proof
of effectiveness, 132–4; scientific
trials, 135–6; triathletes, 145;
types, 127–32; weightlifters,
217
nutritional supplements *see* dietary
supplements; nutritional
ergogenic aids

oils, reducing, 7–14
ornithine, 129
osteoporosis, 55
oxalates, 54

pantothenic acid, 50
peer influence, 277, 288
percentage body fat, 63
percentage fat by energy, 14
percentage fat by weight, 12–13
personal endorsements, of ergogenic
aids, 134–5

Phinney study, *360*
physique, 61–78; *see also* physical
characteristics *under specific
sports*
phytates, 54
pinch test, 63
pole vaulting *see* jumping
post-competition bingeing, 225
potassium, 26, *215*, 224
power to weight ratio, 61
powerlifting *see* strength sports
PR-Bar, *360*
pre-event meals, 87–91; Australian
Rules players, 280; basketball
players, 310; bodybuilders,
224–5; cyclists, 168; distance
runners, 178; hockey players,
299; hurdlers, 201; jumpers, 201;
netball players, 310; rowers,
267; skiers, 355; soccer players,
299, *303–5*; sprinters, 201; tennis
players, *324–5*
pregnancy, energy allowance for,
40
Pritikin, Nathan, *194–5*
Pritikin, Robert, *197*
Pritikin diets, 177, *194–7*
Pritikin restaurants, 339
processed foods, 11–12
protein: cost of supplements versus
food, 133; for bulking-up,
210–11; high-protein diets,
222–3; mixing with
carbohydrate, *228*; nutritional
recovery, 115; powders, 131,
133, *215–17*; sources, 10, 47,
261; vegetarian diets, *259*,
261; *see also* protein
requirements
protein requirements, 44, 46–7;
bodybuilders, *227, 229*; Rugby
League players, 288; strength
sports, 45, 46
psychology, pre-event, 87, 89
puberty: divers, 246; gymnasts, 246;
swimmers, 153
pyridoxine, 50

race preparation *see* competition
nutrition
recipe books, 295
Recommended Dietary Intake (RDI),
49, 123, *205, 216*

recovery: Australian Rules players, 277, 279–80; boxers, 235; cricketers, 343; distance runners, 174; eating for, 107–21, 290; effect of rapid weight loss on, *238*; hockey players, 298–9, 300–1; hurdlers, *205–6*; middle distance runners, 192; Rugby League players, 289; skiers, 354, 358; soccer players, 298–9, 300–1; swimmers, 154; triathletes, 144; wrestlers, 235
recreational skiing, 357–8
refined carbohydrates, 17, 22, 23
relaxation techniques, *194*
restaurants, and good nutrition, 192, *196*, 278, 331–9
riboflavin, 50, 262
Rim, Kerryn, *362–4*
rowing: case studies, 268–74; competition, 264; lightweight, 267–8, *271–4*; making weight, 75; nutrition issues, 265–8; overview, 263; physical characteristics, 264–5, 265; training, 263–4
Rugby League: case studies, *290–5*; competition, 287; nutrition issues, 288–90; overview, 286; physical characteristics, 287–8; training, 286–7
running *see* distance running; middle distance running; sprinting

salt, 26–8, *240*; losses, 109; tablets, 27–8, 280
Saris, Wim, 169
'scientific studies,' *230–3*, *360–1*
scientific theory, and ergogenic aids, 132–4
Scott, Dave, 146
Sears diet, 154–5
secondary amenorrhea, 176
serotonin, 80, 130
Sheffield Shield, 340, 341
shot put *see* strength sports
simple carbohydrates, 16–17, 23
skiing: case studies, *358–64*; competition, 351; nutrition issues, 352–8; overview, 350; physical characteristics, 352; touring, 350–1; training, 350–1

skinfold measurements: AIS skinfold protocol, 63; gymnasts, *253*, *255*, *256–7*; hurdlers, *204*; international standards, 63, 65; rowers, *274*; sites for taking, 64
slalom courses, 351
sleep, 212, *214*, 223
snack foods, 12
soccer: competition, 297; nutrition issues, 298–301; overview, 296; physical characteristics, 297–8; training, 296–7
sodium: blood sodium imbalance, 81; blood sodium levels, distance runners, 81; in fluids, 109; in sports drinks, 102, 103, 105; restriction of, in bodybuilders, 224
sodium bicarbonate, 27
sodium chloride, 26–8
soy milk, 58
'split routines,' 219
sports bars, 20, 97, 99, 124, *360*
sports drinks: adjusting concentration of, 104–5; analysis, 102; as a source of carbohydrate, 99, 101, 103–4, *187*; as a source of fluids, 33, 94, 101; as dietary supplements, 20, 123, 124, 125; Australian Rules players, 280–1; case study, *149–50*; choice of, 105–6; composition, 103–4; development of, 102–3; distance runners, 105; for electrolyte replacement, 27, 28, 102; for recovery, 110; for sodium replacement, 104–5; glucose polymers in, 103–4; hockey players, 300; maintenance of blood volume, 81; retention rate, 109; Rugby League players, 289; skiers, 356; soccer players, 300; tennis players, 318
sprinting: case studies, *202–3*; competition, 199–200; nutrition issues, 200–2; overview, 198; physical characteristics, 200; training, 199
stable isotopes, energy measurement, 71
Stanford Swimming Team, 154, 155
starches, 16

steroids *see* anabolic steroids
stomach-emptying: competition
    nutrition, 93, 94, 97; distance
    runners, 176–7; fluid
    requirements, 101, 110; middle
    distance runners, *194*; recovery,
    110; sports drinks, 102–3, 104,
    356
stomach 'fullness,' 20, 33
strength sports: case studies,
    213–17; competition, 208–9;
    making weight, 75, 212; nutrition
    issues, 210–13; overview, 208–9;
    physical characteristics, 210;
    training, 209
stress, *192–4*; *see also* heat stress
stress fractures, 143–4, *179–80*
sucrose, 21
sugar: overconsumption, 22; prior to
    events, 90–2, *186*; reducing, 26;
    refined carbohydrates, 23; role
    in training diet, 22; simple
    carbohydrates, 16; tooth decay,
    22
supplements *see* dietary
    supplements; nutritional
    ergogenic aids
sweat losses: fluid intake during
    events, 92–4, 95; loss of
    electrolytes, 27; reducing, 117;
    replacing, 80, 100–1, 178–9;
    study of, in cricketers, *347–9*;
    see also dehydration; fluid
    requirements; fluids
sweets *see* desserts and sweets
swimming: case studies, *158–62*;
    competition, 152–3; nutrition
    issues, 154–8; overview, 151;
    physical characteristics, 153;
    training, 151–2

take-away food, 12, 278, 312–14
tannin, 54
tennis: case studies, *323–6*;
    competition, 316; nutrition
    issues, 317–19; overview, 315;
    physical characteristics, 317;
    training, 315–16; travel nutrition,
    319–23
Thai restaurants, 337
thiamin, 50
thirst, 28
throwing *see* strength sports

tocopherols, 129
tooth decay, 22, 26
Tour de France, 163, 167, 168–9,
    169–71
touring *see* travel nutrition
training nutrition, 3–36; basketball
    players, 308–9; boxers, 236;
    cricketers, 343; cyclists, 165–6;
    divers, 247; golfers, 329;
    gymnasts, 247; hockey players,
    298–9; hurdlers, 200–1; jumpers,
    200–1; monitoring fluid balance,
    29–33; netball players, 308–9;
    recovery eating, 107–21; rowers,
    265; skiers, *363*; soccer players,
    298–9; sprinters, 200–1;
    swimmers, 154–6; tennis
    players, 317–18; triathletes, 143;
    wrestlers, 236; *see also*
    competition nutrition
travel nutrition: Australian rules
    players, 278; basketball players,
    310–11; cricketers, 344; distance
    runners, 179; divers, 247;
    golfers, 331; guidelines, 319–23;
    gymnasts, 247; hockey players,
    301; hurdlers, 202; jumpers, 202;
    middle distance runners, 192;
    netball players, 310–11; skiers,
    354–7, *362–4*; soccer players,
    301, *304*; sprinters, 202; take-
    away food, 312–14; tennis
    players, *323–6*
triathlon: case studies, *146–50*;
    nutrition issues, 142–50;
    overview, 140; physical
    characteristics, 141–2; training,
    140–1
triglycerides, 212
tryptophan, 130
twelfth man, *347*

underwater weighing, 62
urinary alkanisers, 127
urine production, and post-exercise
    drinks, 109–10

valine, 130
vegans, *258, 259*
vegetarianism, 177, *257–62*
vitamins: megadoses, 131; nutritional
    recovery, 115; requirements,
    47–52; sources, 49–51;

vitamins (*continued*):
supplements, 125; vegetarian
diets, *259*; vitamin A, 51;
vitamin B$_1$, 50; vitamin B$_2$, 50,
262; vitamin B$_3$, 50; vitamin B$_6$,
50; vitamin B$_{12}$, 51, 261–2;
'vitamin' B$_{15}$, 131, *217*; vitamin
C, 27, 51, 129; vitamin D, 51;
vitamin E, 51, 126, 129;
vitamin K, 51; weightlifters' diet,
215–17

water, 28, 31, 33, 94, 95, 102–3,
145
weight: calculating rate of
dehydration, 108; daily
fluctuations, 246, *255*; effect of
alcohol, 35–6; effect of carnitine,
131; gain during injury, *301–3*;
overweight golfers, 329;
preoccupation with, 245–6,
251–7; *see also* body fat;
muscles, bulking-up of; weight
loss; weight making
weight loss: Australian Rules
players, 278, *282–4*; cricketers,
344–7; divers, 245–6; drastic
weight loss, 75; gymnasts,
245–6, *251–7*; netball players,

311–12; rowers, 267–8, *271–4*;
skiers, 352–3, *363*; swimmers,
153, 156; wrestlers and boxers,
235, 236–7, *237–41*
weight making: choosing a
competition weight, 75, 236–7;
fluid levels, 95; hints for, 75–6;
pre-event meals, 89; rowers,
263, *268–70*; strength sports,
212; wrestlers and boxers, 235,
236–7, *237–41*
weightlifting *see* strength sports
wholesome carbohydrates, 17, 23,
116
women athletes: amenorrhea, 55–6,
71, 143–4, 176, *180*, 247; body-
fat goals, 175, 245; cyclists,
165–6; iron requirements, 52,
259, 266, 309, 353; low-energy
consumers, 70, 73; weight
problems in swimmers, 156
wrestling: case studies, *237–9*;
competition, 235; making
weight, 75, 236–7; nutrition
issues, 236–7; overview, 234;
physical characteristics, 235;
training, 235

zinc, *184*, 261